FORECASTING INFORMATICS COMPETENCIES FOR NURSES IN THE FUTURE OF CONNECTED HEALTH

Studies in Health Technology and Informatics

This book series was started in 1990 to promote research conducted under the auspices of the EC programmes' Advanced Informatics in Medicine (AIM) and Biomedical and Health Research (BHR) bioengineering branch. A driving aspect of international health informatics is that telecommunication technology, rehabilitative technology, intelligent home technology and many other components are moving together and form one integrated world of information and communication media. The series has been accepted by MEDLINE/PubMed, SciVerse Scopus, EMCare, Book Citation Index – Science and Thomson Reuters' Conference Proceedings Citation Index.

Volume 232

ISSN 0926-9630 (print)
ISSN 1879-8365 (online)

Forecasting Informatics Competencies for Nurses in the Future of Connected Health

Proceedings of the Nursing Informatics Post Conference 2016

Edited by

Judy Murphy

IBM Global Healthcare, Washington, DC, USA

William Goossen

Results 4 Care B.V., Amersfoort, The Netherlands

and

Patrick Weber

Nice Computing SA, Le Mont/Lausanne, Switzerland

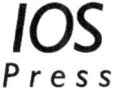

IOS
Press

Amsterdam • Berlin • Washington, DC

ISBN 978-1-61499-737-5 (print)
ISBN 978-1-61499-738-2 (online)
Library of Congress Control Number: 2016963478

Publisher
IOS Press BV
Nieuwe Hemweg 6B
1013 BG Amsterdam
Netherlands
fax: +31 20 687 0019
e-mail: order@iospress.nl

For book sales in the USA and Canada:
IOS Press, Inc.
6751 Tepper Drive
Clifton, VA 20124
USA
Tel.: +1 703 830 6300
Fax: +1 703 830 2300
sales@iospress.com

LEGAL NOTICE

The publisher is not responsible for the use which might be made of the following information.

PRINTED IN THE NETHERLANDS

Preface

The book in front of you arose from a collaboration among nursing informatics experts from research, education and practice settings, from eighteen countries, and from varying levels of expertise – those beginning to forge new frontiers in connected health and those who helped form the discipline. Having participated in several NI post conferences before, each time it is a great pleasure to work in this condensed format of preparing viewpoints, discussing them in person, organizing them into chapters, and then producing the wealth of information into a fine book.

We would like to thank all the participants who attended the NI 2016 Post Conference, as well as all the authors and co-authors who participated but did not attend, for their significant contributions to this NI 2016 Post Conference Proceedings. We appreciate each and every one of you for your time and talent in adding to the wealth of information in this book.

In addition, Patrick Weber must be acknowledged and thanked as organizer of NI 2016, the NI 2016 Post conference, and for his assistance in editing all of the chapters to make them consistent and meet the publisher's requirements.

We are hopeful that this book will help forecast and define the informatics competencies for nurses in practice, and as such, help outline the requirements for informatics training in nursing programs around the world. We are further hopeful that this content will help shape the nursing practice that will exist in the future of connected health, when we believe that practice and technology will be inextricably intertwined. As you read about the concept of Connected Health in this book, consider the wise words from Virginia Henderson to "preserve the essence of nursing in a technological age."

Please be inspired by this book and let it help you achieve the best care possible using health informatics solutions.

Judy Murphy, William Goossen, Patrick Weber

Contents

Section E. Annotated Bibliography

© 2017 IMIA and IOS Press.
doi:10.3233/978-1-61499-738-2-1

Introduction:
Forecasting Informatics Competencies for Nurses in the Future of Connected Health

Judy MURPHY[a, 1] and William GOOSSEN[b]
[a]*IBM, Washington DC, USA*
[b]*Results 4 Care BV, Amersfoort, the Netherlands*

Abstract. This introduction to the book discusses how the topic of competencies for nurses in a world of connected health needs to be addressed at the curriculum level to achieve the specific competencies for various roles, including practicing nurse, nurse teacher, nurse leader, and nursing informatics specialists. It looks back at milestone publications from the international Nursing Informatics post conferences that still serve a purpose for inspiring developments today and looks forward to the way nurses can use connected health to improve the health and health care for their patients. Specific emerging topics in health information technology are addressed as well, such as semantics, genetics, big data, eHealth and social media.

Keywords. Informatics, Competencies, Technology, Education, eHealth, Connected Health, Nursing

1. Background

When asked to be Co-Chairs of the NI 2016 Post Conference and Editors of the Post Conference Proceedings, we of course where honored and enthusiastic at the same time. Besides creating a milestone publication through the work of the eminent participants, it would also pull together various efforts and content on this very important topic into one publication. It is the desire that this work will not only inspire current and future nurse informaticists and educators with concepts that build on the work of our important leaders from the past, but also that it will inspire changes to the current education of nurses, and most importantly, set a vision for where we need to go with nursing education in the next ten plus years.

The ultimate Post Conference goal was to publish a set of informatics competency recommendations for nurses educated in the next decade that cover the informatics skills required for improved, innovative and even transformative health and healthcare delivery. This includes both information management *and* the use of information and communication technology (ICT) such as Electronic Health Record (EHR) systems, medical devices, telemedicine, patient portals, eHealth and mobile applications, and the many more that will emerge. As the work was being completed, the need to focus on positioning these competencies to support care models of the future became more

---

[1] Corresponding author, Judy Murphy, RN, FACMI, FHIMSS, FAAN, Chief Nursing Officer, IBM, Washington DC. Email: murphyja@us.ibm.com.

evident, particularly those that promote patient-centered care and concentrate on connecting health and healthcare across the continuum. The result was the creation of a working organizational model that included three concentric circles, shown in Figure 1, with Patient/Family in the Center, surrounded by Connected Health, and further encompassed by the Informatics Competencies for Nurses to Support Connected Health. The Post Conference participants agreed that informatics competencies for nurses are a critical component for enabling the connectedness needed for the health and healthcare of the future. This concept of Connected Health is referenced in several chapters in this book and is described in depth in Chapter 18.

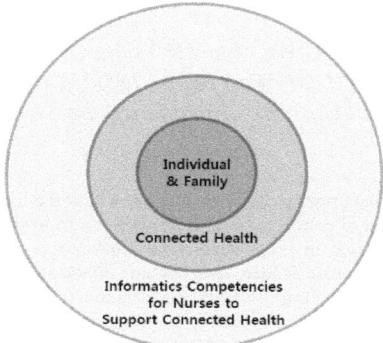

Figure 1. Informatics Competencies for Nurses to Support Connected Health

Nursing informatics has a long history of focus on information management on behalf of the profession, for example Werley and Lang's identification of the nursing minimum data set [1] and Clark and Lang's work for the international classification of nursing practice [2]. Also, nurses have a long history of describing their computer use; see for example work by Saba and McCormick [3], Ball and Hannah [4], and Scholes, Tallberg and Pluyter-Wentink [5] among others from the late seventies and early eighties. However, based on the technical advancements of the past and through the ongoing and consistent changes in healthcare today, we are now challenged to look to the future and help determine what nurses and patients/consumers will need going forward.

2. IMIA-NI Post Conference History

The International Medical Informatics Association - Nursing Informatics (IMIA-NI) Conferences, as a scientific endeavor, have a tradition of inviting leaders in the field to a working post conference. The focus of IMIA-NI is to foster collaboration among nurses and others who are interested in Nursing Informatics to facilitate development in the field [6]. IMIA-NI serves as the working group for nursing informatics from the International Medical Informatics Association (IMIA). IMIA is an independent organization established 1974 and under Swiss law in 1992 [7]. IMIA is the world body for health and biomedical informatics, and works as an 'association of associations', where national health informatics, or research institutes are the members. IMIA has strong links to the International Federation for Information Processing (IFIP - www.ifip.org) from which it evolved from a special interest group into an independent organization and is now an affiliate organization. IMIA also has relationships with the World Health Organization (WHO - www.who.int), the International Federation of Health Information Management (IFHIMA), and is a Liaison-A category organization in cooperation with ISO technical committee TC 215 health informatics.

The IMIA-NI post conferences have each dealt with a specific topic that had gained interest in the NI community, and that required leadership to achieve the next level of application in the field. Examples of post conference publications include the Peterson and Gerdin-Jelger's "Preparing nurses for using information systems recommended informatics competencies" from 1988 [8], Henry, Holzemer, Tallberg & Grobe from 1994 "Use of health information systems to collect and measure patient outcomes" [9], and the Ehnfors, Grobe and Tallberg book on "combining clinical practice guidelines and patient preferences using health informatics" from 1997 [10]. Later, IMIA-NI Post Conferences also published their invited papers for scientific journal theme issues. This was successful for the NI 2003 post conference on patient safety issues and how health informatics can assist in preventing them. Some of these papers, published in the International Journal of Medical Informatics, are still quoted today, because they built upon the best science in health care and adapted it to the nursing profession and applications by nurse informaticists. However, that approach was less successful for other journals, as the rigorous peer review criteria sometimes conflicted with expressing a vision for the NI profession that was not yet evidence based. Hence, despite that some of the excellent contributions were indeed published, some others did not pass and are not published. But whatever their format, the post conference writings can be a good inspiration, and usually last for many years as the concepts expressed and methods applied are timeless and can be used and referenced today, and into the future!

3. 2016 IMIA-NI Post Conference

The topic of *Forecasting Informatics Competencies for Nurses in the Future of Connected Health* was decided by the IMIA-NI Special Interest Group. As described, this post conference activity is a tradition for the IMIA-NI conferences and is part of the bids that members vote on in the years prior to the event. For the NI 2016 post conference the tradition of asking the invited participants to prepare materials was followed again. In fact, participants were asked to write a full chapter before the post conference took place, using the same template that was used for the submissions to the NI 2016 regular conference in Geneva [11]. This approach was based on three goals: 1) to have all the chapters distributed to participants before the post conference so that each had time to review and prepare, 2) to have informed discussion of the topics during the post conference, and 3) to finalize the publication within 60-90 days after the post conference. A reverse order planning schedule was used to stay focused on this outcome.

The goal of the NI 2016 post conference book on informatics competencies for a connected world is to assist nursing instructors/professors with knowledge and examples so that they can expand their capability to integrate eHealth/nursing informatics/health informatics topics into the curricula of basic nursing education. After almost 25 years it is still problematic how few schools of nursing offer education on how the values of patient focused care can be mixed with careful application of health informatics tools and good professional information management.

It may be helpful for all nursing teachers to consider the very wise words on nursing from Virginia Henderson [12]: ... the task of leaders and teachers is ... "preserving the essence of nursing in a technological age." Henderson argues in this paper that technology is inevitable, it requires deep understanding of the technology itself and it requires leadership and faith to adequately use it in a caring environment. She does not define which technology is precisely meant, and that of course is good, as history has shown many expansions of new technologies, systems, applications, methods for data management; the addition of contextual big data to free text and structured data; as well as the growth of cognitive computing and augmented intelligence. In fact, perhaps current technology is only the beginning of our move to connected health in a connected world.

The following topic areas are based on the contributions of the post conference participants, invited experts and leaders, both those new to this work and those with extensive history in the field. All participants worked diligently over the three days of the post conference and delivered input, feedback and content that fit well into the subsequent chapters and overall theme. Every participant authored or co-authored at least one chapter of the NI 2016 post conference book. There were also some chapter co-authors that did not attend the post conference, but were brought in to augment expertise when needed.

4. Organization of the Book

This book handles five core topics in different sections. Section A follows up on both the 1987 work by Ronald and Skiba on Nursing Informatics competencies [13], as well as their chapter in the IMIA-NI guidelines [14] from 1988 to develop nursing informatics education. Hence, the current book starts with Professional Nursing Roles and Nursing Informatics Competencies in this section. It covers the nursing informatics competency work done in the past and moves into the current state, including recommendations for what we need today. The current IMIA guidelines for curricula form the overall landscape for the health informatics profession at large, which function as a point of reference for nursing. Section A ends with looking ahead to plan how nurses and teachers should use informatics competencies to contribute to health and healthcare in a connected world. Recommendations to ensure faculty is competent to integrate the informatics and information management content in curricula for basic nursing education is included, along with specific competencies required for the nurse educators to deliver the new curricula (for basic nursing education) in this connected world. Based on this section, all chapters include recommendations for specific competencies for nurses to master the technology to help patients benefit from its use. But the competencies are not the end part. This work focuses on a growth path that shows the goal for nurses caring for patients in a connected world to achieve desired health outcomes and how these goals can be achieved.

Section B presents an overview of competency-based learning including various national and international initiatives. The authors come from the membership of the IMIA-NI Education Working Group, or have recently started their career in this field. They describe a global view along with each of their own country's status on the development and use of informatics and information management competencies in the education of student nurses. This section concludes with international survey results describing competency recommendations for advancing nursing informatics in the next decade.

Section C moves on from descriptions of various national and international work on nursing competencies to explore current and future trends in health and nursing informatics. Some of these trends are, in fact quite arbitrarily, based on the experience of the participants. One example of new competencies includes semantic content of health informatics technology, which traditionally focused on nursing terminologies, but moves more to data modeling and health informatics architectures. It discusses how facts about patients and nursing care; in particular, inferences for nursing care, patient outcomes and care delivered, can be recorded and reused. Genetics becomes content of Health IT, hence there is a need to define the integration of the genetic, genomics and other 'omics' competencies into the healthcare informatics domain, especially the Electronic Health Record (EHR). Currently, there are also international and interprofessional activities and organizations that have established or are identifying competencies in genetics and genomics. Another topic that was explored included competencies related to data mining, natural language processing and other advanced data analytics techniques. An overview of the rapid and diverse number of developments in Health IT in recent years are described in this section and the move towards more integrated and connected health is described, anticipating on further growth in this area. The evolution of HIT is described as it has increased in complexity, diversity, connectivity, and more recently, the move towards multiple modalities. The section ends with the use of social media in today's life, which also offers new working ways in nursing care. All people, also patients, are increasingly expanding interactions from face-to-face meetings to online ways of communication, networking, searching, creating and sharing information. Nursing Informatics competencies do include taking care of patients/citizens via tweeting care, Facebook care, blogging care, vlogging care, infotainment care, gamification-care, infographic care, for instance. When social media is used effectively and purposefully in health care, it can give all of us a greater choice in how we live, how we take care of our health and how we learn and build our professional competences. Nurses need continuous education and proper tools to take the most of the benefits of social media.

Section D presents the expectations for leadership in the field. It discusses topics related to competencies of nurse leaders related to leadership, transforming models of care, and workforce preparation. In addition, this section discusses the evolving NI specialist role and how the NI specialist contributes to nursing education, practice and research. Increasingly, there is a demand for integrating Health Information Technology Safety into Nursing Informatics Competencies at various levels to include those focused on technology-induced errors and Health IT safety. The section wraps up with content related to continuing education and certification in nursing informatics.

Because one book cannot address all relevant materials, particularly when something of high value has just been published, the post conference attendees decided to include an annotated bibliography. The annotated bibliography includes historical key sources, up to date sources on the subject, and some information on content that, with hindsight, the post-conference team felt relevant to the connected world content of this book.

5. Conclusion

Though we would have loved to provide readers with a single set of recommended competencies that would cover all programs, we discovered early on that no one set would be able to meet all needs. As such, we present here ideas and examples of the types of competencies that may be included, in order to plant ideas and generate discussion regarding competency inclusion in different programs. We sincerely hope you enjoy this book and find it useful as you consider incorporating informatics competencies into your programs for entry-to-practice nurses, for currently practicing nurses, as well as for nurse leaders. It is our belief that the transformation of health and healthcare lies in the innovative and judicious use of health IT by nurses as we care for our patients and families.

References

[1]   Werley, HH., Lang, NM 1988 Identification of the Nursing Minimum Data Set, New York: Springer publishing comp. inc.

[2]   Clark J, Lang NM. Nursing's Next Advance: an International Classification for Nursing Practice. Int Nurs Rev. 1992: 39:109-12.

[3]   Saba V & McCormick K. (1986). Essentials of Computers for Nurses. Philadelphia, Lippincott Williams and Wilkins.

[4]   Ball, MJ. & Hannah, KJ., Using Computers in Nursing,. Reston, V.A., Reston 1984.

[5]   Scholes M, Tallberg M & Pluyter-Wenting E (2000). International Nursing Informatics: a history of the first forty years. Swindon UK, the British Computer Society.

[6]   IMIA NI SIG / International Medical Informatics Association - Nursing Informatics Special Interest Group http://www.imia-medinfo.org/new2/node/151

[7]   IMIA / International Medical Informatics Association http://www.imia-medinfo.org/new2/

[8]   Peterson, HE., Gerdin-Jelger,U., (Eds.), (1988). Preparing Nurses for Using Information Systems: recommended Informatics Competencies.. New York, National League for Nursing.

[9]   Henry SB, Holzemer WL, Tallberg M, Grobe SJ, (Eds). (1994). Informatics; the infrastructure for quality assessment and improvement in nursing. Austin, Texas, IMIA.

[10] Ehnfors M, Grobe SJ, Tallberg M, editors. Nursing informatics: Combining clinical practice guidelines and patient preferences using health informatics. Proceedings of the Sixth International Nursing Informatics Symposium Post-Conference, Lidingö, Sweden, October 1-4 1997. Omvårdnad No: 6, Spri and the Swedish Nurses' Association. Stockholm, Spris förlag, 1998,

[11] NI 2016. Nursing Informatics 2016 Conference, Geneva. http://ni2016.org/

[12] Henderson,VA. (1980). Preserving the essence of nursing in a technological age. Journal of advanced nursing, 3, 245-260.

[13] Ronald,JS., Skiba,DJ. (1987). Guidelines for basic Computer Education in Nursing. New York, National League for Nursing.

[14] Ronald,JS., Skiba,DJ. Computer Education for Nurses: Curriculum issues and guidelines. In: Petersen HE. & Gerdin-Jelger U.,(Eds.), Preparing nurses for using information systems:recommended information competencies, New York, National League for Nursing, 1988, pp.15-23.

Section A

Professional Nursing Roles and Nursing Informatics Competencies

Forecasting Informatics Competencies for Nurses in the Future of Connected Health
J. Murphy et al. (Eds.)
doi:10.3233/978-1-61499-738-2-9

Nursing Informatics Education: From Automation to Connected Care

Diane J SKIBA[1]
University of Colorado College of Nursing

Abstract. The use of health information technologies has evolved over the last 50 years. These technologies have moved from the automation of data and data processing to connected care tools that are part of a health care ecosystem that provides the best care at the point of care. To correspondence with the evolution of technologies and their disruptions within the health care delivery system, there is a need to re-examine the necessary competencies of health care professionals.

Keywords. Connected Care, Competencies, health information technologies

1. Introduction

The education of health care professionals has a long rich history that has evolved since the 1970s. To describe the history, it is important to understand the driving forces pushing the development and implementation of computerized systems across the decades. The evolution also highlights some of the major developments such as the shift from mainframe computer hardware to mobile devices and the increasing reliance on the Internet and web based applications.

2. Early Years 1960s & 1970s: Data Processing & Automation Era

In the early days, the mainframe computer was the computer of choice with the mini-computer being introduced in the 1970s. The focus was on automation of common tasks related to administrative and financial systems [1]. There were relatively few examples of computer applications for clinical care. In nursing, one of the first was Chow's article [2] on physiologic monitoring in 1961. She described how physiological monitoring can be used in nursing and that "some devices are being designed to be labor saving for nurses or to add to the preciseness of nursing procedures." [2 (62)] She also suggested that "Perhaps, being electronically monitored, the patient will need a different type of nursing care." [2 (60)] In the same issue, an editorial introduced the "electronic nurse" [3] and noted "there are powerful pressures on hospitals to look to automation to achieve greater efficiency." [3 (55)] This editorial recommended sorting out the roles of nursing within this new era of electronic monitoring. The majority of the articles written in the 1960s focused on physiological monitoring and the automation of hospitals. Rosenberg and Carriker [4] wrote one of the first articles about

---

[1] Corresponding author: Diane J Skiba, PhD, FACMI, ANEF, FAAN, University of Colorado College of Nursing Aurora Colorado. Diane.Skiba@ucdenver.edu.

the automation of nursing notes. Throughout the 1970s, there was an emergence of articles that examined hospital information systems, nurse scheduling, computer applications in public health and psychiatric nursing. Thus, the initial emphasis on data processing and automation and growing number of applications in the clinical arena served as a catalyst to develop educational opportunities for health care professionals.

Anderson, Gremy & Pages [5] first wrote about informatics education for health care professionals in 1974. Their monograph was published under the auspices of the Technical Committee 4 of the International Federation for Information Processing (IFIP - www.ifip.org). This group was the predecessor of the International Medical Informatics Association (IMIA), an independent organization established under Swiss law in 1989. Anderson, Gremy & Page referred to the state of computers in health care as a large number of "diverse experiments in system development and computing techniques." [5 (1)] These experiments did not always produce the expected results and lack of knowledge about medical computing was one of the main reasons for this failure. Thus, it was important to develop a set of recommendations for educational programs.

In order to address the education of health care professionals about informatics, the group conducted a survey to assess the need for computing in health services across the globe. The survey addressed three difference audiences: physicians, paramedical personnel (nurses, laboratory and other technicians) and hospital or medical community administrative personnel. Although they use the term informatics, data and information processing was the predominate theme. The questions examined necessary computer skills (i.e. operate a teletypewriter, visual display unit and writing small computer programs), knowledge of logic and hardware aspects of computer design and techniques, and methods of using a computer for functions such as medical record, lab data, medical diagnosis, library information retrieval, intensive care monitoring, mathematical models of biomedicine and system analysis. They also asked about standardization of medical terminology, medical & nursing procedures.

Based upon their results, the group recommended three levels of education to meet the needs for medical computing. Here is a brief description of the three levels of education. The first level focused on "a general level of computer education which is necessary to provide general knowledge of computers and data processing for all uses in the health service." [5 (8)] The second level focused on health care professionals that will work with experts in data processing. The third level focused on extensive training for those health care professionals that will spend the majority of their time in computing and data processing. Here are the objectives for the various levels:

Level 1: "how to use basic knowledge about a computer system, organize information about a medical problem, describe the system theory behind the application and investigate special medical applications" [5 (29)] most specific to that professional. Content should include: data processing terminology, computer hardware & software, information management (file structures, file handling procedures, function of computer languages, system analysis, algorithmic thinking, flowcharting), and applications and the relevance of information processing to health care.

Level 2: "will be able to discuss, plan and cooperate with computer scientists developing medical systems, analyze and design a medical system, allow for hardware and software constraints in the design of a system and be able to be active members of a team in designing and implementing systems in their area of health activity." [5 (30)] Content should include: basic information sciences (information and coding theory, logic basic concepts, functions and relationship between hardware components, information flow, basic software functions, programming including proficiency in writing a program, data structure & file organization, system analysis and design, and how to choose a computer system); Medical/Health Applications (broken into three groups: non-numerical methods (medical records), numerical methods (statistical procedures) and real-time applications (monitoring).

Level 3: specialized knowledge in computer sciences (such as a Master's degree) that allows one to design interactive systems for medical diagnosis, medical record systems and using information processing statistical procedures and other mathematical analytical methods. [5 (31)]

In nursing, there were relatively few examples of educational opportunities for nurses to learn about computers in health care. Dr. Judith Ronald [6] was one of the first to offer a course to teach baccalaureate nurses about computers. Her course covered: "1) the importance of technology in contemporary society, 2) basic concepts of computerized data processing, 3) present and potential applications of computers in health, 4) the nurse as a participant in a computerized information system and 5) social/ethical aspects of health data automation." [7 (772)]

3. 1980-1990s: Personal Computer Era

In this decade, we saw the emergence of personal computers (PCs) and software programs that were now addressing more clinical aspects of care. PCs provided more functional devices at nursing stations, doctor offices and on the units than the previous visual display screens. Software programs were emerging for order entry, admission discharge and transfer (ADT) systems, laboratory systems and early documentation systems. Minimum nursing data sets and nursing terminologies began to emerge.

In the 1980s, "Nursing informatics gained momentum." [8 (201)] The first track in nursing was introduced in the Symposium on Computer Applications in Medicine Conference in 1981. The IMIA Nursing working group held its first international meeting in 1982. Professional organizations such as the National League for Nursing and American Nurses Association formed informatics committees. Continuing education workshops and university level courses were being offered. In 1987, Ronald & Skiba [9] published *Guidelines for Basic Computer Education in in Nursing.* In the monograph, they introduced a framework that included cognitive and interactive learning across a continuum from informed user, proficient user to a developer. This informed user was for all beginning nurses. The proficient user was aimed at professional nurses in practice and the developer was aimed at those nurses with advanced degrees in the field. The monograph provided a curriculum development model, content outline and learning activities as well as other resources to facilitate the development of courses. Towards the end of the decade, the first two graduate programs in nursing informatics were established at the University of Utah and University of Maryland.

On the international level in 1988, the IMIA Working Group 8 (Nursing Informatics) Task Force on Education created "broad competency statements about nursing informatics for the practicing nurse, the nurse administrator, the nurse educator, the nurse teacher and the nurse researcher. [10 (4)] At the end of the meeting, recommendations were made for three levels of competencies (user, modifier and innovator) for the practicing nurse, nurse administrator, educator/teacher and researcher. Nursing informatics was defined "as the application of information science to nursing and patient care." [10 (117)] A nurse informatics specialist was defined "as a nurse who has special preparation and experience and uses information science principles for the development of computer applications for nursing and patient care." [10 (117)] For each type of nurse, fundamental knowledge was identified. Below are the broad competencies defined for each nursing role and for each level (user, modifier, innovator)

Broad Competency Areas across Nursing Role			
Practicing Nurse	Nurse Administrator	Nurse Teacher	Nurse Researcher
• Documenting nursing practice • Accessing information • Using a system's data & information • Coordinating information flow	• Directing the organization of info for (financial, patient care, resource personnel, risk management, quality control, safety & infection control) • Accessing information • Using a system's data & information • Communicating & networking inside & outside the organization • Assuring ethical standards & data protection	• Teaching about applications for providing & administering care and conducting research about care. • Teaching with computer-based instructional materials • Deciding from the variety of alternatives what instructional materials should be available and how it should be provided to learners • Performing student assessment & evaluation	• Using search strategies for electronically retrieving bibliographic citations and primary source data • Accessing, communicating and storing data • Managing & manipulating data • Processing text and graphic information

In 1989, Graves and Corcoran published their seminal work to define "nursing informatics as a combination of computer science, information science and nursing science designed to assist in the management and processing of nursing data, information and knowledge to support the practice of nursing and the delivery of nursing care." [11 (227)] The foundation for defining the discipline of nursing informatics was beginning to take shape. There was a shift from talking about computers in nursing to the use of the term nursing informatics.

4. 1990s: The Internet Era

In the 1990s, the computer based patient record was a hot topic fueled by a study conducted by the National Academy of Sciences to improve patients records to meet the need of better information management and harness advances in technology.[12] Computers were not only smaller but faster and telecommunications provided new methods for information exchange and telemedicine. Personal digital assistants (PDAs) and the Internet were changing how health care professionals communicated, accessed and shared information and knowledge. Email and electronic bulletin board systems began to proliferate. As the decade came to a close, the World Wide Web (WWW) provided access to a wealth of information and knowledge. The Internet was no longer just accessible to computer scientists but to citizens. The WWW democratized knowledge access and facilitated patients and families engagement in health care.

In nursing informatics, there was a growing emphasis on the development and testing of nursing classification and terminology systems. The American Nurses Association published the first Scope of Nursing Informatics Practice and Standards of Nursing Informatics Practice in 1994. [13] In the following year, the American Nurses Credentialing Center offered a certification exam for informatics nurses at the generalist level.

There was continued growth in the nursing informatics education. Continuing education opportunities, such as the Weekend Immersion in Nursing Informatics programs and professional conferences (AMIA, HIMSS) provided informatics education to many nurses. To prepare educators to learn more about informatics, the HBO Nurse Scholars program was initiated and successfully educated many faculty across the United States, Canada and the United Kingdom. [14, 15] The European SummerSchool in Nursing Informatics [16] and the Nightingale Project [17] shaped nursing informatics education across Europe. Defining the scope and standards as well as having a certification exam facilitated the development of academic informatics programs. Graduate programs in nursing informatics increased and in the late 1990s, two programs (University of Colorado and Duke University) began to offer their graduate programs online. [18]

During the 1999 AMIA Spring conference, a session was held to examine health care professionals views of informatics education. [19] The results indicated there were core competencies needed for all health care professionals in terms of basic computer knowledge and skills, principles of interface design, principles of privacy, confidentiality & security, ethical use of information & decision-making, knowledge of terminologies, user-driven clinical systems, structured data for evidence based practice, methods for evaluating information, how to critically and efficiently process information and understanding the impact of technology. In addition, there needed to be an interdisciplinary focus and emphasis on teamwork. Many of the competencies echoed those proposed by Association of American Medical Colleges [20], American Association of Colleges of Nursing [21] and the IMIA Recommendations on Education in Health and Medical informatics. [22]

5. 2000s: The EHRs Era

Throughout this decade, there was a convergence of driving forces that served as a major catalyst to move this agenda forward and insure that all health care professionals have the necessary "21st century knowledge and skills for practice in a complex, emerging technologically sophisticated, consumer-centric, global environment." [23 (58)] Here were some of the driving forces:

- Institute of Medicine's (IOM) Reports [24, 25, 26] stressed the importance of health information tools to provide safe and quality care. These reports had impact on patient safety measures around the globe.

- Health Professional Education: A Bridge to Quality [27] recommended the following goal: "All health professional should be educated to deliver patient-centered care as members of an interdisciplinary team, emphasizing evidence-based practice, quality improvement approaches and informatics." [27 (x)] Informatics tools are considered essential for communication, management of information and knowledge, mitigation of error, support for decision-making and health care interventions.
- Creation of the Office of the National Coordinator of Health Information Technology and its federal mandates served as a catalyst for the adoption of electronic health records (EHRs).
- The Technology Informatics Guiding Educational Reform (Tiger) Initiative, where many countries have engaged in.
- Robert Wood Johnson Foundation funded Quality and Safety Education for Nurses (QSEN) initiative. The Quality and Safety Education for Nurses (QSEN) project emphasizes the integration of knowledge, skills and attitudes related to the IOM five core competencies for all pre-licensure programs. [28] Pilot schools are integrating these competencies in their nursing programs and are sharing their work on the QSEN web site (http://www.qsen.org) [29]
- Web-based applications, mobile devices and EHRs were part of the global technology landscape.

Nursing informatics graduate programs continue to evolve and increase in number over this decade. These programs evolved based on two revisions of the ANA's Scope and Standards of Nursing Informatics [30, 31] and the work of Staggers, Gassert and Curran [32,33] In addition, the definition of nursing informatics was evolving as witnessed by ANA's two new definitions, the IMIA Nursing Informatics Working Group definition and the Health Resources & Services Administration (HRSA).

During this decade, the urgency for all health care professionals to have knowledge and skills in informatics blossomed. Although the idea that all healthcare professionals needed knowledge and skills in this area started back in 1974, it was only now being adopted. The driving forces previously mentioned of this decade served as a catalyst for this movement. In particular, the Health Professional Education: A Bridge to Quality [27] and the TIGER Initiative: Collaborating to Integrate Evidence and Informatics into Nursing Practice and Education: An Executive Summary. [34] Professional organizations, particularly related to nursing education began to promote informatics competencies for all levels of nursing education. In 2008, The National League for Nursing released Position Statement on Preparing the next generation of nurses to practice in a technology-rich environment: An Informatics Agenda. [35] The American Association of Colleges of Nursing released their baccalaureate, masters and doctorate of nursing practice essentials documents that outlined the need for all nurses to have information management knowledge and skills. [36,37,38] Nursing began to distinguish the differences between computer and information literacy from information management knowledge and skills. This became particularly apparent when the National League of Nursing surveyed nursing faculty and administrators and there was considerable confusion as to their view of nursing informatics. [39] Similar developments were also occurring in United Kingdom, Canada, Australia, New Zealand and Finland. [40]

6. 2010 to Present: Post EHRs Era

With the establishment of the Health Information Technology for Economic and Clinical Health (HITEC) Act of 2009, hospitals, clinics and physician practices in the United States increased their adoption of electronic health records systems (EHRs). [41] For nursing, health information technologies will fundamental change in how "RNs plan, deliver, document, and review clinical care." [42 (104)] Nurses at all levels will be "expected to use a variety of technological tools and complex information management systems that require skills in analysis and synthesis to improve the quality and effectiveness of care." [42 (7)] In addition, health care professionals need competencies that will allow them to practice as a collaborative interprofessional team as defined by the Interprofessional Education Collaborative Practice (IPEC). [43] These competencies included values/ethics, roles and responsibilities, Interprofessional communication, and teamwork.

The Post EHR era is being fueled by three major trends. [44] These trends are the connected age; transformation of the health care delivery system and the engaged patient. "The connected age is all about everything and everyone being connected." [44] When the connected age is combined with the Internet of Things (connected device and physical objects), it is a very powerful platform for health care and education. [45] In health care, there have been several definitions of connected health [46,47] that include not only digital tools but will connect people (providers to providers, providers to patients and patients to patients) to share ideas and resources as well as to create new communities. The second trend shifts the care from acute to outpatient setting and moves from fee for service models to value-based care. There is also a continuing emphasis on quality of care, population health, transitional care and a continuous learning health system. [48,49] As a part of this trend, there is an increasing reliance on big data and data analytics, precision medicine & genomics, and information governance. The last trend focuses on patient, family, caregivers and consumer engagement [50,51] in their health care. With the growing number of digital tools available to patients, patient centric care is beginning to become a reality. In the United States, two other driving forces are also intersecting with these trends: interoperability (Connecting Health and Care for the Nation A Shared Nationwide Interoperability Roadmap) [52] and the Federal Health IT Strategic Plan. [53]

In terms of informatics education, there were several important events that occurred during this time period. First, AMIA Board White Paper [54] developed a definition of biomedical informatics and delineated core competencies for graduate education in the discipline. This work was build upon previous AMIA work as well as competency endeavors by such professional organizations as the Association of Computing Machinery, International Medical Informatics Association, American Nursing Association, Australian Health Informatics Educational Framework, Canadian Health Informatics Association, TIGER and Commission on Accreditation of Health Informatics and Information Management. Second, accreditation standards were being developed and implemented by organizations such as the Canadian College of Health Information Management (CCHIM) and Accreditation for Health Informatics and Health Information Management Education (CAHIIM). [55] In addition, IMIA implemented a pilot program related to accreditation of medical informatics educational program (http://www.imia-medinfo.org/new2/node/449). Third, The American Board of Medical Subspecialties established clinical informatics as a medical subspecialty. The core content covered in clinical informatics includes: fundamentals, clinical decision-making and care process improvement, health information systems, leadership & change management. [56] The most recent endeavor is an examination of "two prominent disciplines have emerged from the mix of e-health workers employed in health organizations—health informatics and health information management." [55 (164)] This essay defined the convergent evolution of these two disciplines and how they may work together in the future.

As a result of these driving forces and trends, the University of Colorado has begun to rethink the necessary knowledge and skills needed by our advanced practice nurses. To this end, we designed a Connected Care Framework [44] to begin our development of competencies and coursework. This framework builds on the core competencies [43] for interprofessional collaborative practice as well as the concepts of connected health, patient engagement, clinical transformations (Accountable care, Triple Aim, Precision medicine) and new digital tools. These new concepts were framed within the context of the continuously learning health care system and interoperability principles. A diagram of the Connected Care Framework is shown below (Figure 1).

Connected Care Framework

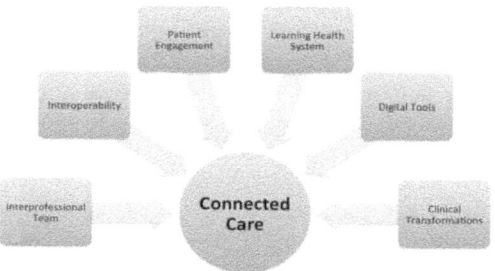

Figure 1. Connected Care Framework.

7. Summary

The delineation of the next generation of informatics competencies for practicing nurses need to examine the following challenges. First, as technology becomes more ubiquitous, is there a need to focus on computer literacy knowledge and skills? Should we be thinking of digital literacy [57] knowledge and skills? Second, is information literacy still important? Does this need to change to health information literacy [58] in the connected care arena? Or perhaps it should be digital health literacy as noted by the European Commission [59]. Third, what are the new communication knowledge and skills practicing nurses need in the connected care era? Do they understand how to use digital tools to communicate with an interprofessional team? Do they understand how to interact with patients, families and caregivers via virtual visits, patient portals, social media, and even personal robotic assistants? Do they know how to maintain a sense of presence and caring in virtual patient visits and through various digital media? Fourth, with the growing deluge of data, are data processing and information management still necessary knowledge and skills? Or do we need to also examine knowledge management and data analytics competencies? What about data visualization competencies? What about the growing amount of personal generated health data from patients, how will that be integrated into care? If we are to create a learning health system, how will we ensure semantic operability so nurses can create evidence based practice by analyzing clinical data? And last but certainly, not least, it is important to re-examine what we expect nurse to know about privacy, confidentiality, and security issues in a connected care ecosystem. What are the new legal, ethical, social and public policy questions once we move beyond the post-EHRs era and into the connected care age?

In summary, the time is now to re-examine the informatics competencies of both practicing nurses as well as informatics specialists. The transformation of health care across the globe demands this re-examination of basic informatics knowledge, skills and attitudes for both practicing nurses, advanced practice nurses, nurse leaders and those specializing in nursing informatics. There is a need to build on the existing foundation and delineate new competencies needed given the changing health care landscape.

References

[1] Ball MJ., Hannah KJ., Using computers in nursing, Reston Publishing Company, Inc: Reston, VA. 1988.
[2] Chow R., Patient Monitoring is more than just a dream, Amer J of Nurs, 61(1961),60-62.
[3] Editorial, From blinking to thinking, Amer J of Nurs, 61(1961,55.
[4] Rosenberger M. & Carriker D., Automating Nurse's Notes. Amer J of Nurs. 66(1966),1021-1023.
[5] Anderson J., Gremy F. & Pages JC, Education in Informatics of Health Personnel. IFIP Medical Informatics Monograph Series: Volume 1. North Holland Publishing: Amsterdam, 1974.
[6] Ronald JS., Computers and undergraduate nursing education: A report of an experimental introductory course. J of Nurs Ed, 18(1978), 4-9.
[7] Ronald JS., Introducing baccalaureate nursing students to the use of computers in health care. In H Heffernan (Ed) Proceedings of the Fifth Annual Symposium on Computer Applications in Medical Care. (1981) 771-775. Available at: http://www.ncbi.nlm.nih.gov/pmc/articles/PMC2581216/
[8] Ozbolt J. & Saba VK, A brief history of nursing informatics in the United States of America. Nurs Outlook,56 (2008) 199-205.
[9] Ronald JS. & Skiba DJ., Guidelines for Basic Computer Education in Nursing. National League for Nursing: New York, 1987.
[10] Peterson HE. & Gerdin-Jelger U. (Eds), Preparing Nurses for Using Information Systems, National League for Nursing: New York 1988.
[11] Graves JR. & Corcoran S., The study of nursing informatics. Image: J Nurs Scholar 21 (1989), 227-31.
[12] Dick RS., Steen EB. & Detmer DE., The Computer-Based Patient Record: An Essential Technology for Health Care, Revised Edition. National Academies Press: Washington, DC, 1997.
[13] American Nurses Association. Scope of Nursing Informatics Practice and Standards of Nursing Informatics Practice. American Nurses Association: Silver Spring, MD. 1994
[14] Skiba DJ., Simpson R. & Ronald JS., HealthQuest/HBO Nurse Scholars Program: A Corporate Sponsorship with Nursing Education. In J. Arnold and G. Pearson (Eds.). Computer Applications in Nursing Education and Practice. National League for Nursing: New York, 1992.
[15] Simpson R., Skiba DJ. & Ronald JS., A Five Year Retrospective of the HBO Nurse Scholars Program. In Grobe S. and Pleyter-Wenting ESP. (Eds.). Nursing Informatics: An international overview for nursing in a technological era. Elsevier: North Holland: Elsevier, 1994.
[16] Wainwright P., First European Summerschool in Nursing Informatics. Information Technology in Nursing. 4(1992), 10-11
[17] Mantas J., Nursing Informatics Educational Issues: The NIGHTINGALE project. In Brender J., Christensen JP, Scherrer JR., McNair P. (Eds). Medical Informatics Europe 1996. IOS Press: Amsterdam, 1996, 804-807
[18] Skiba DJ., The Learning Collaboratory: A Knowledge Building Environment for Nursing Education. In Gerdin U., Tallberg M., & Wainwright P. (Eds.). Nursing Informatics: The Impact of Nursing Knowledge on Health Care Informatics. Proceedings of the Sixth International Conference. IOS Press: Amsterdam, the Netherlands, 1997

[19] Staggers N., Gassert C. & Skiba DJ., Health Professionals' Views of Informatics Education: Findings from the AMIA Spring 1999 Conference, J of the Amer Med Inform Assoc, 7 (2000), 550-558.

[20] Association of American Medical Colleges. Contemporary issues in medicine – medical informatics and population health: report II of the Medical School Objectives Project. Acad Med 74(1999): 130-41.

[21] American Association of Colleges of Nursing, Essentials of baccalaureate education for professional nursing practice. AACN: Washington DC, 1998.

[22] Recommendations of the International Medical Informatics Association (IMIA) on Education in Health and Medical Informatics International Medical Informatics Association, Working Group 1: Health and Medical Informatics Education. Available at: http://www.imia-medinfo.org/new2/rec_english.pdf

[23] Warren J. & Connors H.,(2007). Health information technology can and will transform nursing education. Nurs Outlook, 55(2007), 58-60.

[24] Kohn LT., Corrigan JM. & Donaldson MS. (Eds), To err is human: Building a safer health system. National Academies Press: Washington, DC, 2000.

[25] Committee on Quality Health Care in America, Institute of Medicine. Crossing the quality chasm: A new health system for the 21st century. National Academy Press: Washington DC, 2001.

[26] Aspden P., Corrigan JM., Wolcott J. & Erickson S. (Eds.) for Committee on Data Standards for Patient Safety, Institute of Medicine. Patient safety: Achieving a new standard of care. National Academies Press: Washington DC, 2004.

[27] Greiner A. & Knebel E. (Eds.) Health professions education: A bridge to quality. National Academies Press: Washington, DC , 2003

[28] Cronenwett L., Sherwood G., Barnsteiner J., Disch J., Johnson J., Mitchell P., Sullivan D. & Warren J., Quality and safety education for nurses. Nurs Outlook. 55(2007): 122-131.

[29] Barton AJ., Cultivating informatics competencies in a community of practice. Nurs Admin Quarterly, 29(2005), 323-328.

[30] American Nurses Association. The Scope and Standards of Nursing Informatics. American Nurses Association: Silver Springs, MD, 2001.

[31] American Nurses Association. The Scope and Standards of Nursing Informatics. American Nurses Association: Silver Springs, MD, 2008.

[32] Staggers N., Gassert CA. & Curran C., Informatics competencies for nurses at four levels of practice. J of Nurs Edu, 40(2001).

[33] Staggers N., Gassert CA. & Curran C., A Delphi study to determine informatics competencies for nurses at four levels of practice. Nurs Res, 51(2002), 383-390.

[34] TIGER Initiative: http://s3.amazonaws.com/rdcms-himss/files/production/public/FileDownloads/tiger-report-executive-summary.pdf

[35] Skiba DJ. & Rizzolo M., National League for Nursing's Informatics Agenda. Computers, Informatics & Nursing, 27 (2008), 66-68.

[36] American Association of Colleges of Nursing, Essentials of baccalaureate education for professional nursing practice. (2008) Available at: http://www.aacn.nche.edu/education-resources/essential-series.

[37] American Association of Colleges of Nursing, Essentials of Master's Education in Nursing (2011) Available at: http://www.aacn.nche.edu/education-resources/essential-series

[38] American Association of Colleges of Nursing, The Essentials of Doctoral Education in Nursing (2006). Available at: http://www.aacn.nche.edu/education-resources/essential-series

[39] Thompson B. & Skiba D J., Informatics in the Nursing Curriculum: A National Survey. Nurs Ed Persp, 29 (2008), 312-316.

[40] Honey ML., Skiba DJ., Procter P., Foster J., Kouri P. & Nagle L., Informatics Competencies to Start Professional Life: A Global Perspective. In Sermeus W., Procter PM. Weber P. (Eds) Nursing Informatics 2016 eHealth for All: Every Level Collaboration – From Project to Realization. IOS Press, Amsterdam, the Netherlands, 2016.

[41] Health Information Technology for Economic and Clinical Health (HITEC) Act of 2009. Available at: https://www.healthit.gov/sites/default/files/hitech_act_excerpt_from_arra_with_index.pdf

[42] Institute of Medicine. The future of nursing: Leading change, advancing health. National Academies Press: Washington, DC, 2010.

[43] Interprofessional Education Collaborative Expert Panel. Core competencies for interprofessional collaborative practice. Report of an expert panel. Interprofessional Education Collaborative: Washington, DC,2011.

[44] Skiba DJ., Barton AJ., Estes K., Gilliam E., Knapfel S., Moore G. & Trinkley K.. Preparing the next generation of advanced practice nurses for Connected Care. In Sermeus W., Procter PM. Weber P. (Eds) Nursing Informatics 2016 eHealth for All: Every Level Collaboration – From Project to Realization. IOS Press, Amsterdam, the Netherlands, 2016.

[45] Skiba DJ., The Connected Age: Implications for 2014. Nurs Ed Perspect. 35 (2014), 63-65.

[46] Caulfield BM. & Donnelly SC. What is Connected Health and why will it change your practice? QJM: An Inter J of Med. 2013; 106(8): 703-707.

[47] Iglehart JK., Connected Health: Emerging disruptive technologies. Hlth Affairs.33(2014),190.

[48] Fraher E., Spetz J. & Naylor M.. Nursing in a transformed health care system: New roles, new rules. 2015 Jun. Available from: http://ldi.upenn.edu/brief/nursing-transformed-health-care-system-new-roles-new-rules

[49] Institute of Medicine. Best care at lower cost: The path to continuously learning health care in America. 2012. Available from: http://iom.nationalacademies.org/Reports/2012/Best-Care-at-Lower-Cost-The-Path-to-Continuously-Learning-Health-Care-in-America.aspx

[50] Kish L.. The blockbuster drug of the century: An engaged patient. HL7 Health Standards. 28 August 2012. Available from: http://hl7standards.com/blog/2012/08/28/drug-of-the-century/.

[51] Ricciardi L., Mostashari F., Murphy J., Daniel J. & Siminerio E., A national action plan to support consumer engagement via e-health. Hlth Affairs,32(2013),376-384.

[52] Office of the National Coordinator for Health Information Technology. Connecting Health and Care for the Nation A Shared Nationwide Interoperability Roadmap: DRAFT Version 1.0. 2015. Available from: https://www.healthit.gov/sites/default/files/nationwide-interoperability-roadmap-draft-version-1.0.pdf

[53] Office of the National Coordinator for Health Information Technology. Federal Health IT Strategy Plan 2015-2020. 2015 September. Available from: https://www.healthit.gov/sites/default/files/9-5-federalhealthitstratplanfinal_0.pdf

[54] Kulikowski C., Shortliffe E., Currie L., Elkin P., Hunter L., Johnson T., et al. AMIA Board White Paper: Definition of biomedical informatics and specification of core competencies for graduate education in the discipline. J Amer Med Inform Assoc. 19(2013) 931-938.

[55] Gibson CJ., Dixon BE. & Abrams K., Convergent evolution of health information management and health informatics. A perspective on the future of information professionals in health care. Appl Clin Inform 6(2015),163-184.

[56] Gardner RM., Overhage JM., Steen EB., Munger BS., Holmes JH., Williamson JJ., & Detmer DE., Core content for the subspecialty of clinical informatics. J Am Med Inform Assoc 16 (2009),153-157.

[57] Jones-Kavalier BR. & Flannigan SL., Connecting the digital dots: Literacy for the 21st century. Educause Quart 29 (2006), 8-10. Available at: http://er.educause.edu/~/media/files/article-downloads/eqm0621.pdf

[58] Medical Library Association. Health information literacy: definitions. Chicago, IL: The Association. Available at: http://www.mlanet.org/resources/healthlit/define.html.

[59] European Commission Directorate General Communication Networks, Content and Technology. European Citizens' digital health literacy. European Union 2014. Available at http://ec.europa.eu/public_opinion/flash/fl_404_en.pdf

Forecasting Informatics Competencies for Nurses in the Future of Connected Health
J. Murphy et al. (Eds.)
© *2017 IMIA and IOS Press.*
This article is published online with Open Access by IOS Press and distributed under the terms
of the Creative Commons Attribution Non-Commercial License 4.0 (CC BY-NC 4.0).
doi:10.3233/978-1-61499-738-2-20

IMIA Educational Recommendations and Nursing Informatics

John MANTAS [a,1] and Arie HASMAN [b]

[a] *Health Informatics Lab, Department of Nursing, National and Kapodistrian University of Athens, Greece*
[b] *Department of Medical Informatics, AMC, University of Amsterdam, The Netherlands*

Abstract. The updated version of the IMIA educational recommendations has given an adequate guidelines platform for developing educational programs in Biomedical and Health Informatics at all levels of education, vocational training, and distance learning. This chapter will provide a brief introduction of the recommendations pinpointing aspects for developing and assessing educational programs. We will provide a review of the existing feedback we have acquired during the IMIA site visits of accrediting educational programs at a worldwide level and discuss implementations issues. A brief overview of existing academic programs in Europe, North America and in other regions, especially for programs related to Nursing and to Nursing Informatics is provided. Finally, we will draw conclusions as how the IMIA recommendations may be required to be fitted into the specific needs of the Nursing Informatics and the needs of the Nursing professionals when they apply the recommendations to their academic and/or hospital/professional environments.

Keywords. Educational recommendations, nursing informatics

1. Introduction

Increasingly information systems are installed in hospitals, General Practitioners (GP) practices and other healthcare organizations. More and more activities such as registration of data in electronic health records, order entry, interpretation of images, different types of decision making and searching for medical knowledge are supported by information systems. Since patients are transferred between healthcare organizations communication between information systems is also becoming more important. Communication between these systems is only possible when semantic interoperability can be achieved, which requires standardization of the communicated messages.

Because of the ageing of populations the demand for cure and care will increase to such an extent that future healthcare workers cannot cope with the workload any more. So, it should be investigated how Information and Communication Technologies (ICT) solutions can reduce the workload of healthcare workers. An example is to monitor at home the health status of elderly people. Nurses and physicians usually can evaluate at a distance the condition of patients. This approach has led to less hospital admissions and reduces travel time of healthcare practitioners.

---

[1] Corresponding author. John Mantas, email: jmantas@nurs.uoa.gr

Because of the above noted trends, there is an increasing need for informaticians to develop and design information systems but also to investigate new possibilities for the use of ICT in healthcare. At the same time, health informaticians should further develop the scientific foundation of the field.

The more information systems are installed in healthcare organizations, the more the users of these systems need to be knowledgeable about the benefits, but also the limitations of the use of these systems. In addition, relevant users must be able to express, in terms that are understood by software developers, which inefficiencies they experience in medical practice or where effective solutions for certain types of problems are needed. At least part of the end-users should be able to talk with software developers, understand solutions offered by them and judge the potential of these ICT solutions so that they can discuss the suggestions with their colleagues. This requires education and training. All end-users for example should be given the necessary education in health informatics at the level needed for carrying out their job (those nurses and physicians who in addition will be in contact with system designers will need more education in order to understand them and be able to judge offered solutions).

Usually, information systems are implemented and maintained by technically orientated personnel with a computer science background. They usually have limited insight in the problems of medical practice. It is well known that the communication between these ICT specialists and the medical staff is often not optimal. A solution may be to educate persons who are able to function as intermediaries between ICT specialists on the one side and physicians and nurses on the other. These may be health informaticians but also medical doctors or nurses who via additional education obtained the necessary informatics background (specialized healthcare practitioners). The specialized doctors and nurses may talk on the one side with the end-users and on the other side with health informaticians, who may in turn talk with the technically orientated informaticians. In this case there are two types of intermediaries. In other situations either health informaticians or (less frequently: since health informaticians with a medical or nursing background usually are less knowledgeable in the field) specialized healthcare practitioners may be the sole intermediaries. The International Medical Informatics Association (IMIA) Recommendations, to be discussed later, define the knowledge and skills that each of the above introduced groups should master.

Because of the growing need for health informaticians, educational programs in health informatics (both bachelor and master programs, but there are more master programs) increasingly focus on the professional practice rather than on research. These programs prepare graduates for careers oriented toward the use of best practices with respect to the design and development of information systems, their configuration and deployment in clinical and other settings, their integration into workflows, and the evaluation of their impact. Health informatics Master programs may have different focal points and deliver graduates with different kinds of expertise. These programs not only accept students with a bachelor in health informatics but also students with a background in medicine, nursing, biology, computer science, mathematics, physics, etc.

Especially in the bachelor phase, educational programs in health informatics introduce students extensively to medical and nursing subjects, so that health informaticians have, next to informatics knowledge and skills, also the necessary knowledge to support the medical staff in defining the requirements for new applications. Nowadays, also post-graduate master programs exist that have as goal to specialize medical doctors and nurses in health informatics, sometimes using distance learning. In the United States (US) medical informatics is a medical subspecialty.

Knowledge about the use, benefits and limitations of information systems should be part of undergraduate nursing or medicine curricula.

The Recommendations on Education in Biomedical and Health Informatics of IMIA define the knowledge and skills necessary for creating different types of health informaticians [1]. Educational programs as described above use these recommendations when defining the contents of their health informatics curricula. In doing so, they also take the needs of the labor market into account in order to endow their students with employable skill sets.

When searching for an attractive program in health informatics, students take the international status of the higher education institution into account, because increasingly graduates may go to work in another country than their own. Educational institutions compete for students and therefore invite international experts to evaluate their programs so that they can advertise the results if the judgment is positive. Such an evaluation can become a costly business since usually not only the travel and accommodation costs for the experts have to be paid but also the experts have to be remunerated. IMIA has the potential to serve as accreditation agency [2, 3, 4]. The accreditation process can be less costly when experts from member countries of IMIA agree to carry out the peer review for free (expecting only remuneration of travelling expenses and accommodation).

The IMIA Recommendations on Education in Biomedical and Health Informatics are very important for a number of reasons. As mentioned above, the Recommendations are important for educational institutions when they plan to design a curriculum in Health informatics. The Recommendations allow them to design different types of program depending on the type of graduates they want to deliver. The recommendations are also necessary for enabling an international exchange of students and teachers and for establishing international programs and may encourage and support the sharing of courseware.

But also for accreditation the Recommendations are important. Since the health informatics curricula have various focuses, can be vocational or academic, a framework is necessary to judge whether the curriculum provides enough knowledge and skills for the type of graduates the program is delivering. The Recommendations are, therefore extensively used both for designing programs and for accrediting purposes.

In this book contribution among others the Recommendations and the Accreditation process are presented. We, as authors, have already published a lot about these topics. Therefore, we make use of earlier articles [1-6] to give our current readers a good overview of these topics.

2. Introduction to the IMIA Recommendations

Education in the field of health informatics is not available in all countries. In some countries health informatics curricula, both vocational and academic and for various types of healthcare professionals, are adequately available, in other countries this is hardly the case. It is now well recognised that the availability of specialists in health informatics and end-users who have knowledge of the benefits and limitations of the use of information systems has a positive influence on the quality and effectiveness of healthcare. A framework describing the possible subjects that should be part of health informatics curricula and at which depth therefore will be of help in checking the quality of existing curricula and a guide for designing new curricula is therefore not a luxury. The IMIA recommendations for education [1] were designed just for this purpose. Existing educational programs have different focuses, depending on the type of institution that is delivering the education and the type of healthcare system existing in the country. Nevertheless, there is still quite a lot of overlap in the subjects that are taught. Due to this overlap, the development of a framework for recommendations becomes possible.

Around 2006 it was clear that the original version of the Recommendations had become outdated and should be revised and updated. In 2010, the revised version of the Recommendations [6] was published.

As shown above we can distinguish end-users from specialized nurses and doctors and health informatics specialists. The IMIA Recommendations specify major learning outcomes for the group of end-users and for the group of specialists:

- Learning outcomes for all health care professionals in their role as IT users: these learning outcomes should be included in all undergraduate curricula, leading to a health care professional qualification.
- Learning outcomes for health informatics specialists: these learning outcomes need to be included in all curricula that have the aim to deliver specialists in health informatics, leading to a qualification as specialist in health informatics, be it the group of health practitioners with additional knowledge and skills in health informatics or the group of specialists who follow a master course in health informatics.

Obviously, curricula for specialisation of a health care professional (post-graduate programs) or as a health informatics specialist (graduate programs), will show a varying depth and breadth of their learning outcomes.

The learning outcomes define the levels of knowledge and skills needed at the end of the study. The desired outcomes determine the contents of the educational components either in courses/course tracks in health informatics as part of non health informatics undergraduate programs or in the contents of dedicated programs in health informatics.

In the IMIA Recommendations the knowledge and skills levels are specified for four domain areas:

1. Biomedical and Health Informatics.
2. Medicine, Health and Biosciences, Health System Organisation.
3. Informatics/Computer Science, Mathematics, Biometry.
4. Optional modules from related fields.

Moreover for each of the recommendations it is stated at what level they should be taught (from introductory to advanced) both for the group of end-users and for the group of specialists. The latter group is more variable and therefore for each variety a different curriculum has to be specified.

3. Experiences with accreditation

In 2011, the IMIA General Assembly accepted a proposal to test a suggested accreditation procedure in a trial phase in which five institutions, spread over the IMIA regions, would volunteer to participate. It should be noted that the IMIA accreditation is an addition to national accreditation and does not replace it.

The accreditation procedure in the meantime has been tested and IMIA now offers to accredit educational programs in health informatics. The national accreditation procedures show a lot of commonalities. A quality assurance agency publishes which topics will be assessed and which criteria will be used. The institution prepares a self-assessment report covering the topics specified by the quality assurance agency. Usually a peer review team validates the contents of the report during a site visit and assesses the quality of the program. The peer reviewers usually are experts in the field that is covered by the program.. The IMIA accreditation procedure is similar.

The self-assessment report provides the information needed by the peer review team to evaluate the assessment criteria. According to the IMIA accreditation procedure the self-assessment report should answer the following six main questions:

1. What are the goals of the program for which the institute asks accreditation?
2. How are the goals implemented in a curriculum?
3. What is the size and quality of the staff?
4. Which facilities for teaching are available?
5. How does the institute guarantee the quality of the program?
6. Are the goals routinely reached?

The peer review usually comprises a site visit that may take from one to four days, during which the site-visit the peer review team (called site visit committee in the IMIA accreditation documentation) consults with the various stakeholders. The stakeholders for an educational program may range from the rector and dean to staff and student and alumni representatives, to employers of the graduates of the reviewed programme or institution. The site-visit committee may during the site visit ask for more information when needed.

After the site-visit the committee prepares a report containing an evaluation of the program and the final judgment. The IMIA Accreditation Committee sends the report to the institution or program with the question to correct factual errors if they are present in the report. Then the Accreditation Committee will make the final decision concerning accreditation or not.

During the trial period, IMIA accumulated substantial experience regarding the advantages of the process and ways of improving it. The different levels and orientations of the programs, the variety of cultures encountered, and the differences in implementation and infrastructural possibilities provided enough material to generalize and refine the accreditation procedure to facilitate its routine use in the future.

An assessment of the IMIA Accreditation process is reported elsewhere [2]. In [3] the experiences with the accreditation procedure were reported by the first educational program accredited by IMIA. Here we only mention an example of a change in the documentation that was necessary for theses written in the national language. The peer review team selects a number of theses that should be in their possession before the site visit. Theses usually prepared in the national language could not be understood by the reviewers. It was too time consuming or costly to translate the selected theses into English. Therefore, theses summaries in English were requested. However, the thesis summaries did not provide a sufficient impression of the quality and content of the theses. Therefore, a translation of the Table of Contents was also requested and during the site visit an additional day was devoted to the discussion of the theses with the supervisors.

The common characteristics of all visits were the willingness of the volunteering institutions to accept the costs and time for accreditation, the overwhelming preparation and enthusiasm to participate shown at all levels of their hierarchy, and the acceptance of the final judgment of the committee, which included a number of recommendations for improvement.

An Accreditation Review Committee consisting of three independent IMIA Board members chaired by Reinhold Haux at that time, evaluated the accreditation reports [5] that were written during the trial period. The Committee came to the conclusion that:

- the site-visit committees have carefully studied the respective programs;
- they have documented their reviews and recommendations extensively and well-written in their reports;
- the IMIA Accreditation Review Committee fully supports all the recommendations;
- in case of reaccreditation, the actions for improvement, as expressed in the accreditation report, have to be put in practice. Otherwise, reaccreditation is probably not possible.

4. Educational programs in HI for nurses

There is a number of Biomedical and Health Informatics educational programs at academic institutions across the world. Detailed list of programs for Europe can be found at the EFMI website available at the WG EDU link [8]. The American Medical Informatics Association has a long tradition in establishing a database of educational programs available at US institutions [9]. Unfortunately, the tradition of IMIA to develop and hold a database of educational programs across the world is not available any more in the last ten years; therefore, there is a very important missing link of information available to those interested to have a global view in education in our field. However, from the available information and search, one may deduce that there is an increased number of programs especially in the field of Health Informatics and more lately in the field of Biomedical Engineering and Bioinformatics. Most of the programs are at the Master's level, which is quite reasonable, as you may specialise or convert professionals with different backgrounds to the Health Informatics discipline.

In most countries there is no Nursing Informatics specialisation or certification. So for a Nursing graduate the informatics skills and knowledge may be acquired at their undergraduate studies. From a brief review into the European nursing curricula it is not directly evident that nursing curricula include nursing informatics or health informatics courses/modules. One may find computer skills classes taught from outside the department faculty. Those classes are given to almost every other student at the University or Institution. Therefore, searching in European Institutions nursing curricula very few programs include nursing/health informatics courses. Also at those departments of nursing, where nursing/health informatics courses exist, there are even fewer mandatory courses in nursing/health informatics.

Since very few nurses are pursuing postgraduate studies due to the need either to work immediately, lack of nurses at the healthcare environment not allowing them to take a leave of absence for further studies, and/or sometimes lack of financial resources, emphasis should be given to the undergraduate curriculum to include a nursing informatics module/course as obligatory.

5. Recommendations for Nursing science and Nursing practitioners

So the movement of the 1990's and later, which in many ways was rather successful as Council of Europe provided mandate for health informatics courses implementation to be suggested as obligatory to all Medical, Nursing and other Health Sciences schools curricula, European Commission funded nursing specific actions such as Nightingale [10] and Telenursing/ Telenurse [11], seems now that it is fading out. One reason may be that the curriculum developers think that nowadays all students are already adequate users of computers so there is no need in a clinical school to introduce any more computer courses. This reason is not correct since Nursing/Health Informatics is a scientific discipline part of the Health Sciences curriculum and a computer skills requirement in the curriculum. This important difference has not yet penetrated into the traditional thinking of our fellow colleagues in a number of nursing departments or other health related departments including medicine.

6. Refocusing the Recommendations for Nursing

Studying the Recommendations and trying to view them from a specific professional viewpoint is the usual practice, whenever one wants to acquire a particular perspective.

Nursing is a clinical profession with particular needs and requirements regarding the Biomedical Medical Health Informatics (BMHI) field. It is well known that in both IMIA and AMIA, Nursing plays a very important and strategic role requiring special attention and the specialization of Nursing Informatics has a long history of accomplishments and specialized meetings and Conferences and attract special attention. The same goes with the educational requirements.

Therefore, we truly believe that a special attention should be paid to the IMIA recommendations when looked from a Nursing perspective. We have refocused specific skills in Table 1 where we underline the additional items that should be included to the already required skills.

Table 1. Modified table of Knowledge and Skills focused on Nursing

	Knowledge/Skills – Domain	Level	
		Nurse as User	NI specialist
1	**Biomedical and Health Informatics Core Knowledge and Skills**		
1.1	**Evolution of informatics** as a discipline and as a profession	+	+
1.2	**Need for systematic information processing** in health care, benefits and constraints of information technology in health care	++	++

Knowledge/Skills – Domain		Level	
		Nurse as User	NI specialist
1.3	Efficient and responsible **use of information processing tools,** to support health care professionals' practice and their decision making	++	++
1.4	**Use of personal application software** for documentation, personal communication including Internet access, for publication and basic statistics	++	++
1.5	**Information literacy:** library classification and systematic health related terminologies and their coding, literature retrieval methods, research methods and research paradigms	++	++
1.6	Characteristics, functionalities and examples of **information systems in health care** (e.g. clinical information systems, primary care information systems, nursing information systems, etc.)	+	+++
1.7	**Architectures of information systems** in health care; approaches and standards for communication and cooper- ation and for interfacing and integration of component, architectural paradigms (e.g. service-oriented architectures)		++
1.8	**Management of information systems** in health care (health information management, strategic and tactic information management, NI management, IT governance, IT service management, legal and regulatory issues)	+	+++
1.9	Characteristics, functionalities and examples of **information systems to support patients and the public** (e.g. patient-oriented information system architectures and applications, personal health records, sensor-enhanced information systems)	+	++
1.10	Methods and approaches to **regional networking and shared care** (eHealth, health telematics applications and inter-organizational information exchange	+	++
1.11	Appropriate documentation and **health data management principles** including ability to use **health and medical coding systems,** construction of health and medical coding systems, nursing coding schemes	+	+++
1.12	Structure, design and analysis principles of the **health record** including notions of data quality, minimum data sets, architecture and general applications of the electronic patient record/electronic health record, including nursing records	+	+++
1.13	**Socio-organizational and socio-technical issues,** including workflow/process modelling and reorganization	+	++
1.14	Principles of **data representation and data analysis** using primary and secondary data sources, principles of data mining, data warehouses, knowledge	+	++
1.15	Biomedical **modelling and simulation**		+
1.16	**Ethical and security issues including** accountability of health care providers and managers and BMHI specialists and the confidentiality, privacy and security of patient data	+	++
1.17	**Nomenclatures, vocabularies,** terminologies, ontologies and taxonomies in BMHI	+	++
1.18	Informatics methods and tools to **support education** (incl. flexible and distance learning), use of relevant educational technologies, incl. Internet and World Wide Web	+	+
1.19	**Evaluation and assessment** of information systems, including study design, selection and triangulation of (quantitative and qualitative) methods, outcome and impact evaluation, economic evaluation, unintended consequences, systematic reviews and meta-analysis, evidence-based health informatics		++

	Knowledge/Skills – Domain	Nurse as User	NI specialist
2	**Medicine, <u>Nursing</u>, Health and Biosciences, Health Systems Organization**		
2.1	Fundamentals of **human functioning** and biosciences (anatomy, physiology, microbiology, genomics, and clinical disciplines such as internal medicine, surgery, <u>nursing</u>, etc.)	+	+
2.2	Fundamentals of **what constitutes health,** from physiological, sociological, psychological, nutritional, emotional, environmental, cultural, spiritual perspectives and its assessment	+	+
2.3	Principles of **clinical/medical decision making, <u>nursing assessment</u>,** and diagnostic and therapeutic strategies	+	++
2.4	**Organisation of health institutions** and of the overall health system, interorganizational aspects, shared care	+	+++
2.5	**Policy and regulatory frameworks** for information handling in health care		+
2.6	Principles of **evidence-based practice** (evidence-based medicine, <u>evidence-based nursing</u>	+	+
2.7	**Health administration, health economics,** health quality management and resource management, patient safety initiatives, public health services and outcome measurement	+	++
3	**Informatics/Computer Science, Mathematics, Biometry**		
3.1	**Basic informatics terminology** like data, information, knowledge, hardware, software, computer, networks, information systems, information	+	+++
3.2	**Ability to use personal computers,** text processing and spread sheet software, easy-to-use database management systems	++	+++
3.3	**Ability to communicate electronically,** including electronic data exchange, with other health care professionals, internet/intranet use	++	+++
3.4	Methods of **practical informatics**/computer science, especially on programming languages, software engineering, data structures, database management systems, information and system modelling tools, information systems theory and practice		+++
3.5	Methods of **theoretical informatics**/computer science, e.g. complexity theory		++
3.6	Methods of **technical informatics**/computer science, e.g. network architectures and topologies, telecommunications, wireless technology, virtual reality, multimedia		++
3.7	Methods of **interfacing and integration** of information system components in health care, interfacing standards, dealing with multiple patient identifiers		++
3.8	Handling of the **information system life cycle**: analysis, requirement specification, implementation and/or selection of information systems, risk	+	+++
3.9	Methods of **project management and change management** (i.e. project planning, resource management, team management, conflict management,	+	+++
3.10	**Mathematics:** algebra, analysis, logic, numerical mathematics,		++
3.11	**Biometry, epidemiology,** and **health research methods,** including study		++
3.12	Methods for **decision support** and their application to patient management, acquisition, representation and engineering of medical knowledge; construction	+	+++
3.13	Basic concepts and applications of **ubiquitous computing** (e.g. pervasive, sensor-based and ambient technologies in health care, health enabling technologies,		+

Knowledge/Skills – Domain		Level	
		Nurse as User	**NI specialist**
3.14	Usability engineering, **human-computer interaction**, usability evaluation, cognitive aspects of information processing		++

Nursing ontologies and classifications systems such as North American Nursing Diagnosis Association (NANDA), Nursing Intervention Classification (NIC), Nursing Outcome Classification (NOC), Omaha, and International Classification for Nursing Practice ICNP, and generic health care terminologies such as SNOMED CT should be included into any NI curriculum. Furthermore, nursing management skills is mandatory including change management, whereas patient safety nursing roles and patient advocacy are obligatory to be taught and discussed. Specific nursing information systems should also be added as required by both clinical environments and nursing management. The scientific nursing should be emphasized in relation to the nursing informatics field where osmosis may benefit both academic and clinical work. The need for professional nursing assessment and scientific evidenced based nursing may both gain support from the upcoming Informatics applications.

The additional items may be there at the revised Educational Recommendations but the authors feel that emphasis should be given in such a way that the obscured definitions become more obvious in the refocused for NI Educational Recommendations as mentioned in Table 1.

7. Conclusions and Discussion

We understand that education is a very powerful instrument for change in the society, the scientific domain and in the professional world. For many years Nursing has struggled to attain a scientific status across the world. This may be true for many years at certain countries such as US or Canada. However, for most countries including in Europe only in the last thirty years (almost one generation), Nursing has become and it has been accepted as a scientific field taught at University level.

In most of the Nursing schools modules or courses in IT skills exist, however, it is not evident from the search we have done that all programs in Nursing at undergraduate level teach Nursing Informatics. In addition, very few specific postgraduate programs exist in Nursing Informatics. Most programs at postgraduate level are called Health Informatics where graduate Nurses are accepted along with other interest medical/health sciences graduates. In those programs, specific modules/courses in Nursing Informatics are very rare.

It is therefore, a requirement to revisit the Educational recommendations and emphasize as clearly as possible the required skills and knowledge in BMHI as required from the Nursing scientific and professional viewpoint. In the modified table we have tried to provide a first effort to refocus the skills with nursing perspective.

References

[1]   Recommendations of the International Medical Informatics Association (IMIA) on education in health and medical informatics. Methods Inf Med 2000; 39: 267–277.
[2]   Hasman A, Mantas J, IMIA Accreditation of Health Informatics Programs. Healthc Inform Res, 19,3, (2013), 154-61.
[3]   Hasman A. IMIA Accreditation of Health Informatics Programs. Yearb Med Inform. 7, (2012), 139-43.
[4]   Hasman A, IMIA accreditation of health informatics programs. Stud Health Technol Inform. 2012;174:47-52.
[5]   Mantas J, Hasman A, Shortliffe EH. Assessment of the IMIA educational accreditation process. Stud Health Technol Inform 2013;192:702-6.
[6]   Mantas J, Ammenwerth E, Demiris G, Hasman A, Haux R, Hersh W, Hovenga E, Lun KC, Marin H, MartinSanchez F, Wright G., Recommendations of the International Medical Informatics Association (IMIA) on Education in Biomedical and Health Informatics. First Revision, Methods Inf Med 49, 2 (2010), 105-120.
[7]   Mantas J, Implementation of the recommendations in master's courses in health informatics. Stud Health Technol Inform. 2012;174:57-61.
[8]   European Federation of Medical Informatics (EFMI). Overview of Educational Programs in Health Informatics. Available from: www.efmi.org / https://www.efmi.org/workinggroups/edu-education / http://en.hil.nurs.uoa.gr/wgedu/educational-programs-in-europe.html
[9]   American Medical Informatics Association (AMIA). Education. Available from www.amia.org. / https://www.amia.org/education/programs-and-courses
[10] Mantas J. Advances in Health Telematics Education: A Nightingale Perspective. Amsterdam, IOS Press, 1998.
[11] Mortensen R. ICNP in Europe: Telenurse. Amsterdam, IOS press, 1997.

Forecasting Informatics Competencies for Nurses in the Future of Connected Health
J. Murphy et al. (Eds.)
© 2017 IMIA and IOS Press.
doi:10.3233/978-1-61499-738-2-31

The Shifting Sands of Nursing Informatics Education: From Content to Connectivity

Michelle HONEY[a,1] and Paula PROCTER[b]

[a] *School of Nursing, University of Auckland, Auckland, NEW ZEALAND*
[b] *Sheffield Hallam University, Sheffield , UNITED KINGDOM*

Abstract. This chapter considers the development of nurse education over the past 50 years and ventures a view towards 2020. A link will be made to the introduction of informatics to nursing curricula. It is clear when looking over the recent history of nurse education that it has moved from a medical model and content driven apprentice mode to that of a reflective agile professional mode where autonomous practice allows for collaboration in care and connectivity between health professionals. Parallel to these pedagogical changes are the introduction of informatics across healthcare, starting with computer skills and moving through information management to decision support. The chapter will conclude with some thoughts around the next possible steps forward for nursing informatics education.

Keywords. Nursing education; Learning Theories; Connectivism

1. Introduction

Nursing education has changed over time, from an apprenticeship model approach, to one where nursing education is valued for creating critical thinking, problem solving autonomous practitioners [1]. Nursing competencies have been introduced into nursing education internationally in an attempt to produce nurses who can demonstrate performance against the expected role of a Registered Nurse (RN). Berwick [2] describes this saying "During professional preparation, nurses-in-training should experience, reflect upon, and develop the knowledge, skills, and attitudes that create competence in patient-centred care, teamwork and collaboration, evidence-based practice, quality improvement, safety, and informatics".

This chapter considers the historical development of nursing education, then links the changes in nursing education to the development of nursing informatics education. Learning theories are described, following the evolving approach taken by nursing and nursing informatics education over time. This chapter concludes with identifying some of the challenges facing nursing informatics education towards 2020, and the question of whether post connectivism can support the development of the agile health practitioner needed in an ever-increasing digital world.

---

[1]Corresponding author, Michelle Honey, Senior Lecturer, School of Nursing, The University of Auckland. Private Bag 92019, Auckland, NEW ZEALAND; Email: m.honey@auckland.ac.nz.

2. Changes in the education of nurses

Early nursing education followed an apprenticeship model based in hospitals [1]. Senior nurses and doctors provided the training, along with on-the-job experience supervised by qualified and more senior student nurses. Servicing the needs of hospitals, not the educational needs of the students, was the emphasis in the apprenticeship model of nursing education.

From the early 1970s nursing education started to move to the education sector. The focus shifted to student learning and understanding of nursing. Education that supported the development of nurses' decision-making power was introduced, accompanying a change from task oriented practice, from 'doing' to 'knowing' [3]. The literature describes a paradigm shift that occurred in nursing education coined as a 'curriculum revolution' [4]. Key themes of the 'revolution' included social responsibility, the centrality of caring in nursing, an interpretive stance, reflection and critical thinking [4-6]. It is now well recognized that nursing education needs to provide for lifelong learning including critical thinking ability, communication skills, and information literacy [7-9]. Resulting in part from the information explosion and increased access to information through the Internet, there is less emphasis on what students need to learn as a finite body of knowledge and more on the process of learning [10].

The use of nursing competencies started to appear in literature in the 1970s, being touted as being a way to provide a standard approach to education [11, 12]. Rather than set a core curriculum the preference grew to describe competencies that nurses would develop, which was considered to provide education providers sufficient guidance and also the opportunity to be creative in how their curricula were designed [11]. The Quality and Safety Education for Nurses (QSEN) project [13] describes competencies as including knowledge, skills, and attitudes, highlighting achievement of competencies as indicators of nurses who can provide safe and effective care. The effectiveness of competencies in nursing education is proven, but also highlights the important role of nurse educators [14], which is addressed in section B chapter 1.

The challenge is in preparing nurses for the future, recognizing that most programmes of learning to become a nurse take at least three years, and therefore a forward-looking approach is always needed. It is well known that future nurses will be working in a healthcare environment that is increasingly complex, where change is constant, and with individuals who will be living longer, are more likely to have a long-term condition and multiple co-morbidities [15-17]. In conjunction with this is the view that health should be considered longitudinally, across the lifespan of the person, rather than as episodic, where healthcare intercedes only when the person is sick [18]. This means nurses need a stronger focus on health promotion and disease prevention, rather than a sickness focus and the knowledge, skills and tools to achieve this.

3. Learning theories

Nursing education has always been open to new models of learning and teaching, moving and drawing on behaviorism, cognitivism, constructionism and connectivism, but at each juncture there has been a focus on the teacher rather than always understanding the student needs first. This may reflect early healthcare where historically a paternalistic approach to practice dominated, rather than negotiated care and working in partnership with patients and their families [1].

Behaviorism led into a world of classic conditioning or stimulus-response learning with the underlying concept that behavior was more influential to actions, including learning, than thinking or feeling [19]. Many will have learnt about Pavlov's dogs, where the dogs were conditioned to salivate upon hearing a bell even though there was no food presented, a classic conditioned response [20]. More recently Skinner [21] added further with his concept of operant conditioning where the mind of an individual plays a part in the way in which we do things, so the start of adding 'thinking' to the way in which we learn. Through development of Skinner's work emerged the theory of 'Law of Effect' where rewarded behavior tends to be repeated and behavior unrewarded tends to reduce or go away completely [22]. There remain elements of behaviorism in nurse education today where students follow regime processes such as the essentials of aseptic technique or the use of risk assessment tools whereby selection of responses result in a treatment protocol. However, in today's nursing education additional elements for student learning provide further enhancement which allows for an individualised approach.

The development of individualism allowing for greater conscious thinking came with cognitivism as a learning theory in the 1960s. The main concept behind cognitivism was that the process of learning was more important than the outward response to learning [23]. At the time of emergence of this theory there were significant developments in the uses of computers in different sectors of society which may have led to the theory often being described as concerned with the student as an information processor. Thinking, memory, problem-solving were at the heart of cognitivism where learning was considered as a thought change rather than just a response to stimuli [24]. In application to nurse education this theory heralded the start of the transition to individualised patient care through the understanding of processes with added variance due to individual patient need, which was shown in written nursing care plans.

In the 1980s a further expansion on individual learning was expounded through constructionism theory [25]. Bruner is one of the main theorists of constructionism and he suggests that learning is an active process, stimulated by curiosity [26]. Additionally, learning occurs when the information and experiences are meaningful and specific to the individual [27]. Students are seen as not just responding in a behaviorist way to stimuli, but seeking to understand and find meaning in the stimulation provided by the learning experience. This represents a significant shift away from 'teacher-led' education towards understanding and implementing 'student-led' learning where the activity of educational construction lay with the individual student constructing solutions guided or facilitated by a set of learning objectives which could be attained in more than one way, allowing for diversity of knowledge and thought by the student. Nursing education has drawn extensively from this theory of learning as it allows for individualised patient care whilst acknowledging that the process of learning is also individual and centred on the student, based on what the student needs to know related to gaps in their knowledge.

This brings us to the most recent theory espoused by Siemens called connectivism, which is considered a learning theory appropriate for the digital age [28]. The main thrust of this theory is that learning is moving from the 'know-how' or 'know-what' to the 'know-where', reflecting the need for information literacy skills around information accessing, filtering, and sequencing so the student knows when an appropriate resource has been located. Connectivism has been described as a dynamic state where knowledge is created beyond the individual participants, and is constantly shifting and changing: Knowledge is a shifting phenomenon as information flows across networks that themselves are inter-connected [29]. An obvious example of this is Wikipedia, where information is fluid and evolving. Wikipedia also indicates the need for students to be able to filter, and the need for information literacy to discern the credibility and usefulness of information accessed. Applied to nursing education, learning starts with the individual student who forms networks to aid their learning and extend their personal communities; hence their learning also draws on the experiences and learning of others. The use of social media among today's nursing students emphasizes the place of connectivism.

4. Nursing informatics education

The use of information and communications technology (ICT) in the delivery of healthcare is now usual practice in many countries. However, this occurred because of instrumental nursing informatics pioneers [30]. Now, more than ever, the increased use of ICT is being driven by patients and population demand, with countries looking for ways to improve efficiency with most nations struggling with inadequate resources. In many countries consumers can access and control their care records and participate in their health care. Nursing education prepares students for beginning practice as a RN, and this now includes being ready to act as information management advocates for patients and their families, to help them navigate the masses of accessible information. Moreover, nurses also need to be prepared to act as custodians of health information within a governance framework.

In the early 1960s the World Health Organization arranged international seminars on automatic data processing in health care but nurses were not invited until 1971 [31]. Then in 1982, the first world congress for nursing and ICT was held in London and attracted delegates from all over the world. It was this conference that resulted in the International Medical Informatics Association (IMIA) establishing a Working Group specifically for nursing; this working group continues to be at the forefront of nursing informatics today [30]. At this first nursing informatics conference in 1982, Constance Berg [32] presented a paper entitled 'The importance of nurses' input for the selection of computerized systems' and gave a profound warning:

> "The choice is there and the time to make the choice is now. The decision must be whether to act traditionally and have change thrust upon the profession [nursing] from the outside or to anticipate this revolution in nursing practice, familiarize nurses with it, and prepare them to take an active part in the introduction of computers into the nursing community".

Nursing informatics education builds on essential concepts within nursing education, such as communication skills, teamwork, the importance of nursing documentation, and working within legal and ethical boundaries. Early nursing informatics education followed the broad steps seen in nursing education. Initially the focus was on 'doing' tasks, such as how to use a computer with the aim of nurses developing basic computer skills. Then the emphasis moved to 'knowing' about information management and issues associated with using ICT. Nursing informatics is often presented drawing on the data–information-knowledge-wisdom framework [33, 34]. Over time the importance of nurses understanding how ICT can be used wherever nursing occurs, including patients using ICT, and both nurses and patients developing information literacy skills, has come to the foreground in our increasingly connected world. Nursing informatics frameworks and competencies are seen as one way to encapsulate the knowledge, skills and attitude nurses need.

5. Nursing informatics frameworks

In order to determine the most appropriate nursing informatics competencies it is helpful to understand the focus of various frameworks from different countries, organisations or individuals. An example from each is briefly offered here.

An European Union (EU) and United States (US) collaboration created HITComp - the Health IT competencies [35]. These EU/US health IT competencies were developed as a collaboration under the auspices of the Standards and Interoperability Framework of the US Office of the National Coordinator of Health Information Technology and the EU through the European Commission's Directorate General for Communication. A workgroup of public and private sector industry, ICT and e-health professionals, together with educators and clinicians, created a database. The outcome of this collaboration was published online in May 2015 and is a searchable database of skills and competencies needed across a variety of healthcare roles, including nursing [35].

An organisational example is the Quality and Safety Education for Nurses (QSEN) project which developed knowledge, skills and attitude competencies aimed to prepare nurses to continuously improve the quality and safety of the healthcare systems where they work [13]. QSEN acknowledges nursing informatics and developments such as electronic health records (EHR), social media, the increased role of consumers and their use of technology, mobile-health, smart phones, and health related applications. Additionally, QSEN suggests that ICT "is an enabling tool that links data, information, knowledge, and wisdom and facilitates problem solving and decision making". A further organizational example of nursing informatics frameworks is provided by the Technology Informatics Guiding Educational Reform (TIGER) Initiative [36] and this is described fully in section B chapter 3.

Bond and Procter [37] are individual nurse academics based in the United Kingdom. They proposed a framework to enable all RNs to have an essential understanding of informatics to work effectively in the healthcare information intensive environment. Figure 1 is taken from their work and as an overall view would appear to support many of the leading nursing informatics competency frameworks including, TIGER [38] and the HITComp [35]. The model (Figure 1) attempted to identify various informatics elements considered important for inclusion in a course preparing nurses for registration. The relationship between new knowledge (informatics) and advancing conventional healthcare knowledge was considered crucial in giving contextual meaning to the inclusion of informatics for the students. The original paper contains the 'key' to the various elements, but even looking at a meta level it is the movement in the learning that the student can undertake from bottom left to top right which binds such learning in a larger curriculum [37].

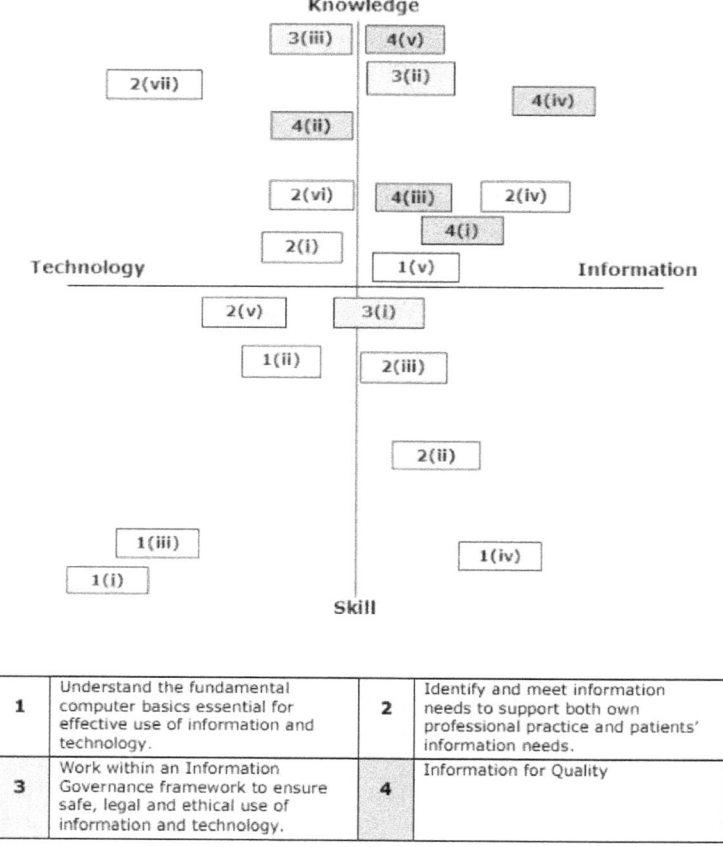

Figure 1: High level scatter chart of nursing informatics competencies across two continuums (Bond and Procter 2009) [37].

6. Challenges facing nursing education

With the changes to the models of nursing education, nursing informatics education has also changed. The changes in nursing education have been driven by societal and professional expectations of high quality nursing. In addition, new nursing roles have emerged, with RNs working at levels of advanced practice, yet all nurses are required to work with technology in their day to day work. While there have been significant changes and improvements in nursing education over the last century, there have also been challenges, which today include the blurring of health professional roles where professional boundaries overlap and sometimes cause increased workload due to duplication whilst the emerging roles find their place [39]. The growing division between service delivery and RN preparation causes a delay between curriculum designs meeting the needs of service improvement. This response delay increases the necessity to construct the education of nurses in a more generalist manner which has a flow on effect regarding a lack of professional identity which has the potential of returning nurse education to the early years where the curriculum design was developed to meet service need [40].

The Horizon Report suggests a number of developments in technology that will impact higher education in the next five years, with two key long-term influencing trends being advancing cultures of innovation and changes in how education providers (universities, colleges) work [41]. These changes and trends equally impact nursing education. For example, this report suggests technological developments as including students bringing their own devices, adaptive learning, augmented and virtual reality, affective computing, and robotics, which are already emerging or present in nursing education [42, 43].

The following competencies were identified as being important; and these are listed with examples for entry-level nurses, those studying to become a RN, and for the nurse educators involved in their education.

- Respect the individual's preference in their use(s) of digital health applications.
- Support individuals and family/carers through available information sources.
- Describe and work within the legal and ethical rules/ regulations associated with managing and sharing patient information.
- Identify, improve, encourage and use new technologies, including remote care from a clinical and community perspective of connected care.
- Find the most reliable sources of information to support evidence based practice.
- Incorporate information and communications technology into consultations.
- Manage the nurse-patient relationship when the nurse is not physically in the same place and/or time as the patient.
- Perform accurate and timely data entry at the point of care which is clinically meaningful.
- Explain the role of technology in the delivery and organization of care.
- Extract data to support decisions, monitor the outcomes of practice and generate knowledge.
- Support other users to identify and use relevant information and communications technologies for connected care.

7. Post connectivism

Earlier nursing informatics education mirrored nursing education, with a focus on tasks associated with using a computer [44-47]. In her chapter on the history of nursing and the computer, Saba in 2001 described 'computer' as an all-encompassing term including the internet [48]. With the increasingly widespread availability and connectivity to the Internet, web-based learning options came to the fore, so that by the late 1990s the focus was more on improving access to learning opportunities and using the technology to enhance learning [8, 49-51]. This change indicated a more cognitive approach to nursing informatics education [52]. More recently the focus has been on using ICT to collaborate, recognizing the power of the internet, electronic communications and social media, heralding a change of focus to connecting and networking amongst nurses.

In 1999 McGuiness and Hardy distinguished between personal, professional and educational technology for health professionals [53]. This synergy between the use of technology by nurses in their personal and professional lives, and for their ongoing education, indicates a blurring of the boundaries between each aspect, and with the ability to connect to other people, resources and ideas we are truly living in what Skiba termed 'The Connected Age' [43]. The Educause Center for Education and Research (ECAR) report of a study involving over 112,000 students from 250 higher education institutions across 13 countries suggests students are connected, with students reporting that technology makes them feel more connected to their school (64%); their teachers (60%), and to each other (53%) [54]. But this report also cautions that although students may be ready to use their mobile devices more in relation to their learning, their education providers need to provide a need to do so; also, that students are rightly concerned about their privacy. This highlights the challenge for educators to keep abreast of recent advancements and to also be cognizant of future developments so that their teaching strategies are suitable to prepare students for the future, rather than just the status-quo.

Is there an argument for considering nursing informatics as a seamless attribute to the nursing role rather than something extra-ordinary? Procter and Woodburn [55] suggest that nurses and the profession have a choice to engage with and lead the development of these technologies to ensure that they can continue providing patients with high quality and safe care, or not. In reality though, nurses must get involved in building their knowledge base and working towards adding information management wisdom to the professional knowledge.

8. Conclusion

The profession of nursing, and therefore the education of nurses, has seen significant changes over time to a place where nursing is now a respected profession. Changes in nursing education have been driven by a greater need for efficiency and safety, and as a response to public expectations. These changes also impact on nursing informatics education, and nursing informatics is now recognized as appropriate for a profession with its own body of knowledge and the ability to regulate itself. One of the changes in nursing, and therefore nursing informatics education is the introduction of competency based education, where knowledge, skills and attitudes are considered important to guide developing RNs. Having internationally agreed, clearly articulated nursing informatics competencies, may address a lack of nursing informatics awareness and skills in the nursing workforce, and the need for continued nursing informatics leadership within the profession.

References

[1] Black BP. Professional nursing: Concepts and challenges. 7th ed. St Louis, MO: Elsevier; 2014.
[2] Berwick DM. Preparing nurses for participation in and leadership of continual improvement. Journal of Nursing Education. 2011;50(6):322-7.
[3] Papps E, Kilpatrick J. Nursing education in New Zealand - past, present and future. In: Papps E, editor. Nursing in New Zealand: Critical issues, different perspectives. Auckland, New Zealand: Prentice Hall Health; 2002. p. 1-13.
[4] Tanner CA. Reflections on the curriculum revolution. Journal of Nursing Education. 1990;29(7):295-9.

[5] Bevis EO, Murray JP. The essence of the curriculum revolution: Emancipatory teaching. Journal of Nursing Education. 1990;29(7):326-31.

[6] Bevis EO, Watson J. Towards a caring curriculum: A new pedagogy for nursing. New York, NY: National League for Nursing; 1989.

[7] Whyte DA, Lugton J, Fawcett TN. Fit for purpose: The relevance of Masters preparation for the professional practice of nursing. Journal of Advanced Nursing. 2000;31(5):1072-80.

[8] Skiba DJ. Transforming nursing education to celebrate learning. Nursing & Health Care Perspectives. 1997;18(3):124-30.

[9] Freeman LH, Voignier RR, Scott DL. New curriculum for a new century: Beyond repackaging. Journal of Nursing Education. 2002;41(1):38-40.

[10] Higgs J, Edwards H, editors. Educating beginning practitioners: Challenges for health professional education. Oxford, United Kingdom: Butterworth-Heinemann; 1999.

[11] Avery MD. The history and evolution of the core competencies for basic midwifery practice. Journal of Midwifery and Women's Health. 2005;50(2):102-7.

[12] Grant G, Elbow P, Ewens T, Gamson Z, Kohli W, Neumann W, et al. On competence: A critical analysis of competence-based reforms in higher education. San Francisco: Jossey-Bass; 1979.

[13] Quality and Safety Education for Nurses (QSEN) Institute. Competencies pre-licensure knowledge, skills and attitudes 2014 [cited 2015 April 25]. Available from: http://qsen.org/competencies/pre-licensure-ksas/#informatics

[14] Wu F, Wang Y, Wu Y, Guo M. Application of nursing core competency standard education in the training of nursing undergraduates. International Journal of Nursing Sciences. 2014;1(4):367-70.

[15] Banerjee S. Multimorbidity—older adults need health care that can count past one. The Lancet. 2015;385(9968):587-9.

[16] Haverhals LM, Lee CA, Siek KA, Darr CA, Linnebur SA, Ruscin JM, et al. Older adults with multi-morbidity: Medication management processes and design implications for personal health applications. Journal of Medical Internet Research. 2011;13(2):e44.

[17] Johnson NB, Hayes LD, Brown K, Hoo EC, Ethier KA. CDC National Health Report: Leading causes of morbidity and mortality and associated behavioral risk and protective factors-united states, 2005-2013. Centers for Disease Control and Prevention: Morbidity and mortality weekly report. 2014;63(4):3-27.

[18] Edelman CL, Kudzma EC, Mandle CL. Health promotion throughout the life span. St Louis, MO: Elsevier; 2014.

[19] Watson J. Psychology as the behaviorist views it. Psychological Review. 1913;20:158-77.

[20] Pavlov IP. Lectures on conditioned reflexes. (Translated by W.H. Gantt). London: Allen and Unwin; 1928.

[21] Skinner BF. The behavior of organisms: An experimental analysis. New York, NY: Appleton-Century; 1938.

[22] Thorndike EL. The psychology of wants, interests and attitudes. Oxford, England: Appleton-Century; 1935.

[23] Ausubel DP. Educational psychology: A cognitive view. New York, NY: Holt, Rinehart and Winston, Inc.; 1968.

[24] Rogers A. Teaching adults. 2nd ed. Buckingham, United Kingdom: Open University Press; 1996.

[25] Papert S. Mindstorms: Children, computers and powerful ideas. Brighton, United Kingdom: Harvester; 1980.

[26] Bruner JS. Towards a theory of instruction. Cambridge, MA: Belknap; 1966.

[27] Entwistle N. The impact of teaching on learning outcomes in higher education: A literature review. Sheffield, United Kingdom: CVCP/USDU; 1992.

[28] Siemens G. Connectivism: A learning theory for the digital age. International Journal of Instructional Technology and Distance Learning. 2005;2(1):3-10.

[29] Bates AW. Teaching in a digital age: Guidelines for designing teaching and learning [Internet]2015 [Available from: http://opentextbc.ca/teachinginadigitalage/

[30] Scholes M, Tallberg M, Pluyter-Wenting ESP. International nursing informatics: A history of the first forty years, 1960-2000. 2nd ed. Swindon, England: British Computer Society; 2000.

[31] Tallberg M, Saba V, Carr RL. The international emergence of nursing informatics. In: Weaver CA, Delaney CW, Weber P, Carr RL, editors. Nursing and informatics for the 21st century: An international look at practice trends and the future. Chicago, IL: Health Information and Management Systems Society; 2006.

[32] Berg CM. The importance of nurses' input for the selection of computerized systems. In: Scholes M, Bryant Y, Barber B, editors. The impact of computers on nursing: An international review. Amsterdam, Netherlands: North-Holland; 1983. p. 42-58.

[33] Matney S, Brewster PJ, Sward KA, Cloyes KG, Staggers N. Philosophical approaches to the nursing informatics data-information-knowledge-wisdom framework. Advances in Nursing Science. 2011;34(1):6-18.

[34] Ronquillo C, Currie LM, Rodney P. The evolution of data-information-knowledge-wisdom in nursing informatics. Advances in Nursing Science. 2016;39(1):E1-18.

[35] HITComp - Health IT competencies. 2015. Available from: http://hitcomp.siframework.org

[36] Technology Informatics Guiding Education Reform (TIGER). About TIGER 2013. Available from: www.tigersummit.com

[37] Bond CS, Procter PM. Prescription for nursing informatics pre-registration nurse education. Health Informatics Journal. 2009;15(1):55-64.

[38] Weaver CA, Skiba D. ANI connection. TIGER Initiative: Addressing information technology competencies in curriculum and workforce. Computers, Informatics, Nursing. 2006;**24**(3):175-6.

[39] Kennedy C, Brooks Young P, Nicol J, Campbell K, Gray Brunton C. Fluid role boundaries: exploring the contribution of the advanced nurse practitioner to multi-professional palliative care. Journal of Clinical Nursing. 2015;24(21-22):3296-305.

[40] Ten Hoeve Y, Jansen G, Roodbol P. The nursing profession: public image, self-concept and professional identity. A discussion paper. Journal of Advanced Nursing. 2013;70(2):295–309.

[41] Johnson L, Adams Becker S, Cummins M, Estrada V, Freeman A, Hall C. NMC Horizon Report: 2016 higher education edition. Austin, TX: The New Media Consortium; 2016.

[42] Honey M, Connor K, Veltman M, Bodily D, Diener S. Teaching with Second Life: Hemorrhage management as an example of a process for developing simulations for multiuser virtual environments. Clinical Simulation in Nursing. 2012;8(3):e79-e85.

[43] Skiba DJ. The connected age: Implications for 2014. Nursing Education Perspectives. 2014;35(1):63-5.

[44] Gassert CA, McDowell D. Evaluating graduate and undergraduate nursing students' computer skills to determine the need to continue teaching computer literacy. MedInfo. 1995;8(2):1370.

[45] Austin S. Baccalaureate nursing faculty performance of nursing computer literacy skills and curriculum integration of these skills through teaching practice. Journal of Nursing Education. 1999;38(6):260-6.

[46] Lindqvist R, Kristofferzon M-L, editors. Computer skills among Swedish nursing students,. Nursing Informatics 2000, One Step Beyond: The Evolution of Technology and Nursing; 2000 April 28-May 3; Auckland, New Zealand: Adis.

[47] Ball MJ, Hannah KJ. Using computers in nursing. Reston, VA: Reston Publishing; 1984.

[48] Saba VK. Historical perspectives of nursing and computers. In: Saba VK, McCormick KA, editors. Essentials of Computers for Nurses: Informatics for the New Millennium. 3rd ed. New York: McGraw-Hill; 2001. p. 9-45.

[49] Billings DM. A framework for assessing outcomes and practices in web-based courses in nursing. Journal of Nursing Education. 2000;39(2):60-7.

[50] Bloom KC, Hough MC. Student satisfaction with technology-enhanced learning. CIN: Computers, Informatics, Nursing. 2003;21(5):241-6.

[51] O'Neil CA, Fisher CA, Newbold SK. Developing an online course: Best practices for nurse educators. New York: Springer; 2004.

[52] Carty B, Phillip E. The nursing curriculum in the information age. In: Saba VK, McCormick KA, editors. Essentials of computers for nurses: Informatics for the new millennium. 3rd ed. New York: McGraw-Hill; 2001. p. 393-412.

[53] McGuiness B, Hardy J. Learning through technology. In: Higgs J, Edwards H, editors. Educating Beginning Practitioners: Challenges for Health Professional Education. Oxford, United Kingdom: Butterworth-Heinemann; 1999. p. 212-8.

[54] Dahlstrom E, Walker JD, Dziuban C. ECAR study of undergraduate students and information technology Louisville, CO: Educause Center for Education and Research; 2013. Available from: https://net.educause.edu/ir/library/pdf/ERS1302/ERS1302.pdf

[55] Procter PM, Woodburn I. Encouraging nurses to develop effective electronic documentation. Nursing Management. 2012;19(6):22-4.

© 2017 IMIA and IOS Press.
This article is published online with Open Access by IOS Press and distributed under the terms
of the Creative Commons Attribution Non-Commercial License 4.0 (CC BY-NC 4.0).
doi:10.3233/978-1-61499-738-2-41

Curricula Challenges and Informatics Competencies for Nurse Educators

Ulla-Mari KINNUNEN[a,1], Elina RAJALAHTI[b], Elizabeth CUMMINGS[c],
Elizabeth M. BORYCKI[d]

[a] *University of Eastern Finland, Department of Health and Social Management, Kuopio, Finland*
[b] *Laurea University of Applied Sciences, Espoo, Finland*
[c] *University of Tasmania, Tasmania, Australia*
[d] *University of Victoria, Victoria, British Columbia, Canada*

Abstract. Nursing informatics competencies are fundamental to nursing practice in all areas of nursing work, including direct patient care, administration and education. The recent activity relating to the development of nursing informatics competencies for beginning level nurses has exposed a paucity of understanding of the requirements for nursing informatics competencies for nurse educators. So, whilst the challenge of educating faculty to teach informatics has been limited, research into such competencies is required to meet this challenge. This paper describes the challenges and issues associated with nursing informatics competency development for faculty, outlines the capabilities of faculty, and presents a vision for the future of informatics education for faculty. The final requirement of the introduction of new competencies is to determine appropriate evaluation measures that reflect the requirements of all stakeholders.

Keywords. Informatics, competency, nurse educator, curriculum, health information technology

1. Introduction

Nurses' informatics competencies have been studied for over ten years [1-3]. There exist several studies that outline expected nursing manager's informatics competencies [4-6]. Also, nutrition informatics competency studies have been published [7]. Different requirements for nursing programs and curriculums have been introduced [8, 9], including those focusing on informatics [10]. Yet, a consensus among nurse educators regarding informatics competencies has not been reached. In addition, the identification of specific competencies, such as informatics competencies, have yet to be connected to specific areas of practice. Finally, the informatics competence of the faculty members has seen limited research, although this is deemed to be a critical factor limiting the development of informatics abilities in the workforce. The objective of this paper is to: (1) describe some of the challenges and issues associated with

---

[1] Corresponding author: Ulla-Mari Kinnunen, Virranniementie 3, 78310 Varkaus, Finland, e-mail: ulla-mari.kinnunen@uef.fi , phone: +358 400 678110 Institution: University of Eastern Finland, Department of Health and Social Management, POB 1627, FIN-70211 Kuopio, Finland, phone +358 40 3553953

nursing informatics competency development among faculty, (2) outline the capabilities of faculty, and (3) present a vision for the future of informatics education for faculty into the future.

We begin by defining the term competency and some of the nursing initiatives aimed at developing nursing informatics competencies. A competency refers to skills, knowledge, values, and attitudes [11]. Early attempts to develop nursing informatics competencies include the TIGER Initiative, Technology Informatics Guiding Education Reform, which began in 2004 to develop strategies and actions to improve nursing practice, education, and care with the aid of health information technology (HIT). The Tiger Summit [12] produced several recommendations for education. These include the need: (1) for informatics competencies for all levels of nursing education including undergraduate and graduate, (2) for nursing informatics competencies for education and practicing nurses, (3) to strike an educational committee to examine the integration of informatics throughout the curriculum, (4) to develop informatics specialty programs, and (5) to evaluate the baseline and the changes in informatics knowledge among nurse educators. It has also been highlighted that nursing education must be enhanced because of a constantly changing health technology environment. This is among the objectives and actions of the IMIA-NI Education Working Group [13] whose mandate is to review the scope of nursing informatics and its implication for nursing education.

The lack of knowledge about eHealth, its advantages and potential benefits for users is a significant educational challenge. The challenge includes teaching and steering not only citizens and patients, but also health care professionals [14]. Teaching health informatics and using electronic health record systems in education cannot be dependent on a teacher's or other faculty members' competencies alone. There is a need for investment by professional associations, universities and colleges in providing the educational opportunities and tools (e.g. electronic health records) so that faculty and students can learn about informatics [15, 16]. This is essential for nurse educators to develop informatics as a core competency [17, 18]. In addition to this, there is a need for nurse educators' informatics competencies to be more fully attended to [9, 19]. The final documents of specific nurse educator competencies have not been published by Tiger Initiative [20].

2. Challenges for nurse educators in nursing informatics

In informatics, the issues of state education and competence have been touched upon in studies examining competence in informatics or linking informatics to nursing curricula [21]. This has occurred in conjunction with an expanding focus on simulation pedagogy [21]. Curran [21] highlighted a concern in practicing new nursing skills, such as entering data into a patient record system and related competence in education and nursing. A number of nursing skills are emphasized in the field of nursing, but nursing informatics has not gained an independent domain where nursing education is concerned. Informatics has traditionally been treated as separate in terms of knowledge and skills.

Studies of health educators' have primarily focused on comprehensive work as educators and been concerned with examining the area of expertise in teaching or central fields of competence, such as leadership and cooperation skills. Several studies present the challenges for nursing and health care education, which should be paid attention to in order to receive high-quality teaching and patients' customer-oriented safe care [20, 22, 23]. The adoption of new knowledge and education for changes in electronic systems and used programmes in health care require new nurse educator skills in informatics, the development of an informatics knowledge base, information retrieval and information management competencies [19, 23]. To illustrate this, Rajalahti's 2014 extension of Curran's framework is useful (see Table 1).

Table 1. Curriculum work and health educator's area of required competencies in informatics and competencies with an emphasis on informatics [19]

Curran's framework (2008)	Evidence (studies and reports) supporting decision-making	The area of competencies in informatics and areas of competencies with an emphasis on informatics
Theoretical background	Theoretical background of informatics	Area of competencies in informatics
Skills and knowledge in applying informatics	Skills and competence of informatics	a) Knowledge base of informatics b) Adoption of informatics tools and devices
Competence in integrating knowledge of informatics	Informatics integration	c) Nursing information integration management
Caring	Patient safety care	Patient-centered care
Implementation of learning and teaching	Evidence based working, investigative work	Research, development and innovation activities
Implementation of learning and teaching	Knowledge management, self-management	Leadership and curriculum work
Human personal activities and competence, such as cooperation skills	Networking	Work in networks and management of network processes
Learning how to learn.	eLearning and teaching in different environments	Environments for implementing eLearning, different environments for learning nursing.

First, attention must be paid to the continuous changes in information management, where digital data in information systems, e-health solutions in the mobile systems, and health technology devices set the requirements. It is imperative that health educators understand the importance of, and are supported in, keeping pace with informatics related change and the implications for their students in practice. Secondly, education should produce new methods and models efficiently, economically and effectively [23]. Third, research and development competence sets challenges for health educators in a situation in which new applications and techniques are constantly being developed [22-24]. Competence in using research is the challenge [23, 24]. Constantly regenerated research data set up a challenge for the knowledge-intensive nature of health care. Rajalahti's [19] literature review and dissertation research have led to the development of competency recommendations in informatics and informatics competencies that focus on the nurse educator (Table 1).

In summary student nurses need to learn about health information technology (HIT) as part of their education and practice. Informatics must be a fixed part of today's nursing curriculum. For nursing students to be prepared to use HIT, faculty must require the use of current technology as part of class work. To meet these required informatics competences and rapid changing challenges in health care, nursing education programs and curriculum work as well as nurse educators working in university and college settings must have flexible model of dynamically building new informatics competences.

3. Should we be talking about competencies or capabilities for Nurse Educators?

Bromley states [25 (110)]: "the terms competent, competence, competency and competencies have often been interpreted as the same thing. It has been implied that competency 'is', whereas competencies are the skills to be assessed and, if successful in demonstrating these competencies, the nurse can be deemed competent". This is confirmed by Phelps et al.'s [26] work that suggests that competencies represent a simplicity of task, are prescriptive and best suited to less challenging and more stable environments than those experienced by advanced nurses or nurse educators. Watson [27] describes competencies as descriptions of abilities that do not necessarily require a high level academic achievement and considers this to potentially be an inappropriate term for nursing education skills [27]. So, whilst university undergraduate curricula must account for the core competencies it remains essential that informatics competencies are considered at a minimum level and higher level skills are incorporated, particularly in advanced education [28].

The current debate in nursing education tends to use the term capability for advanced nursing skills, including nursing education. The term capability can be used to reflect or measure the expertise of nurses who demonstrate skill levels above the entry level. Capability reflects individual's demonstrating self-efficacy and taking responsibility for their actions and education [29, 30]. According to Bromley [25 (110)] capability also "promotes the pursuit of excellence in the development, acquisition and application of knowledge and skills".

In Europe, the competences have been defined in accordance with the recommendation of EQF (European Qualification Framework) [31]. The base of the framework is the competence comparability with 8-level criteria. EQF and these levels make qualifications more readable and understandable across different countries and systems in Europe. The European higher education structure emphasizes a holistic view of competence. The base of the definition for competences lies in the knowledge, skills and qualifications, which can be seen as a result of learning (a learning outcome). These point of view emphasize understanding, values, knowledge and its application. The perspective of competence required is based on the profession and society that are part of working life; i.e. the individual's ability to take advantage of their knowledge, different skills, and a combination of qualifications [19, 31].

4. Next steps

Irrespective of whether we are establishing nurse educator informatics competencies or capabilities, it is essential that effort now turns to the design and development of an evidence-based informatics curriculum for nurse educators. Currently, many nurse educators are under prepared in the requisite skills to use or demonstrate informatics technologies. Whilst they are familiar with a wide range of educational technologies, these educational technologies differ significantly from the technologies that are associated with HIT and nursing informatics. The nursing educators' challenge of incorporating informatics into curricula was observed in 2010 by Flood and colleagues [32]. However, there continues to be a lack of research on strategies to effectively teach informatics.

As was experienced when learning technologies were introduced into nursing education, there is significant interest from educators about including informatics in their curricula, but time constraints and confidence can limit active adoption. Universities and colleges need to invest in building the skills required by the nursing faculty [33], and this work should be motivated by and supported by national nursing faculty organizing bodies (e.g. Canadian Association of Schools of Nursing, Australian Nursing and Midwifery Advisory Council) [34]. Therefore, development of faculty's skills in informatics education must be supported by the educator's department as part of standard professional development requirements.

Health takes place in the everyday lives of individuals so the importance of connectivism, as described by Honey and Proctor in section A chapter 3, is elementary in that nurses need to know how to relate context to their information acquisition and sharing to ensure relevancy for their clients. This skill needs to be conveyed throughout undergraduate nursing education and so it is important that educators have expertise in assisting individual students to form networks for learning and to draw upon others' experiences, including their clients. It is also important that new graduates appreciate the diversity of clients and their wide range of understandings and desires in relation to informatics. For example, some clients will embrace new technologies in their health care whilst others may shun them. It is the nurse's role to support their client in their personal choices. Therefore, the nurse educator needs to include advocacy in relation to the use of technology as part of nursing education.

5. Implementing and evaluating education

Related to this is the need to develop a means of measuring and understanding the impact of nurse educator education on the teaching of nursing informatics students and ultimately outcomes in practice etc. There currently exist several projects internationally that attempt to support faculty development and integration of nursing informatics competencies into curricula. For example, the Canadian Association of Schools of Nursing [34] has developed nursing informatics competencies, educational resources and a national faculty peer-leader network that has conducted group (i.e. workshops, presentations) and individual learning activities with nursing faculty (individualized educational and one-on-one support sessions) across Canada. The work has been evaluated using surveys of participating faculty.

In Finland, nationally the 100% of electronic patient record system coverage and the implementation of National Patient Data Repository has influenced demands for integrating nursing informatics competencies in both nursing and nurse educator education. Documentation and general informatics for nurse educators was enhanced and training conducted in 2008-2010 through the eNNI project (Electronic Documentation of Nursing Care – Research and Development for Creation of Nursing Informatics Competences in Cooperation with Education and Work life). Based on the project, a national network for nurse educators was established to develop nursing informatics competences [19].

In Australia, whilst the recent Registered Nurse Standards for Practice [35] and Continuing Professional Development [36] support the Australian Nursing and Midwifery Accreditation Council mandate that all undergraduate curricula must include nursing informatics [37], there has been limited engagement in the development of policies around the requirement for nurse educators to have informatics skills. In fact, the first set of informatics competencies for nurses was released through the Australian and Nursing and Midwifery Federation National Informatics Standards for Nurses and Midwives in early 2016 [38]. Whilst these standards have merit and provide direction regarding expectations for competence of nurses in informatics they are not yet ratified by any of the national professional nursing bodies. However, individual universities have commenced the development of courses for nurse educators in nursing informatics [39].

Ultimately the result of nurse educator competencies in nursing informatics needs to be measured in terms of all stakeholder groups. This involved evaluation of not only the faculty responses or increased confidence and capacity to teach informatics skills to their students. There must be concurrent research and evaluation of changes in new graduate knowledge and capability in using HIT when entering the workforce, and evaluation of whether the employing organizational needs are being met by the new graduate skills.

6. Conclusion

Progress in the development and implementation of nursing informatics competencies for nurses has gained increasing traction in most countries, but the teaching of these competencies and their inclusion in curricula is dependent upon the skills and knowledge of the faculty members who teach these components. Attention needs to shift to the development of faculty to deliver the informatics skills to assist their students to meet the required competencies. Rajalahti [19] has proposed a set of competencies for nurse educators to assist them in becoming confident and capable of delivering the nursing informatics knowledge to ensure their students achieve the appropriate level of competencies. Education for faculty must agile to enable them to cover the range of rapidly changing HIT and must be supported by their organizations. The final requirement is an evaluation strategy that considers all stakeholders in the evaluation. Evidently once nurse educator competencies have been finally agreed the subsequent piece of research required is to develop a robust evaluation framework to ensure the needs of all parties is being met.

References

[1]   Staggers N, Gassert CA, Curran C. Informatics Competencies for Nurses at Four Levels of Practice, Journal of Nursing Education 40 (7) (2001), 303-316.
[2]   Staggers N, Gassert CA, Curran C. A Delphi Study to Determine Informatics Competencies for Nurses at Four levels of Practice, Nursing Research November/December 51 (6) (2002), 383-390.
[3]   TIGER   2010.   The   TIGER   Nursing   Informatics   Competencies.   Available: http://www.himss.org/ResourceLibrary/genResourceDetailPDF.aspx?ItemNumber=44660 (24.3.2016)

[4] Bickford CJ. Informatics competencies for nurse managers and their staffs, Seminars for Nurse Managers Jun;10 (2) (2002), 110-3

[5] Westra B, Delaney CW. Informatics Competencies for Nursing and Healthcare Leaders, AMIA Annual Symposium Proceedings 2008; 804–808. Available: http://www.ncbi.nlm.nih.gov/pmc/articles/PMC2655955/

[6] Yang L, Cui D, Zhu X, Zhao Q, Xiao N, Shen X. Perspectives from Nurse Managers on Informatics Competencies, The Scientific World Journal 2014 (2014), Article ID 391714, http://dx.doi.org/10.1155/2014/391714 http://www.hindawi.com/journals/tswj/2014/391714/

[7] Ayres EJ, Greer-Carney JL, Fatzinger McShane PE, Miller A, Turner P. Nutrition informatics competencies across all levels of practice: a national Delphi study, Journal of the Academy of Nutrition and Dietetics 112 (2012), 2042-2053

[8] Drummond-Young M, Brown B, Noesgaard C, Lunyk-Child O, Maich NM, Mines C, et al. A comprehensive faculty development model for nursing education, Journal of Professional Nursing May-Jun;26(3) (2010), 152-61. doi: 10.1016/j.profnurs.2009.04.004.

[9] Rajalahti E, Heinonen J, Saranto K. Developing nurse educators' computer skills towards proficiency in nursing informatics, Informatics Health Social Care 39 (1) (2014), 47-66.

[10] Mantas J, Ammenwerth E, Demiris G, Hasman A, Haux R, Hersh W, et al. Recommendations of the International Medical Informatics Association (IMIA) on Education in Biomedical and Health Informatics. First Revision, Methods of Information in Medicin 49 (2010), 105–120. doi: 10.3414/ME5119.

[11] Pijl-Zieber EM, Barton S, Konkin J, Awosoga O, Claine V. Competence and competency-based nursing education: Finding our way through the issues, Nurse Education Today 34 (2014), 676-678.

[12] TIGER 2007. The TIGER Initiative. Evidence and Informatics Transforming Nursing: 3-Year Action Steps toward a 10-Year Vision. Available: http://www.aacn.nche.edu/education-resources/tiger.pdf (24.3.2016)

[13] IMIA-NI Education Working Group 2016. Strategic Plan. Available: https://sites.google.com/site/imianiedwg/Strategic-Plan (24.3.2016)

[14] European Commission 2012. Communication from the commission to the European parliament, the council, the European economic and social committee and the committee of the regions. eHealth action plan 2012-2020 - innovative healthcare for the 21st century. Available: http://ec.europa.eu/digital-agenda/en/news/ehealth-action-plan-2012-2020-innovative-healthcare-21st-century (24.3.2016)

[15] Borycki E, Joe RS, Armstrong B, Bellwood P, Campbell R. Educating health professionals about the electronic health record (EHR): Removing the barriers to adoption, Knowledge Management & E-Learning: An International Journal, 3 (1) (2011), 51-62.

[16] Cummings E, Borycki EM, Madsen I. Teaching nursing informatics in Australia, Canada and Denmark, Studies in Health Technology and Informatics 218 (2015), 39.

[17] WHO 2013. Transforming and scaling up health professionals' education and training. World Health Organization Guidelines 2013. Available: http://whoeducationguidelines.org./sites/default/files/uploads/WHO_EduGuidelines_20131202_web.pd f (26.3.2016)

[18] Kowitlawakul Y, Chan S, Pulcini J, Wang W. Factors influencing nursing students' acceptance of electronic health records for nursing education (EHRNE) software program, Nurse Education Today, 35 (1) (2015), 189-194.

[19] Rajalahti E. Reforming the expertise of health sector teachers' information management. [Terveysalan opettajien tiedonhallinnan osaamisen uudistaminen.] Publications of the University of Eastern Finland. Dissertations in Social Sciences and Business Studies. No 89, (2014) Abstract in English. Available: http://epublications.uef.fi/pub/urn_isbn_978-952-61-1611-2/urn_isbn_978-952-61-1611-2.pdf

[20] Hebda T, Calderone TL. What Nurse Educators Need to Know About the TIGER Initiative, Nurse Educator 35 (2) (2010), 56-60.

[21] Curran CR. Faculty development initiatives for the integration of informatics competencies and point-of-care technologies in undergraduate nursing education, Nursing Clinics of North America 43 (4) (2008), 523-33.

[22] Dixon BE, Newlon CM. How do future nursing educators perceive informatics? Advancing the nursing informatics agenda through dialogue, Journal of Professional Nursing 26(2) (2010), 82-89.

[23] Skiba DJ. On the Horizon: Emerging Technologies for 2011, Nursing Education Perspectives 32(1) (2011), 44-46.

[24] Elomaa L. Research evidence implementation and its requirements in nursing education. University of Turku. Serie D Medica-Odontologica 2003 (532).

[25] Bromley P. Clinical competence of neonatal intensive care nursing students: How do we evaluate the application of knowledge in students of postgraduate certificate in neonatal intensive care nursing? The Journal of Neonatal Nursing, 20 (4) (2014),140-146

[26] Phelps R, Hase S, Ellis A. Competency, capability, complexity and computers: exploring a new model for conceptualising end-user computer education, British Journal of Educational Technology 36 (1) (2005), 67–84.

[27] Watson R. Is there a role for higher education in preparing nurses? Nurse Education Today 26 (2006), 622–626.

[28] Sasso L, Bagnasco A, Watson R. Competence-sensitive outcomes, Journal of Advanced Nursing (2016) doi: 10.1111/jan.12941

[29] O'Connell J, Gardner G, Coyer F. Beyond competencies: using a capability framework in developing practice standards for advanced practice nursing, Journal of Advanced Nursing 70 (12) (2014), 2728–2735. doi: 10.1111/ jan.12475

[30] Stephenson J, Weil S. Four themes in educating for capability. Quality in Learning. A Capability Approach in Higher Education. London: Kogan Page, 1992.

[31] European Comission. Learning Opportunities and Qualifications in Europe. Available: https://ec.europa.eu/ploteus/documentation#documentation_75 (25.4.2016)

[32] Flood L, Gasiewicz N, Delpier T. Integrating information literacy across a BSN curriculum, Journal of Nursing Education 49 (2) (2010), 101-104

[33] Talcott K, O'Donnell JM, Burns HK. Technology and the Nurse Educator Are You ELITE? Nurse Educator, 38 (3), May/June 2013.

[34] Nagle L, Borycki E, Donelle L, Frisch N, Hannah K, Harris A, et al. Nursing informatics: Entry to practice competencies for registered nurses. Canadian Association of Schools of Nursing, Ottawa. 2012.

[35] Nursing and Midwifery Board of Australia (2016) Registered nurse standards for practice. Available: http://www.nursingmidwiferyboard.gov.au/News/2016-02-01-revised-standards.aspx (6.4.2016)

[36] Nursing and Midwifery Board of Australia (2016) Registration Standard: Continuing Professional Development. Available: http://www.nursingmidwiferyboard.gov.au/News/2016-02-01-revised-standards.aspx (6.4.2016)

[37] ANMAC. (2012). Australian Nursing and Midwifery Accreditation Council Registered Nurse Accreditation Standards. Available: http://www.anmac.org.au/sites/default/files/documents/ANMAC_RN_Accreditation_Standards_2012.pdf (23.7.2013)

[38] ANMF (2015) National Informatics Standards for Nurses and Midwives, Available: http://anmf.org.au/documents/National_Informatics_Standards_For_Nurses_And_Midwives. (6.4.2016)

[39] Cummings E, Shin EH, Mather C, Hovenga E. (2016) Embedding nursing informatics education into an Australian undergraduate nursing degree, Forthcoming presentation at NI2016 The 13th International Congress in Nursing Informatics, Geneva 25-29 June.

Section B

Overview of National and International Initiatives

Forecasting Informatics Competencies for Nurses in the Future of Connected Health
J. Murphy et al. (Eds.)
© 2017 IMIA and IOS Press.
This article is published online with Open Access by IOS Press and distributed under the terms
of the Creative Commons Attribution Non-Commercial License 4.0 (CC BY-NC 4.0).
doi:10.3233/978-1-61499-738-2-51

Nursing Informatics Competencies for Entry to Practice: The Perspective of Six Countries

Michelle L.L. HONEY[a], Diane J. SKIBA[b], Paula PROCTER[c], Joanne FOSTER[d], Pirkko KOURI[e], and Lynn M. NAGLE[f]
[a]The University of Auckland, NEW ZEALAND; [b]University of Colorado College of Nursing, Aurora, Colorado, USA; [c]Sheffield Hallam University, Sheffield , UNITED KINGDOM; [d]Queensland University of Technology, Brisbane, Queensland, AUSTRALIA; [e]Savonia University of Applied Sciences, Unit of Health Care, Kuopio, FINLAND; [f]University of Toronto, Ontario, CANADA.

Abstract. Internationally, countries are challenged to prepare nurses for a future that has ever increasing use of technology and where information management is a central part of professional nursing practice. There has been a growing trend to move nursing to competency-based education, especially for those students undertaking their first nursing qualification. This first nursing qualification may be linked to pre-registration, pre-licensure or undergraduate education; the term used depending on the country. The authors are drawn from the International Medical Informatics Association special interest group, Nursing Informatics (IMIA-NI) Education Working Group and represent New Zealand, the United States of America, England, Australia, Finland and Canada.

Keywords. Nursing education; undergraduate; pre-licensure

1. Introduction

Every country faces the challenge of preparing nurses for entry to practice in a changing world where an ageing population, shortage of qualified nurses, increased longevity and incidence of long term conditions occurs alongside technological developments and opportunities for effective use of information and communication technologies to support nursing care. The use of competency based nurse education is seen as a move to ensure future nurses are prepared to be active participants in complex health care systems. Each country struggles to satisfy demand within an environment of reduced funds and resources. With the requirement to maximize effectiveness the focus is drawn to effective information management and the use of technology to become part of daily nursing practice.

The initial educational preparation of nurses varies between countries in relation to the length of the course or programme of education, place of education and the mix of theory and clinical within the curriculum. Additionally, the initial nursing education is known by different terms depending on the location and country. For example, the United States uses the terms pre-licensure and baccalaureate, where New Zealand uses the terms undergraduate. While the terms may vary, the focus is on the early education that allows for entry to practice that culminates in becoming a registered nurse.

Competency-based education has attracted renewed attention and is a growing trend internationally. It is defined as "education that derives a curriculum from an analysis of a prospective or actual role in modern society and that attempts to certify student progress on the bases of demonstrated performance in some or all of the aspects of that role" [1]. The Quality and Safety Education for Nurses (QSEN) project describes competencies as including knowledge, skills, and attitudes that are necessary to continuously improve the quality and safety of the healthcare systems within which they work [2]. Nursing informatics competencies are explicitly described in some countries curricula [3, 4], while others are less clearly stated [5].

The authors are drawn from members of the International Medical Informatics Association special interest group, Nursing Informatics (IMIA-NI) Education Working Group and presents a global view as each briefly describes their representative country's status on the development and use of informatics competencies in their education of student nurses.

2. New Zealand

New Zealand is a small country with 4.7 million people and nearly 50,000 registered nurses [5]. In New Zealand there are 17 schools offering three year Bachelor of Nursing programmes and these are accredited by the national nursing statutory and regulatory body, Nursing Council of New Zealand [5]. At the undergraduate level nursing informatics has been recognised as important since the early 1990s when Jan Hausman wrote the national nursing informatics curriculum [6]. The current competencies identified by the Nursing Council are broadly stated as "Demonstrate the skills needed to acquire, understand and assess information from a range of sources" and "the use of information technology and health information management" [7]. However, the way these competencies are incorporated into each school's nursing curriculum varies, with some being more explicit than others, with an integrated curricula approach being more common. Evidence based practice is seen as a fundamental attribute of a Registered Nurse, and resources to support evidence based practice are accessible through schools of nursing, clinical intranets and the internet. Additionally, each School of Nursing provides a description of the profile of their graduate and information literacy is commonly identified as a degree programme core competency.

A more pressing concern in New Zealand has been nurses developing informatics knowledge and skills post registration. Health Informatics New Zealand (HiNZ), as the independent national health informatics organization, established a working group who, drawing on international guidelines and experience, developed a list of health informatics competencies for New Zealand health professionals [8]. Core competences identified were: health domain knowledge, social/ethics/legal aspects of health information technology (HIT), basic computer science, basic data management, clinical information systems (IS), basic health IS/IT management and health informatics concepts [8, 9]. Free introductory health informatics workshops for clinicians, sponsored by the government, and conducted by HINZ, have been offered around the country with the aim of raising awareness of the importance of the field of health informatics, the competencies involved and the requirements and opportunities for upskilling or advancing learning in this area.

3. United States of America

As of 2016, there were over 3.1 million registered nurses active in the workforce [10]. Most recent estimates, there are approximately 150,000 new registered nurse graduates per year [11]. Approximately 55% of the nursing population hold baccalaureate degrees or higher [12]. Associate degree nurses represent the remaining percentage [12]. The US has set a goal that 80% of all registered nurses will have a baccalaureate degree by 2020. Yet, in 2014 close to 69,000 suitably qualified potential students were turned away from nursing baccalaureate and graduate programs due to faculty shortage, lack of clinical sites and preceptors [13].

Nursing informatics competencies have evolved since the early days of computer literacy. Although there were several studies identifying the necessary knowledge and skills needed by nurses there was very little momentum to incorporate these into nursing education. Several driving forces helped to facilitate the adoption of informatics competencies in the nursing curriculum. An Institute of Medicine report [14] documented the need for all health care professionals to have the following five core competencies to practice in today's health care system: provide patient-centered care, work in interdisciplinary teams, employ evidence based practice, apply quality improvement and utilize informatics. In this report, informatics tools are considered essential for communication, management of information and knowledge, mitigation of error, support for decision-making and health care interventions.

In 2004, the establishment of the federal Office of the National Coordinator of Health IT, created the "decade of Health IT" in the United Sates. This initiative to promote the widespread adoption of Electronic Health Records, foster health information exchanges and advance consumer engagement in their health care served as a foundation for the development of the Technology Informatics Guiding Education Reform (TIGER) initiative [15]. The goal of TIGER is to ensure that all nurses, in current practice as well as the next generation, will have the necessary knowledge and skills to fully engage in the unfolding digital era of health care [16]. A corresponding initiative funded by Robert Wood Johnson was The Quality and Safety Education for Nurses (QSEN) project [2]. Both the TIGER and QSEN initiatives paved the way for professional nursing organizations, such as the National League for Nursing and the of American College of Nursing, to examine the necessary knowledge and skills needed for the preparation of future nurses. The National League for Nursing released a position statement, Preparing the next generation of Nurses to Practice in a Technology-Rich Environment: An Informatics Agenda [17], calling upon educators to incorporate the necessary informatics knowledge and skills within nursing curricula. To do this, it was important to prepare faculty to gain competencies in informatics. To this end, the Division of Nursing, Department of Health and Human Services, funded nine Faculty Development Collaboratives to prepare faculty to incorporate technologies into their curriculum including informatics and telehealth.

The American Association of Colleges of Nursing (AACN) sets standards for nursing education and informatics criteria is written for all levels including Baccalaureate, Master's and Doctorate of Nursing Practice (DNP). For those preparing at the prelicensure level, the Essentials of Baccalaureate Education for Professional

Nursing Practice [3] delineates competencies related to the use of patient care technologies to support care, the use of decision support systems to guide practice, understand and use standardized terminologies to reflect nursing's unique contribute to patient outcomes, and to ethically manage and process data, information and knowledge to support safe and quality patient care. As a standard for pre-licensure competencies, this document serves as one of the foundational component of accreditation of a nursing education program.

4. England

The United Kingdom (UK) is divided into four countries, England, Wales, Scotland and Northern Ireland. England is the largest of the four countries with a population of more than 60 million. There are around 308,000 nurses (including midwives and health visitors) in England [18]; student nurses attend a three year undergraduate programme at one of the 56 accredited universities, annually there are around 30,000 undergraduate student nurses. The UK Nursing and Midwifery Council (NMC) is the statutory and regulatory body which sets pre-registration (undergraduate) competences required to be met to register as a nurse in the UK; the most recent competency requirements are set out in the NMC Standards for pre-registration nursing education [19]. Two relevant core competencies are highlighted in the standards: those around record keeping and information governance, with the latter mandatory from 2014. In addition, the use of appropriate evidence to support practice is widely included. By December 2016 it is expected that there will be the introduction of a new information, data and technology knowledge and skills framework which will be aimed at all levels of the health, care and social care workforce to enable enhanced use of digital technologies to commission, deliver, support, evaluate and audit health and social care [20].

In May 2016 a framework for nursing, midwifery and care staff was published by NHS England titled 'Leading Change, Adding Value' [21]. Within the framework there are ten commitments and one of these identifies the need for nurses, midwives and care staff to "champion the use of technology and informatics to improve practice". There are also associated education measures to support this commitment, namely:

- Provide learning that enables staff to maximize the benefits of innovations in technology and informatics;
- Construct training and education to build the knowledge and confidence to utilize technology;
- Raise awareness of the benefits that telehealth, telecare and information management can bring to improve effectiveness; and to
- Consider developing new roles in the leadership of informatics such as a career pathway for nurse informaticians leading to chief nurse information officer roles.

The framework provides a national strategic direction and operational guidance which will enable this commitment to be realised with education, from undergraduate through to continuing professional development, taking a leading role.

5. Australia

The increasing focus on Australia's e-health agenda requires a national approach to the development of competencies in informatics for nurses and the integration of these into nursing curricula. With an estimated 344,190 registered nurses in Australia [22], nursing is the largest single group of health professionals who directly influence the quality and outcomes of health services. A study of Australian nurses and information technology reported that nurses generally are poorly prepared to engage with information technology in their practice. The study reported that almost two thirds of nurses had not received any formal training in basic software applications and of the 90% of nurses who used computers or other information technology applications, only one third had any formal training [23]. These outcomes supported the urgent need for nurses to have nursing informatics professional competency standards developed with a project (2009-2011) being funded by the Australian Government Department of Health and Ageing (DOHA) and managed by the Australian Nursing Federation (ANF). Queensland University of Technology (QUT) was contracted to undertake the research and development of the Australian Nursing Informatics Competency Standards. These Standards were published in 2015 by the Australian Nursing and Midwifery Federation (ANMF) [24].

There are 31 accredited universities offering a three year Bachelor of Nursing degree which are to meet the national accreditation standards of the Australian Nursing and Midwifery Accreditation Council (ANMAC) [25] which is part of the Nursing and Midwifery Board of Australia (NMBA) [26] which is governed by the Australian Health Practitioner Regulation Agency (AHPRA) [27]. Currently in Australia, 'health informatics and health technology' (Standard 4: Program content supports the development and application of knowledge and skills) is the only aspect included as part of the national standards for accreditation by all schools of nursing leading to a Bachelor of Nursing degree. The 2006 national Registered Nurse Standards [28] have been reviewed and the new Registered Nurse Standards come into effect from June 1st 2016. However from the viewpoint of nursing informatics, in the 2006 Registered Nurse Standards there were only two criteria that broadly related back to nursing informatics; a) "accurately uses health care technologies in accordance with manufacturer's specification and organisational policy" and b) "records information systematically in an accessible and retrievable form" [28]. The reviewed Registered Nurse Standards for Practice [29] have no mention of any specific aspects of nursing informatics, hence the critical need for the Australian Nursing Informatics Competency Standards [24] to provide the profession with a set of standards that all registered nurses in Australia must meet. All educational courses in Australia have to meet the Australian Quality Framework (AQF) Standards and Criteria(30] with all Australian Bachelor Degrees meeting AQF Level 7 criteria. Therefore, Bachelor of Nursing degrees have to meet AQF, AHPRA and NMBA standards and criteria for registration as a Registered Nurse in Australia.

6. Finland

Finland has about 5.5 million people and nearly 51,000 registered nurses. There are 23 schools offering three and half year Bachelor of Nursing programmes and these are based both on the statutory and European (EQF) and National Qualification Framework

(NQF). The framework provides an instrument for the classification of qualifications according to a set of criteria for specified levels of learning achieved which aims to integrate and coordinate national qualifications subsystems and improve the transparency, access, progression and quality of qualifications in relation to the labour market. Nursing informatics is included in the Innovation and Working Community Competency. Each nursing school implements nursing informatics studies into sub-competencies and there are variations in curricula. At the bachelor level nursing informatics penetrates the whole nursing curriculum, as themes e.g. information management, documentation, electronic patient records, data security and data protection. There are also practice focused master programmes in nursing informatics and health technology content is included. The Finnish Nursing Association (FNA) aims to increase the standing of the profession of nursing by offering services that help develop professional skills and expertise in the field of nursing informatics and e-Health. The FNA's e-services provide effective tools to carry out evidence-based nursing and access to various databases. In mid-2015 the FNA studied nurses' (n=464) use of and attitudes related to technology use. Over 90% used technology in their work, most commonly within electronic patient records, decision making systems and various medical devices [31]. The newest innovations like games for health, virtual clinics or robotics are gradually coming part of nurse's work. There is a constant need and also a challenge to offer updated education for nurses. The FNA enhances nursing informatics and e-Health by providing the opportunity for nurses with many-sided 'e-health - working experience' to apply for the diploma of Special Qualifications in Nursing Informatics and eHealth [32]. FNA celebrated its 90th anniversary in 2015 and in January 2016, the FNA launched their first National e-Health Strategy for Nurses [32]. Finnish nurses are keen to keep abreast of the times in developing the digitalisation in health. The FNA's eHealth strategy includes informatics competencies. Furthermore, there are three aspects of expertise: knowledge, skills and competence. Nurses' training involves five areas of expertise: learning, ethics, workplace skills, innovations, and internationalisation. The production of eHealth services concerns all these areas. More specifically, workplace skills refer to smooth operations in workplace communications and interaction, as well as the ability to utilise many aspects of Information and Communication Technology (ICT) and networks. Innovation expertise means that nurses are able to develop creative problem solving and work methods, the proficiency to work on diverse programmes and know-how to carry out research and development projects. Nurses also know how to apply existing knowledge and methods in their field and know how to look for financial and client-oriented solutions.

7. Canada

The vast geography of Canada is home to more than 34 million people and more than 360,000 regulated nurses (Registered Nurses, Registered Practical Nurses, and Registered Psychiatric Nurses). Of those regulated nurses, more than 270,000 are registered nurses and graduates of one of 135 schools of nursing. In 2003 less than 30% of all schools reported having any informatics content, theoretical or applied, integrated into their basic entry to practice programs [33]. A decade later, anecdotal evidence suggests that the lack of informatics integration remains relatively the same. In 2011 the development of nursing informatics competencies for new graduates was initiated with the support of the Canadian Association of Schools of Nursing (CASN) and funding from Canada Health Infoway. Rationale for this included: 1) limited informatics content in existing nursing curricula, 2) the need for entry-to-practice nursing competencies reflecting the skills and knowledge needed to work in Health Information Technology (HIT) enabled practice environments, 3) the lack of shared understanding and consensus among educators on required informatics competencies for entry level practice and 4) the need to better prepare registered nurses to practice in increasingly data, information and technology rich environments. In 2012, CASN published national, consensus-based entry to practice informatics competencies for adoption by all Canadian Schools of Nursing, and followed this with the development of a Faculty Learning Resource and Teaching Toolkit to support the integration of informatics into core curricula [34]. Additional details of these development activities have been described elsewhere [35].

An underlying premise of the competencies is that students entering schools of nursing at the undergraduate level will possess basic computer literacy as it relates to the use of generic applications and devices (e.g., word processing, email, smart phones and computers). The competencies are subsumed by a single over-arching competency statement: *Uses information and communication technologies to support information synthesis in accordance with professional and regulatory standards in the delivery of patient/client care.* The following three competencies have been identified:

1) **Information and knowledge management** - Uses relevant information and knowledge to support the delivery of evidence-informed patient care.,

2) **Professional and regulatory accountability** - Uses ICTs in accordance with professional and regulatory standards and workplace policies.

3) **Information and communication technologies** - Uses information and communication technologies in the delivery of patient/client care.

Each of these competency domains has been further elucidated with specific outcome indicators which can be used to determine whether each competency has been achieved. For example: a) *Performs search and critical appraisal of on-line literature and resources (e.g., scholarly articles, websites, and other appropriate resources) to support clinical judgement, and evidence-informed decision making and b) Demonstrates that professional judgement must prevail in the presence of technologies designed to support clinical assessments, interventions, and evaluation (e.g., monitoring devices, decision support tools, etc.).*

The entry-to-practice informatics competencies for registered nurses and the associated toolkit have been widely disseminated to all Canadian schools of nursing, are available on the CASN web-site for free download [34], and have also been shared as an online resource to subscribers of the TIGER (Technology Informatics Guiding Education Reform) Virtual Learning Environment (VLE).

Efforts to continue the dissemination and integration of the informatics competencies into the undergraduate curricula of Canadian schools of nursing are currently underway. An initiative launched in the winter of 2015 included nursing faculty outreach and mentoring by the designation of ten digital health faculty peer leaders from the east to west coast of Canada. Each faculty peer leader led a variety of educational sessions, webinars, workshops and one-on-one mentoring with nursing faculty. In addition, a faculty resource for the teaching of Consumer Health Solutions was developed, published and disseminated to schools of nursing. Data were gathered from peer leaders and their mentees pre and post-implementation of this initiative and indicate the merits of continuing the peer leader strategy to advance curricula integration of informatics.

8. Discussion

The above description provides an overview of how informatics competencies are addressed in six countries. These examples have the potential to be a useful resource for informatics professionals and nursing curriculum developers as they strive to meet the challenge of including, and then ensuring students meet the nursing informatics competencies in their entry to practice education.

While the reports from six countries shared above indicate variety in how nursing informatics competencies are articulated and implemented in nursing education, it also highlights that despite the differences between the countries there is also a shared concern on how to educate and prepare nurses for a technology rich healthcare environment. The differences in the nursing informatics competencies vary considerably. For example, the American Association of Colleges of Nursing, under the item they identify as Essential IV: Information Management and Application of Patient Care Technology state, "Graduates must have basic competence in technical skills, which includes the use of computers, as well as the application of patient care technologies such as monitors, data gathering devices, and other technological supports for patient care interventions. In addition, baccalaureate graduates must have competence in the use of information technology systems, including decision support systems, to gather evidence to guide practice" [3]. This detailed requirement is in marked contrast to the brief statement from New Zealand regarding nurses needing to be competent in "the use of information technology and health information management" [7]. Both of these differ again with the European Health Information Technology Competencies [36] which under the heading of General Knowledge/System Use have the baseline competency for the nurse of "Being able to use technology appropriate to your role and work environment" and being "aware of the various types and components of health information/eHealth systems". Furthermore, these three examples of competencies are difficult to assess. Some suggest that assessment drives learning [37], and so the challenge is how can educators measure or assess attainment of nursing informatics competencies.

Despite having created, document and shared nursing informatics competencies within a country or region, the competencies may not be fully adopted and taught in all schools of nursing. This issue highlights the need for suitably qualified faculty who will champion nursing informatics as a subject and are available to teach students [38, 39].

An international approach to health is well recognized as important for future developments due to the commonalities in issues such as meeting the increasing demand for health care services and reducing the rising cost of those services [40]. This can be extended to healthcare education, which may also benefit from collaboration with a global approach through sharing insights, educational opportunities and resources [41, 42]. The notion of having an internationalised nursing curriculum has been raised [43, 44], and if this was ever to come to fruition, nursing informatics would ideally be included. The concept that nursing informatics is a concern beyond the borders of any one country has some appeal as having such a standardised approach may help to ensure that nurses throughout the world are prepared to the highest levels, and are well placed to support global health.

9. Conclusion

This chapter presents six country's use of informatics competencies for student nurses and as such shows a range of approaches. The use of international networking, information share and learning among nurses is still in its infancy. What remains clear is that much work remains to achieve full integration of core informatics competencies into nursing curricula. Additionally, the challenge to engage nursing faculty in this work requires multi-faceted approaches to develop the competency and comfort of a majority of nurse educators. The state of nursing informatics within each country varies, and it would seem that no one approach is better than another. Rather the challenge is finding a way forward that fits with local drivers and initiatives to strengthen the early stages of nursing education so that nurses are well prepared for their career which includes making best use of available technology to support their practice.

References

[1] Grant G, Elbow P, Ewens T, Gamson Z, Kohli W, Neumann W, et al. On competence: A critical analysis of competence-based reforms in higher education. San Francisco: Jossey-Bass; 1979.

[2] Quality and Safety Education for Nurses (QSEN) Institute. Competencies pre-licensure knowledge, skills and attitudes 2014 [cited 2015 April 25]. Available from: http://qsen.org/competencies/pre-licensure-ksas/#informatics

[3] American Association of Colleges of Nursing. The essentials of baccalaureate education for professional nursing practice. Washington DC: AACN; 2008.

[4] College of Nurses of Ontario. National competencies in the context of entry-level Registered Nurse practice. Toronto Canada: College of Nurses of Ontario; 2009.

[5] Nursing Council of New Zealand. Annual Report 2015. Wellington, New Zealand: Nursing Council of New Zealand; 2015.

[6] Hausman JP. Guidelines for teaching nursing informatics. Wellington, New Zealand: Ministry of Education; 1989.

[7] Nursing Council of New Zealand. Competencies for registered nurses [Internet]Wellington, New Zealand: Nursing Council of New Zealand; 2012 [Available from: http://www.nursingcouncil.org.nz/Nurses/Continuing-competence

[8] Parry D, Hunter I, Honey M, Holt A, Day K, Kirk R, et al. Building an educated health informatics workforce – the New Zealand experience. Studies in Health Technology and Informatics. 2013;188:86-90.

[9] Parry D, Hunter I, Honey M, Holt A, Day K, Kirk R, et al. Health informatics community priming in a small nation:The New Zealand experience. Studies in Health Technology and Informatics. 2013;192:950.

[10] The Henry J Kaiser Family Foundation. Total number of professionally active nurses in the United States. 2016.

[11] American Nurses Association. FAST FACTS: The nursing workforce 2014: Growth, salaries, education, demographics and trends. 2014.

[12] Health Resources and Services Administration Bureau of Health Professions National Center for Health Workforce Analysis. The U.S. nursing workforce: Trends in supply and education. 2013.

[13] American Association of Colleges of Nursing. Amid calls for a more highly educated RN workforce, new AACN data confirm enrollment surge in schools of nursing: Press Release March 2015. 2015.

[14] Greiner AC, Knebel E, editors. The Institute of Medicine Committee on the Health Professions Education Summit: Health Professions Education: A Bridge to Quality. Washington DC: The National Academies Press; 2003.

[15] Technology Informatics Guiding Education Reform (TIGER). About TIGER 2013. Available from: www.tigersummit.com

[16] Technology Informatics Guiding Education Reform (TIGER). Informatics competencies for every practicing nurse: Recommendations from the TIGER collaborative [Internet]: The TIGER

Initiative;   2009   [July   14,   2014].   Available   from: http://www.thetigerinitiative.org/docs/
TigerReport_InformaticsCompetencies.pdf

[17] National League for Nursing Board of Governors. Position Statement: Preparing the next generation of
nurses to practice in a technology-rich environment: An informatics agenda. New York: National League
for Nursing; 2008.

[18] Nursing Times. English nursing posts down by a 1,000 in a month2013;July. Available from:
http://www.nursingtimes.net/nursing-practice/clinical-zones/management/english-nursing-posts-down-
by-1000-in-a-month/5061570.article

[19] Nursing and Midwifery Council. Standards for education 2015 [cited 2015 April 28]. Available from:
http://www.nmc.org.uk/education/standards-for-education/

[20] National Information Board, Department of Health. Personalised health and care 2020: Using data and
technology to transform outcomes for patients and citizens - A framework for action. Leeds, England:
NHS; 2014.

[21] NHS England. Leading change, adding value. NHS Publication.; 2016.

[22] Australian Institute of Health and Welfare. Nursing and midwifery workforce in 2013 2015 [cited 2015
April 28]. Available from: http://www.aihw.gov.au/workforce/nursing-and-midwifery/

[23] Hegney D, Buikstra E, Eley R, Fallon T, Gilmore V, Soar J. Nurses and information technology: Final
report. 2007.

[24] Australian Nursing and Midwifery Federation. National Informatics Standards for Nurses and Midwives.
2015.

[25] Australian Nursing and Midwifery Accreditation Council (ANMAC). Registered Nurse accreditation
standards. 2012.

[26] Nursing and Midwifery Board of Australia. Regulating Australia's nurses and midwives. 2015.

[27] Australian Health Practitioner Regulation Agency (AHPRA). Regulating Australia's health practitioners
in partnership with the National Boards. 2015.

[28] Nursing and Midwifery Board of Australia. National competency standards for the registered nurse.
2006.

[29] Nursing and Midwifery Board of Australia. Registered nurse standards for practice. 2016.

[30] Department of Education and Training. Australian quality framework. 2013.

[31] Finnish Nurses Association. Sairaanhoitajat suhtautuvat myönteisesti teknologiaan (Nurses' attitude to
technology   is   positive)   2015   [31   July,   2015].   Available   from:
https://sairaanhoitajat.fi/2015/sairaanhoitajat-suhtautuvat-myonteisesti-teknologiaan/

[32] Finnish Nurses Association. eHealth strategy of the Finnish Nurses Association 2015-2020 2016 [cited
2016 Octobe 25]. Available from: http://www.nurses.fi/nursing_and_nurse_education_in_f/ehealth-
strategy-of-the-finnish-/

[33] Nagle L, Clarke H. Assessing the informatics education needs in Canadian schools of nursing. 11th
World Congress on Medical Informatics; 7-11 September; San Francisco, California, USA. Amsterdam:
IOS Press; 2004.

[34] Canadian Association of Schools of Nursing (CASN). Nursing informatics entry to practice
competencies   for   Registered   Nurses   2015   [cited   2016   October   25].   Available   from:
http://www.casn.ca/wp-content/uploads/2014/12/Nursing-Informatics-Entry-to-Practice-Competencies-
for-RNs_updated-June-4-2015.pdf

[35] Nagle L, Crosby K, Frisch N, Borycki E, Donelle L, Hannah K, et al. Developing entry-to-practice
nursing informatics competencies for registered nurses. Studies in Health Technology and Informatics.
2014;201:356-63.

[36] HITComp - Health IT competencies. 2015. Available from: http://hitcomp.siframework.org

[37] Wormald BW, Schoeman S, Somasunderam A, Penn M. Assessment drives learning: an unavoidable
truth? Anatomical Sciences Education. 2009;2(5):199-204.

[38] Borycki E, Joe RS, Armstrong B, Bellwood P, Campbell R. Educating health professionals about the
Electronic Health Record (EHR): Removing the barriers to adoption. Knowledge Management & E-
Learning: An International Journal. 2011;3(1):51-62.

[39] Mantas J, Ammenwerth E, Demiris G, Hasman A, Haux R, Hersh W, et al. Recommendations of the
International Medical Informatics Association (IMIA) on Education in biomedical and health
informatics. Methods of Information in Medicine. 2010;49(2):105-20.

[40] Deloitte. Global health care outlook: Common goals, competing priorities. London, England: Deloitte
Touche Tohmatsu Limited 2015.

[41] Garnera BL, Metcalfe SE, Hallyburton A. International collaboration: A concept model to engage
nursing leaders and promote global nursing education partnerships Nurse Education in Practice.
2009;9(2):102-8.

[42] Rosenberg ML, Hayes E, McIntyre M, Neill NW. Real collaboration: What it takes for global health to
succeed. Berkeley, CA: University of California Press; 2010.

[43] Green W, Whitsed C. Critical perspectives on internationalising the curriculum in disciplines: Reflective narrative accounts from business, education and health. Rotterdam, Netherlands: Sense Publishers; 2015.
[44] Kain VJ. Internationalisation of the curriculum in an undergraduate nursing degree. In: Green W, Whitsed C, editors. Critical perspectives on internationalising the curriculum in disciplines: Reflective narrative accounts from business, education and health. Rotterdam, Netherlands: Sense Publishers; 2015.

Forecasting Informatics Competencies for Nurses in the Future of Connected Health
J. Murphy et al. (Eds.)
© *2017 IMIA and IOS Press.*
doi:10.3233/978-1-61499-738-2-62

The Professional Association's Perspective on Nursing Informatics and Competencies in the US

Carol J. BICKFORD[a]
[a] *American Nurses Association*

Abstract. The American Nurses Association (ANA) recognized nursing informatics as a nursing specialty in 1992, developed the first scope and standards of nursing informatics practice in the mid-1990s, and remains the custodian and steward of each document revision. Over the past two decades, the definition of nursing informatics, scope of practice statement, and framework of the standards of practice have evolved to now include a collection of competencies for the informatics nurse and informatics nurse specialist. The American Nurses Credentialing Center (ANCC), an ANA subsidiary, created and maintains a nursing informatics certification program that offers a board certification credential to qualified applicants, including international nurse colleagues. Such a certification program is intended to assess and publicly recognize competence of the informatics nurse.

Keywords. Nursing informatics, scope of practice, standards of practice, competence, certification

1. Introduction

The American Nurses Association (ANA), the professional organization representing the interests of the 3.6 million nurses in the U.S., provided leadership in development of the specialty practice of nursing informatics by engaging nursing leaders from academia, practice, and research in thoughtful dialogue about the future of health care and how best to assure nursing's contribution could be identified, evaluated, and improved. Because this perspective demanded the knowledge and expertise of those nurses interested in the acquisition, codification, analysis, transformation, and dissemination of data, information, knowledge, and wisdom, ANA supported the development and formal recognition of the nursing specialty practice of nursing informatics in 1992.

2. History of the Nursing Informatics Scope and Standards Documents

ANA convened a workgroup to develop the 1994 *Scope of Practice for Nursing Informatics* that included a definition identifying that "Nursing informatics is the specialty that integrates nursing science, computer science, and information science in identifying, collecting, processing, and managing data and information to support nursing practice, administration, education, research, and the expansion of nursing knowledge. It supports the practice of all nursing specialties, in all sites and settings of care, whether at the basic or advanced level." [1] Further detailing of the answers to the "who", "what", "when", "where", "how", and "why" questions addressed in specialty nursing scope of practice statements, confirmed the informatics nurse attended to the development and evaluation of applications, tools, processes, and structures that assist nurses in managing data associated with patient care or the infrastructure supporting nursing practice. Nursing informatics practice included adapting or customizing existing technology to meet nursing requirements. Interprofessional collaboration with other healthcare and informatics professionals was expected in the development of informatics products and standards.

The informatics nurse was expected to hold a bachelor's degree in nursing and have additional knowledge and experience in the field of informatics. Eighteen delineated competencies, such as systems analysis, systems design, use of applications software, and employment of computer programming tools and utilities in the accomplishment of nursing informatics work, were included. The informatics nurse specialist's preparation included a masters' degree in nursing with graduate-level courses in the field of informatics. Seven competencies were identified for this advanced level, including developing and teaching theory and practice of nursing informatics, consultation practice in the field of nursing informatics, and development of strategies, policies, and procedures for introducing, evaluating, and modifying information technology applied to nursing practice. [1]

The following year, ANA published the product of another workgroup, *Standards of Practice for Nursing Informatics*, to further describe nursing informatics practice with a detailed framework of standards and accompanying measurement criteria.[2] Six standards of practice reflected the implementation of the nursing process of assessment, diagnosis, identification of outcomes, planning, implementation, and evaluation in nursing informatics practice. In addition, eight standards of professional performance addressed characteristics of how nursing informatics was to be conducted, including quality of nursing informatics practice, performance appraisal, education, collegiality, ethics, collaboration, research, and resource utilization. This resource also included five domain standards for the informatics nurse addressing the information system life cycle, principles and theory, information technology, communication, and databases. [2] Each standard statement had associated measurement criteria that could be used as part of a personal performance appraisal and could also inform development of a position description.

ANA convened a new expert panel in 2000 to review and revise the first nursing informatics scope and standards documents, resulting in a 2001 combined document, *Scope and Standards of Informatics Practice*. The revised definition of nursing informatics reflected evolution of the specialty: "Nursing informatics is a specialty that integrates nursing science, computer science, and information science to manage and communicate data, information, and knowledge in nursing practice. Nursing informatics facilitates the integration of data, information, and knowledge to support patients, nurses, and other providers in their decision-making in all roles and settings. This support is accomplished through the use of information structures, information processes, and information technology."[3] Note the attention to management and communication of data, information, and knowledge in nursing practice that moves beyond the original identification, collection, processing, and management activities. Changes in focus addressed integration of data, information, and knowledge into decision-making processes that now were completed by patients, nurses, and other providers.

The 2001 scope of practice content more than doubled the content recorded in 1994, included a new figure and discussion addressing the transformation of data to information to knowledge, and introduced ethics content. The section about the diverse roles of the informatics nurse and informatics nurse specialist identified the new roles of entrepreneurs and executive level positions in provider and vendor organizations. The description of the published Delphi study research of Staggers, Gassert, and Curran identifying computer skills, information literacy skills, and overall informatics competencies of the beginning nurse, experienced nurse, and informatics nurse was another key addition.[4] However, these competencies were not detailed in the standards component of this scope and standards edition.

The 2001 standards only addressed the informatics nurse specialist and included new names for the five standards of practice: identify the issue or problem, identify alternatives, choose and develop a solution, implement the solution, evaluate and adjust solutions. The actual standard of practice statements significantly differed from the earlier edition, as did the accompanying measurement criteria. The standards of professional performance carried the same titles, included new Standard IX Communication, and retained standards statements essentially congruent with the 1995 edition. The accompanying measurement criteria, not yet identified as competencies, were revised to reflect the changing nursing informatics environment.

The next revision of the document, *Nursing Informatics: Scope and Standards of Practice* (2008), bore an entirely new title in order to better align with the format of other contemporary specialty nursing scope and standards publications. [5] The definition of nursing informatics remained unchanged except for the addition of wisdom in the series "data, information, knowledge, and wisdom" and inclusion of consumers in the list of those supported by the informatics nurse in their decision-making. Rather than identify roles, the workgroup authors elected to discuss the evolving and expanding nursing informatics practice within discrete functional areas of administration, leadership, and management; analysis; compliance and integrity management; consultation; coordination, facilitation, and integration; development; educational and professional development; policy development and advocacy; and research and evaluation. Inclusion of a two-page competencies matrix addressed the competencies identified by Staggers, Gassert, and Curran [4], other authors, and the American Nurses Credentialing Center (ANCC) 2007 certification examination test content outline.

The 2008 standards of nursing informatics practice and professional performance section presented a new numbering format and revised standards names. The standards of practice names again reflected the nursing process steps of assessment, problem and issues identification, outcomes identification, planning, implementation [with associated standards addressing coordination of activities, health teaching and health promotion and education, and consultation], and evaluation. The standards of professional performance were reordered and now included education, professional practice evaluation (new name), quality of practice, collegiality, collaboration, ethics, research, resource utilization, and new standards of advocacy and leadership. Accompanying measurement criteria for each standard, not competency statements, also addressed additional measurement criteria for the informatics nurse specialist for select standards.

In 2008 ANA published a position statement about professional role competence that served to inform the thinking and decision-making of those developing future nursing scope and standards resources and other professional documents. The position statement, *Professional Role Competence*, was reaffirmed in 2014 by ANA's Board of Directors, including the following statements:

- 'An individual who demonstrates "competence" is performing successfully at an expected level.'
- 'A "competency" is an expected level of performance that integrates knowledge, skills, abilities, and judgment.'
- "Knowledge encompasses thinking; understanding of science, humanities, and professional standards of practice; and insights gained from practical experiences, personal capabilities, and leadership performance."
- "Skills include psychomotor, communication, interpersonal, and diagnostic skills."
- "Ability is the capacity to act effectively. It requires listening, integrity, knowledge of one's strengths and weaknesses, positive self-regard, emotional intelligence, and openness to feedback."
- "Judgment includes critical thinking, problem solving, ethical reasoning, and decision-making."[6]

These definitions and concepts guided development of the 2010 *Nursing: Scope and Standards of Practice, Second Edition* [7], the professional nursing resource that served as the template for future specialty nursing scope and standards documents, including the 2015 *Nursing Informatics: Scope and Standards of Practice, Second Edition.* [8]

3. Current Nursing Informatics Scope and Standards Document

Nursing Informatics: Scope and Standards of Practice, Second Edition (2015) provides a new definition of nursing informatics: "*Nursing informatics (NI)* is the specialty that integrates nursing science with multiple information and analytical sciences to identify, define, manage, and communicate data, information, knowledge, and wisdom in nursing practice. NI supports nurses, consumers, patients, the interprofessional healthcare team and other stakeholders in their decision-making in all roles and settings to achieve desired outcomes. This support is accomplished through the use of information structures, information processes, and information technologies."[8]

The workgroup authors for this edition identified the informatics nurse to be a registered nurse with an interest or experience in an informatics field, most often identified as nursing informatics. The informatics nurse specialist is a registered nurse with formal graduate-level education in informatics or a related field. [8]

This edition retains the description of nursing informatics practice categorized as a framework of functional areas. These detailed sections include discussion of administration, leadership, and management; systems analysis and design; compliance and integrity management; consultation; coordination, facilitation, and integration; development of systems, products, and resources; educational and professional development; genetics and genomics; information management/operational architecture; policy development and advocacy; quality and performance improvement; research and evaluation; and safety, security, and environmental health. A discussion of several organization's directives, publications, research initiatives, and repositories identifying nursing informatics competencies followed.

The inclusion of a section discussing ethics in nursing informatics affirms the responsibility and accountability of the informatics nurse and informatics nurse specialist to adhere to the *Code of Ethics for Nurses with Interpretive Statements*. [9] Each of the nine provisions is cited and further enhanced with a short discussion of specific examples of its application in the specialty practice of nursing informatics. Because a new edition of the *Code of Ethics for Nurses with Interpretive Statements* was published in 2015, each informatics nurse and informatics nurse specialist is now expected to adhere to those provisions and accompanying interpretive statements. [10]

The 2015 Standards of Nursing Informatics Practice follow the architecture of earlier editions with:

Standards of Practice for Nursing Informatics:

Standard 1.   Assessment — The informatics nurse collects comprehensive data, information, and emerging evidence pertinent to the situation.

Standard 2.   Diagnosis, Problems, and Issues Identification — The informatics nurse analyzes assessment data to identify diagnoses, problems, issues, and opportunities for improvement.

Standard 3.   Outcomes Identification — The informatics nurse identifies expected outcomes for a plan individualized to the healthcare consumer or the situation.

Standard 4.   Planning — The informatics nurse develops a plan that prescribes strategies, alternatives, and recommendations to attain expected outcomes.

Standard 5.   Implementation — The informatics nurse implements the identified plan.

Standard 5A. Coordination of Activities — The informatics nurse coordinates planned activities.

Standard 5B. Health Teaching and Health Promotion — The informatics nurse employs informatics solutions and strategies for education and teaching to promote health and a safe environment.

Standard 5C. Consultation — The informatics nurse provides consultation to influence the identified plan, enhance the abilities of others, and effect change.

Standard 6.   Evaluation — The informatics nurse evaluates progress toward attainment of outcomes.

Standards of Professional Performance for Nursing Informatics:

Standard 7.   Ethics — The informatics nurse practices ethically.

Standard 8.   Education — The informatics nurse attains knowledge and competence that reflect current nursing and informatics practice.

Standard 9.   Evidence-Based Practice and Research — The informatics nurse integrates evidence and research findings into practice.

Standard 10. Quality of Practice — The informatics nurse contributes to quality and effectiveness of nursing and informatics practice.

Standard 11. Communication — The informatics nurse communicates effectively in a variety of formats in all areas of practice.

Standard 12. Leadership — The informatics nurse demonstrates leadership in the professional practice setting and the profession.

Standard 13. Collaboration — The informatics nurse collaborates with the healthcare consumer, family, and others in the conduct of nursing and informatics practice.

Standard 14. Professional Practice Evaluation — The informatics nurse evaluates his or her own nursing practice in relation to professional practice standards and guidelines, relevant statues, rules, and regulations.

Standard 15. Resource Utilization — The informatics nurse employs appropriate resources to plan and implement informatics and associated services that are safe, effective, and fiscally responsible.

Standard 16. Environmental Health — The informatics nurse supports practice in a safe and healthy environment. [8]

Unlike earlier editions, each standard includes accompanying competency statements for all informatics nurses and in many instances additional competencies for the informatics nurse specialist. The competencies have been constructed to include only one verb to facilitate easier evaluation that confirms the informatics nurse or informatics nurse specialist demonstrates competence.

As part of its responsibility to update specialty nursing scope and standards resources, ANA will convene a new workgroup in 2019 to review and revise the scope and standards document to describe the scope of contemporary nursing informatics practice, standards of practice and professional performance, and requisite competencies. The expert workgroup will complete an environmental assessment of nursing informatics practice and confirm the standards and appropriate competencies to include in the next edition.

4. Nursing Informatics Certification Program

While ANA developed and then formally recognized nursing informatics as a nursing specialty with an identified scope of practice statement and standards of nursing informatics practice, its subsidiary, the American Nurses Credentialing Center (ANCC) engaged in parallel efforts to develop a nursing informatics certification program. These efforts included creation of an expert panel, test content outline, pool of test questions, and a valid and reliable examination for qualified applicants to become board certified in nursing informatics. Such certification was intended to assess and publicly recognize professional competence. The initial cohort of nursing informatics applicants sat for the first ANCC computer-based test in December 1995 and received notification of their exam status in the first quarter of 1996.

ANCC now uses regularly scheduled role delineation studies to assess the characteristics of contemporary nursing informatics practice, convenes its content expert panel of volunteer certified informatics nurses to review and revise the test content outline, recruits qualified item writers, maintains a secure repository of test items, and contracts with an external testing center to manage the security, administration, and scoring of the nursing informatics exam.

Over the past two decades, ANCC has expanded eligibility for the computer-based testing to qualified international applicants and has developed various types of review materials for purchase. Numerous review courses are now available. As of December 31, 2015, ANCC reported 1,837 nurses maintain their nursing informatics certification (http://www.nursecredentialing.org/Certification/FacultyEducators/FacultyCategory/St atistics/2015-CertificationStatistics.pdf).

5. Summary

Development of the scope and standards formalized the description of the specialty practice of nursing informatics. Concurrent efforts by nursing informatics leaders and other visionary educators continue to focus on confirming what informatics competencies are applicable and merit inclusion in undergraduate and graduate nursing education and professional development programs as connected health becomes a framework for contemporary health care. To assure safe, quality nursing practice and care, all nurses today must demonstrate understanding of the relationship and impact of data, information, knowledge, and wisdom in professional and healthcare consumer decision-making. Please examine additional chapter section B components that present nursing informatics competencies described by other entities.

References

[1]   American Nurses Association, Scope of Practice for Nursing Informatics, American Nurses Publishing, Washington, DC, 1994.
[2]   American Nurses Association, Standards of Practice for Nursing Informatics, American Nurses Publishing, Washington, DC, 1995.
[3]   American Nurses Association, Scope and Standards of Nursing Informatics Practice, Nursebooks.org, Silver Spring, MD, 2001.
[4]   N. Staggers, C. A. Gassert, C. Curran, Informatics competencies for nurses at four levels of practice, Journal of Nursing Education 40(7) (2001), 303-316.
[5]   American Nurses Association, Nursing Informatics: Scope and Standards of Practice, Nursesbooks.org, Silver Spring, MD, 2008.
[6]   American Nurses Association, Professional Role Competence position statement, http://nursingworld.org/position/practice/role.aspx, 2014.
[7]   American Nurses Association, Nursing: Scope and Standards of Practice, Second Edition, Nursesbooks.org, Silver Spring, MD, 2010.
[8]   American Nurses Association, Nursing Informatics: Scope and Standards of Practice, Second Edition, Nursesbooks.org, Silver Spring, MD, 2015.
[9]   American Nurses Association, Code of Ethics for Nurses with Interpretive Statements, Nursesbooks.org, Silver Spring, MD, 2001.
[10] American Nurses Association, Code of Ethics for Nurses with Interpretive Statements, Nursesbooks.org, Silver Spring, MD, 2015.

Forecasting Informatics Competencies for Nurses in the Future of Connected Health
J. Murphy et al. (Eds.)
© *2017 IMIA and IOS Press.*
doi:10.3233/978-1-61499-738-2-69

International Evolution of TIGER Informatics Competencies

Joyce SENSMEIER[a,1] Christel ANDERSON[a] and Toria SHAW[a]

[a] *HIMSS*

Abstract. The TIGER Initiative aims to explain how to equip practicing nurses with informatics competencies. This chapter describes a collaborative effort to identify global informatics requirements in relation to core competencies and to match them with national and regional needs. Recommendations from the TIGER Informatics Competency Synthesis Project, described here, have implications for an international framework of informatics competencies for all types of health care professionals including nurses.

Keywords. Informatics, Competencies, Technology, Education

1. Introduction

The Technology Informatics Guiding Education Reform (TIGER) Initiative is focused on education reform and interprofessional community development. The spirit of TIGER is to maximize the seamless integration of technology and informatics into nursing practice, education and research.

In order to equip every practicing nurse with informatics competencies, TIGER developed recommendations in the areas of basic computer competencies, information literacy and information management. The TIGER International Competency Synthesis Project aims to investigate global informatics requirements in relation to core competencies to match them with national and regional needs [1].

2. History of TIGER

In 2006, TIGER convened a Summit of nursing stakeholders to develop, publish, and commit to an action plan to make healthcare safer, more effective, efficient, patient-centered, timely and equitable. As an outcome of the Summit, topic-focused collaborative teams were formed to advance the action plan. Each team worked on identifying best practices from education and practice, so that this collective body of knowledge could be shared. As a grass roots effort, TIGER built upon and recognized the work of individuals from many organizations, programs, and related initiatives who contributed their expertise in academia, practice, research and government while working towards a common goal [2].

---

[1] Corresponding author. Joyce Sensmeier MS, RN-BC, CPHIMS, FHIMSS, FAAN, HIMSS, 33 West Monroe Street, Suite 1700, Chicago, IL 60603; E-mail: jsensmeier@himss.org

The TIGER Informatics Competencies Collaborative was formed to develop informatics recommendations for all practicing nurses and graduating nursing students. Following a review of the literature and survey of nursing informatics education, research, and practice groups, the TIGER Nursing Informatics Competencies Model was developed consisting of three parts: 1) Basic Computer Competencies; 2) Information Literacy; and 3) Information Management (including use of an EHR). In 2011, the group published a landmark report titled *Informatics Competencies for Every Practicing Nurse: Recommendations from the TIGER Collaborative* [3]. As part of a changing and dynamic environment, the goal of this original report was to influence stakeholders in order to advance the adoption of informatics competencies through existing education, research, and practice groups. This work synthesized an extensive list of competencies into three components that were realistic for the nearly 3 million practicing nurses in the United States.

2.1. Recommendations for Basic Computer Competencies

Basic Computer Competencies (see Table 1) include the informatics competencies that are foundational for all practicing nurses and graduating nursing students in order to achieve the advanced informatics competencies.

Table 1: Basic Computer Competencies

Hardware	File Management	Using the Web
Software	Utilities	Web Outputs
Networks	Print Management	Electronic Communication
Security	Using the Application	Using e-mail
Law	The Internet	e-mail Management
Operating System	Using the Browser	

2.2. Recommendations for Information Literacy

Information literacy builds on computer literacy, and includes the ability to identify information needed for a specific purpose, locate pertinent information, evaluate the information and apply it correctly. Information literacy competencies (see Table 2) are critical for incorporating evidence into nursing practice. Evaluating the information also involves critical thinking and the ability to determine the validity of the source.

Table 2: Information Literacy Competencies

1.	Knowledge to determine the nature and extent of the information needed
2.	Access needed information effectively and efficiently
3.	Evaluate information and its sources critically and incorporate selected information into his or her knowledge base and value system
4.	Individually or as a member of a group, use information effectively to accomplish a specific purpose
5.	Evaluate outcomes of the use of information

2.3. Recommendations for Information Management Competencies

Information management involves collecting data, processing the data, and presenting and communicating the processed data as information or knowledge. Nurses need information management competencies (see Table 3) to carry out their fundamental clinical responsibilities in a safe, effective and efficient manner.

Table 3: Information Management Competencies

Using an EHR, the nurse can manage:
1. Demographic/patient information
2. Consents and authorizations
3. Medication administration
4. Planning care
5. Orders/results
6. Care documentation
7. Decision support
8. Notifications
9. Facilitating communications

3. TIGER International Competency Synthesis Project

The informatics competencies conversation has now expanded to include an interprofessional and international focus. The TIGER International Committee has completed the first phase of an innovative competency synthesis project that highlights recommended core international informatics competencies. The TIGER International Competency Synthesis Project aims to investigate global informatics requirements in relation to core competencies to match them with national and regional needs. In 2015 the TIGER International Committee, with representatives from 21 countries, began comprehensive activities to compile recommended core international informatics competencies reflective of many countries, scientific societies, and research projects.

A survey was deployed in November, 2015 to evaluate and prioritize 24 core competencies in clinical informatics, which were rated based on their relevance to five nursing roles:

1. Clinical nursing (e.g. care planning),
2. Nursing management (e.g. ward or hospital management),
3. Quality management (e.g. organizational development),
4. IT management in nursing (e.g. introduction of new IT systems), and
5. Inter-professional coordination of care (e.g. case management).

As an outcome of this effort, TIGER is creating a competency harmonization matrix that outlines shared and country-specific competencies (including the United States) to provide guidance to the TIGER community and the industry at large. The Committee is taking a unique approach with this project as it is the first to collect various competencies across countries to identify global commonalities and differences. This harmonization effort will help determine how the Committee moves forward in the future [1].

Committee members also submitted and compiled case studies from Austria, Finland, Germany, Ireland, New Zealand, Philippines, Portugal, and Switzerland that reflect country-specific competencies based on country requirements, curriculum, and education. All of the core competencies listed in the case studies were also reflected in the survey, but described with greater detail. Several of these case studies are summarized below.

3.1. Case Study: Australian Nursing and Midwifery Federation Informatics Standards

The Australian Nursing and Midwifery Federation (ANMF) has released the national informatics standards for nurses and midwives. These national informatics standards clearly articulate the activities required for all nurses and midwives in practice [4] and encompass the following three domains:

1. Computer Literacy
    Applies knowledge and skills in computer basics for effective use of information and communication technologies
2. Information Literacy
    Uses fundamental knowledge and skills to identify, locate, access, evaluate and apply information
3. Information Management
    Uses knowledge and skills to ensure safe, legal and ethical management of health information for professional practice and lifelong learning, appropriate to context of practice

3.2. Case Study: Healthcare Informatics Society of Ireland

From an Irish perspective, the integration of informatics competencies in nursing and midwifery is in the early stages of development. A significant milestone is the inclusion and future integration of nursing informatics competencies into the nursing and midwifery undergraduate program. Within Ireland, the Health Informatics Training System (HITS), a dedicated healthcare competencies program, was developed by the Irish Computer Society, in partnership with the Health Informatics Society of Ireland - Nurses & Midwives Group (HISINM). It is acknowledged that the range and scope of competencies across healthcare practitioners can differ greatly. The HISINM Group provided the Irish perspective conceptualized at three levels ranging in broad competencies [5].

Competency Level One: Undergraduate and novice practitioners

*   Knowledge and understanding of the health, life and behavioral sciences and their applied principles which underpins a competent knowledge base for contemporary nursing and healthcare practice

Competency Level Two: Intermediate

*   Concepts of health informatics covering topics ranging from data processing and electronic record keeping to decision-support systems and security

Competency Level Three: Advanced expert practitioner

*   Advanced informatics skills focusing on the integration of data, information, knowledge and wisdom to support patients/clients, nurses and other healthcare professionals in their decision making in all roles and settings

Integration of nursing informatics competencies is referenced in the draft undergraduate requirements and standards report published in February 2015, and is now in the final submission phase by the National Nursing Board of Ireland. Existing policy on Nursing and Midwifery Informatics Competencies will be delivered as part of a coordinated national strategy, specifically in line with eHealth Ireland and National Service Plan agendas.

3.3. Case Study: Defining Informatics Competencies in Austria, Germany and Switzerland

There is a wealth of excellent recommendations concerning medical and nursing informatics competencies including the TIGER recommendations. The competencies, however, vary from country to country and from nursing culture to nursing culture [6]. The nursing informatics workgroups in Germany, Austria and Switzerland agreed to compile a consolidated set of recommendations that:

- Complies with the relevant literature,
- Makes use of existing national recommendations of other healthcare professionals, and
- Is based on a comprehensive survey of selected experts in this field from the three countries.

In all, 120 experts were invited to participate and received a link to the questionnaire and by May 2015, 83 experts responded. The results revealed that the following competencies received the overall highest rating:

1. Project Management
2. Quality Assurance and Quality Management
3. Nursing Documentation
4. Process Management
5. Privacy and Data Security

These results demonstrate that the nursing informatics competencies most needed are more generic than specialized. The group will continue specifying the competencies in more detail in the coming months.

3.4. Case Study: Nursing and Health Informatics in Finland

The development of nursing informatics in practice, industry and education has become increasingly relevant as the role of IT has advanced. The main supporting actors in Finland have been the Finnish Nurses Association (FNA) and the National Development Center for Welfare and Health as well as the International Medical Informatics Association Special Interest Group of Nursing Informatics (IMIA-SIGNI).

In 2012, the FNA launched the standards for special competences of nursing informatics specialty certificate. The certification may be awarded to a registered nurse working in nursing informatics that demonstrates the required accreditation via an electronic portfolio. The requirements are consistent with the Clinical Practice Nursing Certification design for nurses working in a designated clinical area [7].

3.5. Case Study: Country Specific Competencies for New Zealand

In 2006, a report on the health informatics capability in New Zealand noted a need for a significant increase in people trained in health informatics [8]. This same report identified the need for greater co-operation between institutions and for increased awareness of the domain in the health and IT communities. Health Informatics New Zealand, as the independent national health informatics organization, established an education working group, comprising academics from all interested New Zealand universities. Based on the 2006 report and International Medical Informatics Association (IMIA) guidelines, a list of required competencies was developed [9].

Core competences identified were: Health domain knowledge, social/ethics/legal aspects of health IT, basic computer science, basic data management, basic health IS/IT management, clinical information systems and health informatics concepts [10]. It is these competencies that are now being considered in relation to the TIGER Initiative for synthesizing international nursing informatics competencies.

3.6. Case Study: Nursing Informatics Core Competencies for Portugal

Upon admission to a nursing program, all Portuguese students have a basic set of computer competencies developed during high school that overlap with the TIGER Informatics Competencies recommendations. However, during graduate programs, nurses are further prepared to achieve Information Literacy Competencies and Information Management Competencies.

From the analysis of multiple resources, Nursing Informatics Core Competencies have been identified related to Portugal's needs. The following Information Literacy Competencies are necessary and fundamental for EHR use for nurses in Portugal [11]:

- Determine the nature and extent of the information needed;
- Access needed information effectively and efficiently;
- Evaluate information and its sources critically and incorporate selected information into his or her knowledge base and value system;
- Individually or as a member of a group, use information effectively to accomplish a specific purpose; and
- Evaluate outcomes of information usage.

3.7. Case Study Summary

The TIGER International Competency Synthesis Project has deployed a mixed methods approach to investigate global informatics requirements [12]. These requirements leverage regional and national-specific core competencies by using a global survey and country specific case studies. All of the core competencies listed in the case studies are also reflected within the survey. Survey results include opinions from 21 countries; North and South America (four countries), Europe (10 countries), Asia (five countries) and Australia/Pacific (two countries). An average of two in-country experts rated the relevance of 24 informatics core competencies within five domains in nursing. Table 4 shows the top six competencies per domain.

Table 4. Top six core competencies in the five domains

Role/ domain	Top 1	Top 2	Top 3	Top 4	Top 5	Top 6
Clinical nursing	Nursing documentation	Information knowledge management	Principles of nursing informatics	Data protection and security	Ethics and IT	Information communication systems
Quality management	Quality management	Process management	Nursing documentation	Information knowledge management	Information communication systems	Principles of nursing informatics
Inter-professional coordination	Data protection and security	Information knowledge management	Nursing documentation	Process management	Information communication systems	Ethics and IT
Nursing Management	Nursing documentation	Principles of management	Strategic management and leadership	Quality management	Human resource management	Change management. stakeholder management

Role/ domain	Top 1	Top 2	Top 3	Top 4	Top 5	Top 6
IT Management	Information communication systems	Principles of nursing informatics	Data protection and security	IT risk management	Project management	Process management AND information knowledge management

4. Conclusion

The TIGER initiative represents a grass roots effort that brings together experts from around the world to explore informatics-related issues and concerns. There is much to gain when multiple ideas, perspectives and innovations are shared in the spirit of collaboration. The TIGER International Competency Synthesis Project is but one example of such an effort. Recommendations from this work will be widely disseminated to initiate a global discussion with implications for implementation of an international framework that will help health care professionals achieve the informatics competencies of the modern age.

References

[1] Hübner U., Shaw T., Ball MJ.. The TIGER Initiative. Hospital Healthcare Europe 2016, pp. 174-177. Available from: http://www.hospitalhealthcare.com .

[2] Bal MJ., Douglas JV. et.al., Nursing Informatics: Where Technology and Caring Meet, 4th Edition, London: Springer-Verlag; 2011.

[3] TIGER Initiative. Informatics Competencies for Every Practicing Nurse: Recommendations from the TIGER Collaborative. [Internet]. Chicago: Healthcare Information and Management Systems Society (HIMSS); 2015. http://www.himss.org/informatics-competencies

[4] Australian Nursing and Midwifery Federation. National informatics standards for nurses and midwives, Australian Nursing and Midwifery Federation, Federal Office; 2015.

[5] Healthcare Informatics Society of Ireland. Response to TIGER International Group on the creation of Informatics Competencies Relating to Nursing and Midwifery. [Internet] Chicago: Healthcare Information and Management Systems Society (HIMSS); 2015. file:///C:/Users/jsensmeier/Downloads/TIGER_HIMSS15_VLE_IrelandCaseStudy_11022015.pdf

[6] Hübner U. Towards defining nursing informatics competencies in Austria, Germany, and Switzerland. [Internet] Chicago: Healthcare Information and Management Systems Society (HIMSS); 2015. file:///C:/Users/jsensmeier/Downloads/TIGER_HIMSS15_VLE_AustriaGermanySwitzerlandCaseStudy_11182015.pdf

[7] Rajalahti E. and Saranto K.. Nursing and health informatics in Finland 2015. [Internet] Chicago: Healthcare Information and Management Systems Society (HIMSS); 2015. file:///C:/Users/jsensmeier/Downloads/TIGER_HIMSS15_VLE_FinlandCaseStudy_11182015.pdf

[8] Kerr K., Cullen R., Duke J., Holt A., Kirk R., Komisarczuk K., and Wilson S.. Health informatics capability development in New Zealand: A report to the Tertiary Education Commission. Wellington, New Zealand: National Steering Committee for Health Informatics Education in New Zealand. Retrieved from http://homepages.mcs.vuw.ac.nz/~peterk/healthinformatics/tec-hi-report-06.pdf; 2006.

[9] Mantas J., Ammenwerth E., Demiris G., Hasman A., Haux R., and Wright G.. Recommendations of the International Medical Informatics Association (IMIA) on Education in biomedical and health informatics. Methods of Information in Medicine, 49(2), 105-120; 2010.

[10] Parry D., Hunter I, Honey M., Holt A., Day K., Kirk R., and Cullen R.. Health informatics community priming in a small nation: The New Zealand experience. Studies in Health Technology and Informatics, 192, 950; 2013.

[11] Cardoso A. and Sousa P. Nursing informatics core competencies for Portugal. [Internet] Chicago: Healthcare Information and Management Systems Society (HIMSS); 2015. file:///C:/Users/jsensmeier/Downloads/TIGER_HIMSS15_VLE_PortugalCaseStudy_11182015.pdf

[12] Hübner U., Ball MJ., Anderson C., Chang P., and Marin H. Towards implementing a global competency-based nursing and clinical informatics curriculum: Applying the TIGER initiative. NI2016, Geneva, Switzerland; 2016.

© *2017 IMIA and IOS Press.*
This article is published online with Open Access by IOS Press and distributed under the terms
of the Creative Commons Attribution Non-Commercial License 4.0 (CC BY-NC 4.0).
doi:10.3233/978-1-61499-738-2-77

Competencies Related to Informatics and Information Management for Practicing Nurses and Nurses Leaders in Brazil and South America

Sayonara de Fatima Faria BARBOSA[a]
[a] *Federal University of Santa Catarina, BRAZIL*

Abstract. Informatics and information management competency has an important role for nursing. However, these competencies in Brazil and South America lack definition, and are just beginning to develop in these regions with different realities. This chapter presents information related to the development of informatics competencies for nursing in these areas.

Keywords. Digital competencies, nursing professional practice, nursing education

1. Introduction

Nursing informatics competence is extremely important, considering its potential of different applications for health outcomes. However, with regards to training of nurses able to work in this area in Brazil and other countries in South America, the process has been slow. It is important to define what nurses need to know about health information technology, so they can practice autonomously, provide safer care and achieve better health indicators. The World Health Organization (WHO) has recognized the use of information and communication technologies (ICT) as a core competency of the 21st century healthcare workforce to support patient care [1]. Thus, professionals well-trained in the use of ICT are highly needed [2].

2. Overview of Brazil and South America

Brazil is the largest country in South America, the fifth largest country by both area and population, and is the largest country to have Portuguese as an official language, the only one in the Americas. According to Brazilian Institute of Geography and Statistics, Brazil has 206,030,000 habitants, which represents 2.81% of world population and covers almost half (47.3%) of the South American continent.

3. Development of Nursing Informatics

In Brazil, the first steps in nursing informatics started in 1985, when faculty of nursing from Federal University of Rio Grande do Sul presented their experience in the use of computers to teach nursing activities in home care [3]. In the next year, the Brazilian Society of Health Informatics (SBIS) was founded, and three years later, in 1990 during the third Congress of the Brazilian Health Informatics Society, a dedicated session for nursing informatics was organized. During the same year, the Nursing Informatics Group at the Federal University of São Paulo was established, and in 1991, the group hosted the Inter-American Symposium in Nursing Informatics with over 200 participants. At this seminar, Brazil became a member of the International Medical Informatics Association, Nursing Informatics, Special Interest Group (IMIA, NI SIG) [4]. Currently, similar groups at universities across the country and several schools of nursing have established nursing informatics as a discipline in the nursing curriculum and have organized nursing informatics research groups [5].

However, a growing research movement in this field can be observed with several groups having been established in the last years across the country. In 2002, SBIS granted the creation of the Nursing Informatics Working Group (SBIS-NI), integrating nurses from several states within the country, with the established goals: (1) develop a national strategy for NI education, research, management, and clinical practice, (2) determine priorities for implementing nursing informatics educational programs, (3) develop by consensus a definition of nursing informatics according to Brazilian education and professional regulations, (4) recommend NI competencies for clinical nurses, managers, faculty, and researchers, (5) develop innovative care models and standards balanced by human and technological resources, and (6) promote development of next generation electronic health records to facilitate patient-centric care at bedside, clinical research, and public health [5]. In November 2003, the SBIS-NI founded the TeleNursing Department at the Brazilian Telemedicine and Telehealth Council [5]. Over the last 13 years, nursing informatics and telenursing have advanced considerably in the Brazilian healthcare environment, following global trends. Some of the strategies defined by the nursing informatics groups continue to make contributions to the health of Brazilian populations. The primary focus of those strategies is to develop a safer healthcare environment and to stimulate research regarding redesign of professional practice according to the new technological trends [5].

Since 2006, an important ICT project named RUTE network (Telemedicine University Network) has been deployed in the country. The project was led by The Brazilian National Research and Educational Network and was funded by the Brazilian Ministry of Science and Technology through the Brazilian Innovation Agency's research and projects financing.

RUTE implements communication infrastructure in university and teaching hospitals in the largest 53 cities in Brazil, enabling the establishment of telemedicine and ehealth centers with investments on equipment, connectivity and ambience preparation. The goal of the project is allowing all participating hospitals to use the National Network for Education and Research in order to operate applications on telemedicine and telehealth, including video and webconference for exchanging information, talks, continuing education, formative second opinion and teleconsultation, in order to create a base for collaboration among hospitals and to train them for remote collaboration. Several special interest groups (SIGs) were created, and SIG-Telenursing was the first nursing group created in 2007, aiming the integration of informatics and ehealth in intensive care and emergency, as well as research and education [6].

In addition, RUTE handles the multiprofessional integration in the healthcare of the community, and this infrastructure has improved access to healthcare and health information for the populations that live in regions that are remote and difficult to reach. The RUTE project also opened an ongoing channel for the development of research studies and interchange of specialized health knowledge, that has resulted in the growth of scientific collaboration, increased enrollment in healthcare training courses, and improved access to continuing education with the introduction of the e-learning, m-learning, and the integrated evolution of telenursing procedures on a national level [5].

4. CurricularGuidelines for Nursing Undergraduate Courses

The practice of nursing is based on the collection, storage, retrieval and use of data, information, and knowledge. Nurses must be competent in these areas in order to provide safe and effective patient care. Often times, technologies are used in practice to help with the management of information and clinical decision making. The development, implementation, and use of technology are integral to the practice of nursing. However, the use of technology in practice creates new educational needs for nurses in regards to possessing knowledge, behavior, and skills for practice [7]. It is important that nursing professionals and other healthcare providers are educated and competent in the proper use of technology as it applies to the various disciplines in healthcare.

To be competent means to possess specific behaviors, knowledge, skills, and/or capacity within defined areas [8, 9, 10]. Nurses, especially, must possess competence in nursing practice to provide safe and effective care.

In Brazil, curricular structures of Higher Education Institutions are organized according to the Curricular Guidelines for undergraduate nursing education. These guidelines establish a profile of graduated professionals who are capable of knowing and intervening in the most prevalence health-disease problems/situations in the national epidemiological profile [11].

Decision making in Brazil is highlighted in the National Curriculum Guidelines of Nursing Undergraduate Courses as one of the general competencies that determine the training of nurses, composed of clinical and managerial activities [12]. The same guideline proposes that health workers' practice must be based on the capacity for decision making, be them clinical or managerial. To that end, these professionals must possess competencies and abilities to assess, systematize and decide the most adequate actions, based on scientific evidence. Article 5 of the guideline also states that one of the objectives of nursing education is to provide students with the knowledge required to practice competences and skills for the adequate use of new information and communication technologies [13, 14]. Nursing informatics therefore challenges the faculty to produce nurses who are prepared to use information technology to improve the patient care process and change health care [15].

In this context, since 2001, the field of ICT is a core competence, listed on the National Curriculum Guidelines for undergraduate courses in Nursing [12]. In the document, the item "expertise and skills" states that nurses should "properly use new technologies, both information and communication, as tip for the care of nursing."

More than a decade later, we see yet little emphasis on the development of this competence in undergraduate nursing courses in Brazil, at public or private universities [16]. Recently, in a research about computer education in nursing graduate courses in public educational institutions in Brazil [17], it was noted that are offered few informatics courses. In fact, less than half (41.1%) of the federal institutions and less than a third (27.3%) of state institutions offered courses related to information and communication technologies in the curriculum.

Another study [16] verified the knowledge of nursing freshmen and senior students regarding their ability to use informatics resources. The results revealed a low rate of informatics knowledge among the freshmen. However, regarding the applications that students had the most difficulty to operate, between the two periods, seniors had the worst performance, which shows it is necessary to include computer classes in the preparation of these new professionals, in order to prepare them for the work market.

5. Nursing informatics competency development and professional nursing practice

As competence may be defined as the possession of behavior, knowledge, skill, and/or capacity, consequences to competence within the scope of nursing include safe care and safe practice, the ability to create and implement appropriate interventions, and knowing one's limitations: knowing when to ask for assistance [18].

A critical area of nursing competency is that of Nursing Informatics, which can be defined as possessing the appropriate knowledge, behavior, and skills required for nurses to collect, store, retrieve, and process information. In order for nurses to effectively manage patient care, they must understand how to appropriately manage information; thus, possessing informatics competency is elemental to practicing as a professional nurse. Many lists and guidelines exist to identify the specific informatics competencies needed for nurses to provide effective patient care [7].

Informatics competencies are essential for nursing practice, and are critical to providing safe and effective patient care. As a profession that depends on the use of technology, the need for appropriate collegiate and continuing education programs in nursing with a focus on informatics competency is crucial to the development and maintenance of safe and effective practice [7, 19].

To possess competence in nursing informatics, one must possess the ability to obtain, store, retrieve, and communicate data, information, knowledge, and wisdom, which is essential to nursing practice. Many various lists and guidelines exist to address the distinct competencies that nurses must possess; however, very few resources are available to assess the degree to which one is competent in a specific area. The interaction of one's knowledge, experience, environment, and motivation shapes the development of competency within the personal domain, depending on the profession in which one works [7].

In support of competency development, a variety of educational programs exist, ranging from university degrees, continuing education programs, and professional education initiatives such as the TIGER initiative [20]. However, despite the variety of educational programs, in Latin America there is still a lack of educational programs in the area.

Opportunities to build NI competencies are not restricted to formal academia. The United States' Technology Informatics Guiding Educational Reform [21] initiative developed a national informatics education strategy for its existing nursing workforce.

At NI 2012 Conference held in Montreal, TIGER launched its new internationalization phase, complete with an international board including representation from Canada, Asia, South America and Europe. See section B chapter 3 for a description of the TIGER initiative.

Another strategy is the International Network of Nursing Informatics, created in 2008 within the Pan American Health Organization (PAHO) and WHO, a network of technicians and nurses from Latin American countries and the Caribbean. It is based on a strategy for coordination and scientific and technical cooperation for the development and exchange of experiences, information and knowledge that in a voluntary and supportive way with information technology and communications support works based on the universal health coverage. The International Network of Nursing Informatics, uses ICT and the development of specialized virtual networks for information and knowledge exchange, permanent training, research and development of good practice, contributing to human resources and integrated services of excellence in health care. Latin-American countries like Argentina, Brazil, Chile, Colombia, Peru, Uruguay and Venezuela are members of this network, together with Mexico, Cuba, El Salvador and Spain.

Nursing informatics competence is an essential element of nursing practice, especially in the provision of care [7] and ranges from simple clinical skills to complex application based knowledge. Competence in nursing informatics can be defined as the knowledge, behavior, and skills required for nurses to collect, store, retrieve, and process and use information [22]. Nursing informatics is facilitated through the use of technology, and competence in this technology is required for effective nursing practice. With the integration of technology and information science into the field of nursing, there is an increased need for the existence of nursing informatics competencies; thus, nursing informatics competence is a key element to the professional nurse's body of knowledge.

In Brazil, there are few publications that assess skills in the use of ICT by teachers in undergraduate nursing courses. Peres and Kurcgant in a study at a Brazilian federal education institution [23] mention difficulties to use ICT in academic activities by teachers, as they come from a generation that has not grown in touch with the digital technologies.

Since the initial activities in nursing informatics in Brazil, nurses have faced many challenges. Nursing informatics is not completely integrated into the nursing curriculum and the nursing informatics competencies are not established at national level [24].

In a study to identify and analyze the nursing informatics competencies regarding their relevance to the Brazilian reality on Nursing Informatics [25] competencies should be classified accordingly to the level of nursing informatics practice: novice, expert, specialist and innovator. According to this study, validated nursing informatics competencies are divided into the following nursing practice areas: information, data , education, impact , privacy and security , research, regulation, systems, data access , management, usability, project management, communication, monitoring, quality improvement, basic software, fiscal management, simulation, analysis, design and development, evaluation , data structure, management , programming, testing, training, maintenance, implementation, role, practice, system selection systems and requirements. These competencies include skills for computers use, computer knowledge and computer skills [26].

The curriculum content and definition of informatics competences in nursing has been discussed in scientific literature. Although the importance of these competences has been recognized globally, they have not been widely incorporated into undergraduate or graduate nursing curricula in different countries [25]. It was identified that subjects about informatics in undergraduate nursing programs at Brazilian public education institutions are mostly offered as an elective discipline (57%) in the first and second year (80%), with an average workload of 47 classroom hours. The low supply of this undergraduate subject goes against job market trends and the National Curriculum Guidelines for Undergraduate Nursing Programs [17].

In Brazilian studies, several authors describe that faculty and students' knowledge on informatics resources remains deficient, impeding them from using information and communication technologies in the different dimensions of nursing relations, in teaching, research, management and care delivery [27, 28].

According to Yang et al [29], several studies have presented necessary informatics competencies for nurses and nursing students. The first study to present a master list of informatics competencies for nurses to span four levels of nursing practice (beginning nurse, experienced nurse, informatics specialist, and informatics innovator) was proposed by Staggers et al [26] and cover competencies in computer skills, informatics knowledge, and informatics skills; many researchers have used this master list. In a study that proposed a list of nurse practitioner competencies, some competencies related to evidence-based practice were added, and some items were extracted [30]. To determine if informatics competencies were included in the curriculum of a baccalaureate program, the master list was also used by [31].

One study focused on an emerging "avant-garde executive leadership competency" recommended for today's health leaders to guide health system transformation [32]. Specifically, this competency is articulated as "state of the art communication and technology savvy"", and it implies linkages between nursing informatics competencies and transformational leadership roles for nurse executive. The study proposes that distinct nursing informatics competencies are required to augment traditional executive skills to support transformational outcomes of safe, integrated, high-quality care delivery through knowledge-driven care. International trends involving nursing informatics competencies and the evolution of new corporate informatics roles, such as chief nursing informatics officers (CNIOs), are demonstrating value and advanced transformational leadership as nursing executive roles that are informed by clinical data [32].

NI competencies are not necessarily new. The American Nurses Association (ANA) in 1995 was one of the first nursing professional bodies to endorse NI through a formal certification program and a published NI scope and standards of practice [33]. Chapter 7a provides a complete description of the ANA NI specialty certification and standards development. NI competencies are increasingly recognized as a new essential skill set, enabling contemporary nurse executives to support and advance healthcare system transformation evidenced by a number of nursing and health professional associations that endorse NI and health informatics competencies [21, 33, 34]. Understanding the distinction between generic health informatics competencies and NI competencies is necessary for all nursing executives to recognize points of alignment, but also the points where nursing is unique and specifically requires a nursing perspective [32].

Different authors [35, 36, 37] recommended that studies about NI competencies must offer examples of their insertion in nursing practice, making their use more visible, and help faculty to become aware of the real use of them and guide their students with efficiency. Overall, authors recommend that faculty in educational institutions must focus on the development of competencies in informatics, and that competencies should be grouped by complexity throughout the nursing curriculum [37].

There is still a continued interest in NI competencies today, explained by the transition and the concern that nurses must be prepared to perform effectively in safety-focused, integrated and patient-centered environments, in which they are being requested not only to register, retrieve data, search quality information, but also to use technology as an important resource for planning, making informed decisions, and transforming nursing practice [38]. Nursing education programs and their faculty must be able to prepare nursing students, in all levels, to respond to this demand.

6. Next Steps to improve informatics and information management competencies for nurses

In Latin-America there are few leaders and educators with NI skills. It is necessary to invest in NI training for our leaders and educators in the different South America countries. In order to make that happen, it is important to increase awareness in the nursing schools regarding the importance of nursing informatics courses in undergraduate and graduate programs. The use of ICT to connect different regions of Latin-American to regular courses with skilled teachers, including those from areas where NI is more developed, may improve and increase the faculty number, and encourage new professionals.

References

[1] World Health Organization. Preparing a Health Care Workforce for the 21st Century: The Challenge of Chronic conditions. Geneva: WHO, 2005.http://www.who.int/entity/chp/knowledge/publications/workforce_report.pdf (accessed 19 Nov 2010).

[2] World Health Organization. Health Technologies: The Backbone of Health Services. Geneva: WHO, 2007. http://www.who.int/eht/en/Backbone.pdf.

[3] Marin HF. Informática em Enfermagem. Sao Paulo: EPU; 1995:3-20

[4] Marin HF. Nursing Informatics in Brazil. A Brazilian experience. Comput Nurs 1998 Nov-Dec;16(6):327-32.

[5] Marin, HF, Silveira DT, Sasso GTM, Peres HHC. Evolution: Nursing Informatics in Brazil. In: Ball MJ, Douglas J, Walker P. (Org.). Nursing Informatics Where Technology and Caring Meet. 4ed.London: Springer-Verlag, 2011: 401-410.

[6] Coury WB, Messina LA, Filho JLR, Simões N, Sasso GD, Barbosa S, Behring LP, Aguiar G, de-Campo JCL. Implementing RUTE's Usability - the Brazilian Telemedicine University Network. Online braz j nurs [Internet]. 2010 December; 9 (3): Available from: http://www.objnursing.uff.br/index.php/nursing/article/view/3176.

[7] Greer H. 2012. Nursing Informatics Competencies: Implications for Safe and Effective Practice. Honors Theses. Paper 1775. http://scholarworks.wmich.edu/honors_theses/1775

[8] American Association of Colleges of Nursing (AACN). (2008). The Essentials of baccalaureate education for professional nursing practice, 1-63. Washington, DC: AACN.

[9] Cronenwett L, Sherwood G, Barnsteiner J, Disch J, Johnson J, Mitchell P, Sullivan DT, Warren J. Quality and Safety Education for Nurses. Nurs Outlook 2007 May-Jun;55(3):122-31

[10] Nagelsmith L. Competence: an evolving concept. J Contin Educ Nurs. 1995. Nov-Dec;26(6):245-8.

[11] Resolução CNE/CES nº 3 de 7 de novembro de 2001 (BR). Institui Diretrizes Curriculares Nacionais do Curso de Graduação em Enfermagem. Diário Oficial da União [Internet]. 9 nov 2001. [acesso 9 set 2013]. Disponível em: http://portal.mec.gov.br/cne/arquivos/pdf/CES03.pdf

[12] Brasil. Ministério da Educação; Conselho Nacional de Educação. Resolução n. 3, de 07 de novembro de 2001. Institui as Diretrizes Curriculares Nacionais do Curso de Graduação em Enfermagem [Internet]. Brasília; 2001. Available from: Disponível em: http://portal.mec.gov.br/cne/arquivos/pdf/CES03.pdf

[13] Conselho Nacional de Educação (BR). Câmara de Educação Superior. Resolução CNE/CES 3/2001. Diretrizes Curriculares Nacionais do Curso de Graduação em Enfermagem. Diário Oficial da União. Brasília, 09 nov. 2001. Seção 1, p. 37. Brasília; 2006. Available at http://portal.mec.gov.br/cne/arquivos/pdf/CES03.pdf

[14] Peres HHC, Duarte YAO, Maeda ST, Colvero LA. Exploratory study about the use of informatic resources by undergraduate nursing students. Rev Esc Enferm USP 2001;35(1):88-94

[15] Évora YDM. O paradigma da informática em enfermagem [tese livre-docência]. Ribeirão Preto: Escola de Enfermagem de Ribeirão Preto, Universidade de São Paulo; 1998.

[16] Cruz Nathalia Santos da, Soares Danielle Karen Socorro, Bernardes Andrea, Gabriel Carmen Silvia, Pereira Marta Cristiane Alves, Évora Yolanda Dora Martinez. Nursing undergraduates' technical competence in informatics. Rev. esc. enferm. USP 2011 Dec; 45(spe):1595-1599.)

[17] Sanches LMP, Jensen R, Monteiro MI, Lopes MHBM. Informatics teaching in undergraduate nursing programs at Brazilian public institutions. Rev. Latino-Am. Enfermagem 2011 Dec; 19(6):1385-1390.

[18] American Association of Colleges of Nursing (AACN). The essentials of baccalaureate education for professional nursing practice [Internet]. Washington: AACN; 2008 [cited 2015 May 26]. Available from: Available from:http://www.aacn.nche.edu/education-resources/BaccEssentials08.pdf

[19] Hwang JI, Park HA. Factors associated with nurses' informatics competency. Comput Inform Nurs. 2011 Apr;29(4):256-62.

[20] TIGER. Evidence and informatics transforming nursing: TIGER summit summary report. 2006. Retrieved from: http://tigersummit.com/uploads/TIGER_Final_Summit_Report.pdf.

[21] The TIGER Initiative. (2006). Informatics competencies for every practicing nurse: recommendations from the TIGER collaborative. Technology Informatics Guiding Education Reform. Retrieved on November 20, 2014 from http://www.tigersummit.com

[22] Gugerty, B., Delaney, C., DuLong, D. (2012). The TIGER initiative, informatics competencies for every practicing nurse: recommendations from the TIGER collaborative. Technology Informatics Guiding Education Reform. 1-33. Retrieved from http://www.tigersummit.com.

[23] Peres HH, Kurcgant P. Being a nursing teacher in an informatized world. Rev. Latino-Am. Enfermagem 2004 Jan-Feb; 12(1):101-108.

[24] Marin HF. Nursing informatics education in the South: a Brazilian experience. Yearb Med Inform. 2010:68-71.

[25] GONÇALVES, L.S. Informatics competencies required to nurses in the Brazilian professional practice. Thesis [PhD in Nursing]. Curitiba: Universidade Federal do Parana, 2014.

[26] Staggers N, Gassert CA, Curran C. A Delphi study to determine informatics competencies for nurses at four levels of practice. Nurs Res. 2002 Nov-Dec;51(6):383-90.

[27] Silva ISA, Marques IR. Expertise and barriers in the use of resources of Information and Communication Technology by nursing faculties. J Health Inform 2011;3(1):3-8

[28] Cogo ALP, Silveira DT, Pedro ENR, Tanaka RY, Catalan VM. Undergraduated nursing student's opinion about group work in online project. Rev Gaúcha Enferm 2010;31(3):435-41.

[29] Yang L, Cui D, Zhu X, Zhao Q, Xiao N, and Shen X. Perspectives from Nurse Managers on Informatics Competencies. The Scientific World Journal 2014, Article ID 391714, 5 pages. doi:10.1155/2014/391714

[30] Curran CR. Informatics competencies for nurse practitioners. AACN Clin Issues.2003 Aug;14(3):320-30.

[31] Ornes LL, Gassert C. Computer competencies in a BSN program. J Nurs Educ. 2007. Feb;46(2):75-8.

[32] Remus S, Kennedy MA. Innovation in transformative nursing leadership: nursing informatics competencies and roles. Nurs Leadersh (Tor Ont). 2012 Dec;25(4):14-26.

[33] American Nurses Association, *Nursing Informatics: Scope and Standards of Practice, Second Edition,* Nursesbooks.org, Silver Spring, MD, 2015.

[34] COACH 2009. Health Informatics Professional Core Competencies. (Version 2.0). Retrieved Nov 12, 2012 from: http://coachorg.com/en/publications/resources/CoreCompetencies-New_Matrix_Nov_09.pdf

[35] Carter-Templeton H, Patterson R, Russell C. An analysis of published nursing informatics competencies. Stud Health Technol Inform. 2009;146:540-5.

[36] Nelson R, Staggers N. Implications of the American Nurses Association Scope and Standards of Practice of nursing informatics for nurse educators: a discussion. Nurs Outlook 2008:56(2) 93-4.

[37] Graves JR, Corcoran S. The study of nursing informatics. Image J Nurs Sch 1989 Winter;21(4):227-31.
[38] Gonçalves LS, Wolff LD, Staggers N, Peres AM. Nursing informatics competencies: an analysis of the latest research. NI 2012 (2012). 2012 Jun 23;2012:127.

Forecasting Informatics Competencies for Nurses in the Future of Connected Health
J. Murphy et al. (Eds.)
© 2017 IMIA and IOS Press.

doi:10.3233/978-1-61499-738-2-86

Competencies Related to Informatics and Information Management for Practicing Nurses in Select Countries in Asia

Ying WU[a], Yanling WANG[a], and Meihua JI[a]
[a]*School of Nursing, Capital Medical University*

Abstract. The advancement of information and communication technology have enabled nurses to practice more effectively, efficiently, and safely. This chapter introduces nursing informatics competency and information management competency for nurses in China (including Mainland China, Hong Kong and Taiwan), India, Japan, Korea, and Singapore. Most countries in Asia are still in the process of developing and standardizing competences that are relevant to nurses and those specialized in nursing informatics. The level and content of nursing informatics offered in entry-to-practice nursing education programs varies greatly. There is a growing need to adopt more comprehensive curriculum for entry-to-practice nursing education programs, as well as offer continuing education to help nurses to develop knowledge, skill, and attitude related to nursing informatics and information management in the world of connected health.

Keywords. Nursing informatics; Nursing; Competency; Information management

1. Introduction

The advancement of information and communication technology (ICT) and its wide use in nursing practice as well as in the whole healthcare system have enabled nurses to practice more effectively, efficiently, and safely. However, in order to take the full advantage of modern ICT in nursing practice, and create more effective, efficient, and safer nursing information system, it requires nurses to be competent in nursing informatics and information management in their daily practice. This chapter will introduce nursing informatics competency and information management competency for nurses in some Asian countries such as China (including Mainland China, Taiwan and Hong Kong), India, Japan, Korea, and Singapore.

2. Competencies related to informatics and information management for nurses in China

2.1   Mainland China

2.1.1   Evolution of nursing informatics in practice sector

The computer was first introduced into hospitals in the late 70s in Mainland China for the processing of basic administrative tasks and became more extensive in the 80s. It was introduced into nursing practice in late 80s to the 90s.[1-3] Three stages were observed through our profound literature review.

The first stage was a stand-alone system, mainly in office management. Computers were operated independently and there was no data sharing at all. In meeting the needs of nursing practice and management, nurses in some hospitals work with information technicians (ITs) to develop more complicated functions such as unit management and nursing error analysis [4, 5] to assist nursing practice.

The second stage started in late 1990s, along with the rapid development of computer technology, especially broadband and multimedia technology. In 1993, the *"Creation of Chinese Hospital Information System Project"* was launched as the 8th five-year National Key Science and Technology Project, which developed the "China Hospital Information System" named as "Military Health No 1" in 1997. It was recognized as the first integrated clinical hospital information system developed in China [3, 6] and was widely implemented among large tertiary hospitals in China thereafter. [7] It enabled an inpatient nursing workstation system to be built based on that. This second stage was characterized by the utilization of broadband networking and hospital information system focused on three areas: health care management mainly order entry, billing management, and supply management; where data were shared only within the institution. An integrated nursing record information system (mainly free text) was included in this system. [7] In 2002, Peking University People's Hospital developed a nursing record system which included four modules: collection of medical and nursing history data, nursing care planning, printing the nursing record, and a nursing knowledge database.[8]

The third stage was characterized by the wide use of a mobile information system along with the development of wireless network technology in nursing practice (since 2010). Mobile nursing information technologies were first introduced to nursing practice as pilot projects and sporadically emerged at the beginning of this century. One such example is a PDA and mobile nursing information system based on the Hospital Information System (HIS) introduced at Peking Union Hospital in 2002, and then at the People's Liberation Army (PLA) General Hospital and the PLA 251 Hospital in 2005. The popularity of mobile nursing was accompanied with improvement of various mobile information technologies. With advancements in the functions of China's HIS, increased speed of wireless WiFi, adoption of Radio-Frequency Integration Technology (RFIT), mobile nursing carts and mobile devices, the use of mobile electronic nursing records became one of the most important parts in nursing practice. In 2011, The Third Hospital of Peking University reported using mobile nursing carts based on their clinical nursing information system. Since then, the use of PDA and mobile nursing carts to provide bedside nursing care has become more and more popular in a vast majority of hospitals in Mainland China.[9] The functions of the mobile nursing information system cover many aspects of nursing practice, such as input and retrieval of patients' demographic and clinical data, patient identification, entry of assessment data and documentation at the point-of-care, as well as the implementation and management of doctors' orders, nursing quality control, nursing workload tracking etc.[10, 11] In particular, closed-loop medication management, dynamic tracking, quality control and quality improvement are used widely functions in more recent years.

2.1.2   Nursing Informatics Organization in Mainland China

China Medical Informatics Association (CMIA) was established in 1980, eleven years later, the CMIA Nursing Informatics Committee (CMIA-NI) was inaugurated in 1991. However, because the driving force of the implementation of NI in the practice sector was the hospital management bodies instead of nurses themselves in those early years, few NI activities and academic conferences were organized or held by CMIA-NI until 20 years later.

Starting in 2012, the second term of the CMIA-NI board was formed with 48 members. The first academic event hosted by CMIA-NI, the Nursing Informatics Forum, was held on October 24th, 2012, along with the 7th Asia Pacific Association for Medical Informatics (APAMI) Conference. Since then, nursing informatics has developed dramatically in both the practice and academic (mainly research) sectors. In 2013, the 1st China National Nursing Informatics Conference (CNNIC), which is an annual conference hosted by CMIA-NI, was held in Beijing. The 4th CNNIC attracted 264 attendees and was held in September, 2016 in Xiamen, where the 16th World Congress on Medical and Health Informatics (Medinfo 2017) will be held in 2017. Along with the 4th CNNIC, the new term of CMIA-NI Board (4th term) was elected and the number of CMIA-NI members had increased from 48 in 2012 to 249 in 2016. With collaborative efforts from CMIA-NI members, and support from CMIA as well as other local organizations, CMIA-NI won the bid for hosting NI 2020 during NI 2016 GA meeting. It will be held in June, 2020 in Beijing. It was recognized as a new milestone in the history of CMIA and CMIA-NI.

2.1.3   Nursing informatics competencies in Mainland China

With the rapid development of NI in the practice sector, the need for nurses to have informatics and information management competency increased dramatically. In some hospitals, positons for nurses to translate nursing practice needs between bedside nurses and information technology department emerged to close the gap between clinical practice and technology (hereafter, this position will be referred to as "informatics nurse"). Therefore, nursing schools in Mainland China began providing nursing informatics courses or related content to nursing students, mainly at the baccalaureate level, in addition to courses such as "Introduction to Computer Science" and "Literature Searching" which are mandatory for all bachelor degree students in Mainland China. Some nursing schools of universities in Mainland China have established master's programs to prepare nurses working in the practice sector as an informatics nurse or in the academic sector as a NI educator and researcher. In order to provide adequate training on knowledge, skills, and ability related to NI for entry-to-practice nursing graduates, a competency model or a set of nursing informatics competencies for graduates who will work as bedside nurses are an urgent need.

Research on nursing information competency emerged in the early 21st century. Early studies mainly focused on information literacy, and various studies viewed this concept differently. Some authors considered information literacy as the awareness, ability, and ethics of using information, [12] while others considered it as the acquisition, recognition, identification, evaluation, processing, transmission and the ability to create information.[13-15] Liu [16] and Shi [17] considered information literacy as the ability of using information and applying ICT to facilitate problem solving in their workplaces.

Studies have also been conducted on the purpose of identifying the contents and standards for nursing information literacy. In 2008, Capital Medical University School of Nursing developed a core nursing competency model for baccalaureate degree graduates, which included the item "search and retrieve information through electronic data bases" as one of the six core competencies under the domain of "professionalism".[18] In another study, Jiang et al [12] initiated a theoretical model of information literacy for undergraduate nursing students through structural analysis and Delphi method in 2004. They proposed that nursing information literacy consisted of 3 elements: information awareness, information capabilities and information ethics. Through theoretical evaluation and experience analysis, Wang et al. [14] constructed a set of nursing information literacy evaluation standards for vocational nursing students. They summarized that the evaluation standard for nursing information literacy should include four domains: information awareness, information knowledge, information capability, and information ethics. Eleven sub-dimensions were identified under these four domains. In 2012, the Ministry of Education Steering Committee for Higher Nursing Education developed the *Essentials of National Undergraduate Nursing Education Standard*, in which the requirements of having basic skills in searching and retrieving literature, collecting data, as well as effectively acquiring, evaluating and applying nursing informatics skills via modern ICT are included.

Xu [19] conducted a study related to NI competency among undergraduate nursing students by using questionnaire survey, factor analysis, and three rounds Delphi in 2012. A framework for NI competency was developed in which four domains with 13 categories and 33 items were identified. The four domains are information knowledge, information skills, information management ability, and information attitude. Because there was no nationally recognized nursing informatics or nursing information management competency model for nurses in Mainland China, CMIA-NI launched a research project to identify nursing informatics and nursing information management competencies for nurses and informatics nurses to inform nurse professionals from both the educational sector and the practice sector nationwide. The project was based on NI competency and NI management competency described by the American Nurses Association [20, 21] and the Nursing Informatics Competencies Model from the Technology Informatics Guiding Education Reform (TIGER) initiative [22] and was carried out in four stages. During the first stage, an initial pool of nursing informatics and information management competency items was developed through extensive literature review. In the second stage, semi-structured in-depth interviews of bedside nurses, "informatics nurses" (coordinating and communicating with ITs regarding the needs for clinical nursing information system as part of their daily responsibility), and nursing managers were conducted, and the initial pool of competency items was revised. A questionnaire named Chinese NI and information management competency (NIAIMC) was developed based on the revised competency items using Delphi method during the third stage. Finally, a national survey of more than 1,000 nurses across Mainland China was conducted and an exploratory factor analysis was used to generate the NI competency and NI management competency model for nurses in Mainland China. The model includes four domains (with total of 36 items) and explains 74% of the total variance. The identified four domains are basic computer knowledge, computer and network operating ability, information literacy, and operating ability of health information system.

2.2   Hong Kong

The Hong Kong Society of Medical Informatics (HKSMI) was established in 1987 to promote the use of information technology in healthcare. The eHealth Consortium was formed to bring together clinicians from both the private and public sectors. Medical informatics professionals and the IT industry worked collaboratively to further promote IT dissemination and implementation in healthcare in Hong Kong. Since 1994, a computerized patient record system called the Clinical Management System (CMS) has been developed by the Hospital Authority (HA). This system has been deployed at all sites of the Authority (40 hospitals and 120 clinics), and is used by 30,000 clinical staff on a daily basis, with daily transactions up to 2 million. The comprehensive records of 7 million patients are available on-line in the Electronic Patient Record (ePR), with data integrated from all sites.[23]

Despite the fast development and vast utility of health informatics in Hong Kong, the training of nursing informatics has not been required in entry-to-practice level nursing education program in Hong Kong. All nurses currently working in the Health Informatics team of HA are trained on their job. Healthcare staff (including nurses) are sponsored to attend some post graduate or certificate courses offered by universities or school of continuing education on part-time basis. One example of that is the **Postgraduate Diploma in e-Health Informatics** which is organized by the Hong Kong Polytechnic University. It provides health professionals with the theoretical knowledge and practical skills that enable students to take leadership roles within the emerging field of Health Informatics. It focuses on the increasing role and potential of information technology and advanced telecommunication technology for effective and efficient health services. Another example is the **Applied Clinical Informatics** course which is offered through collaborative effort between Department of Health Technology and Informatics (HTI) and School of Professional Education and Executive Development (SPEED), at Hong Kong Polytechnic University, as well as Hong Kong Society of Medical Informatics (HKSMI). The objectives of this course are described as: 1) enhance eHealth capabilities of health care providers including nurses in the Asian Pacific region, including the Greater Mainland China and other Asian countries; 2) promote the acquisition of health informatics knowledge for healthcare professionals in the region; 3) offer practical training for healthcare IT professionals to facilitate their work; and 4) cultivate the best practice and knowledge sharing in the industry.[23, 24]

There are also some graduate education programs (Master and PhD) focusing on Health informatics, which cover a wide range of informatics subjects and are not nursing specific. For example, the postgraduate program "**Master of Science in Health Informatics**' organized by Hong Kong Polytechnic University offers an opportunity for professionals in health care and related disciplines to "develop the knowledge, skills, and attitudes necessary to function more effectively in addition to mastering the advanced skills of information technology in healthcare settings". [23]

For registered nurses, there are some basic requirements on nursing informatics. For example, in order to be registered as mental health nurses, one should have a minimum 20 hours of theoretical introduction on information technology applied to nursing and healthcare.[23]

2.3   Taiwan

In 1988, Taiwan conducted a project called the National Health Information Network (HIN 1.0) to improve the quality of health and medical care. The HIN 1.0 involved collecting accurate and useful administrative information, improving the timely and quality handling of public requests, and providing information for the formulation of health policies.[25] In 1998, the National Health Information Network 2 (HIN 2.0) was established to address the problems encountered with HIN 1.0, such as insufficient bandwidth, low interoperability, and the fact of only a few medical applications being developed and used.[25] In 2005, initiated by the Department of Health in Taiwan, a 5-year plan called the National Health Informatics Project (NHIP) was established to achieve a healthcare system with better efficiency and efficacy and targeting on population health, personal health, patient safety, quality care, and HIT industry.[26, 27] The rapid and extensive use of new information technology in healthcare in Taiwan created a need for the development of NI.[28]

In 1996, hospitals in Taiwan began the transition from a process of paper medical records system to a computerized health care record system, which further facilitated the growth of NI. In 2006, the Taiwan Nursing Informatics Association (TNIA) was established, which promoted the rapid development of NI both in nursing practice and nursing academics. [29] By 2012, nearly 23 medical centers had created informatics nurse specialist positions. [30]

For entry-to-practice nursing education programs such as associate degree and baccalaureate degree programs in Taiwan, nursing informatics courses are not compulsory. [31] There are some graduate programs specialized in nursing informatics open for registered nurses. For example, the Department of Nursing, National Yang Ming University provides both Master's degree and Phd programs on health informatics. [32] [33, 34]

A study conducted by Chang et al. [35] identified nursing informatics competencies required for practicing nurses in Taiwan by using the Delphi method. The Nursing Informatics Competencies Questionnaire (323-item plus 45 additional items), based on the Information Management Framework described by Stagger et al. [36], was sent to experts (nursing educators and administrators) and finally 360 items remained. It concluded that the NI competencies for both beginning nurses and experienced nurses in Taiwan were computer skills, informatics knowledge and informatics skills in various areas depending on the levels of practice. [35] Additional information about nursing informatics in Taiwan can be found in section B chapter 6.

3. Competencies related to informatics and information management for nurses in India

Health informatics was fully recognized in India with the conception of the Indian Association of Medical Informatics (IAMI) in 1993.[37] As the recognition of health informatics continues to grow in the Indian healthcare system, nurses are starting to expand their role to include clinical nursing informatics as a field of nursing practice. However, nursing informatics has not yet been recognized as an independent nursing specialty in India despite the fact that they have been practicing informatics in healthcare settings. [38]

Several studies have been conducted in India to investigate the knowledge, attitude and application of internet technology among nurses, nursing students and nurse scholars. The majority of them determined that nursing informatics was a necessary field for nursing profession and it was rapidly developing in clinical settings. [39-41] However, Nursing informatics is only recognized as a sub-topic and included under various Bioinformatics or Health informatics courses in India. [38]

The basics of computer science have been included in the curriculum for undergraduate nursing education programs. An example of the nursing syllabus from All India Institute of Medical Sciences (AIIMS) includes : 1) Introduction to computer science & its application to health care system; 2) Disk Operating system; 3) Microsoft windows & Microsoft office & its applications, including MS Word, Power point, Excel; 4) Introduction to internet and email; 5) Graphics Introduction to Data base; 6) Use of statistical packages; 7) Computer assisted teaching and testing.[42]

Certain aspects of computer applications are also included in postgraduate programs in nursing at AIIMS. The topics include: 1) MS DOS, Windows, Microsoft word, power point; 2) Internet, literature search; 4) Excel, statistical packages, Health care delivery computer programs; 5) Use of computers in teaching, learning, research and nursing practice.[43]

Topics related to nursing informatics are also included at the PhD level, such as nursing management information system, networking institutions through literature search, knowledge about basic computers, computer systems, NI theory, clinical information systems, and application of NI in research, education, practice, and administration etc.[44]

A well defined role of Nursing Informatics Specialist (NIS) has been described by AIIMS to assist in dissemination of information among healthcare providers through implementing best practices and workflow change by using information technology, digital media, educational programs, etc. However, NISs are trained within the work settings and no additional qualification is required. A full description of NIS job responsibilities can be obtained from AIIMS website. [45]

Currently, there is no defined competency for entry-to-practice nurses in India, and very few educational institutes provide nursing students with formal training to understand the information systems being used in clinical settings in detail. Such kind of training only happens "on the job" in clinical settings. [38]

4. Competencies related to informatics and information management for nurses in Japan

The Japanese Association of Medical Informatics (JAMI) was founded in the 1980s. With Medinfo 1980 being held in Tokyo in 1980, a special interest group on NI was included in the congress, which marked the beginning of NI in Japan. [46] Before the turn of 21st century, NI in Japan was seen more in the applied clinical practice setting, rather than in the academic settings, due to the nature of nursing schools being vocationally oriented. In 2003, JAMI started the certification system for Healthcare Information Technologists (HITs) which evaluates knowledge and skills on health information system, information technology and healthcare, and nurses started to be certified as HITs through this system in 2004. [47, 48] However, with limited resources on NI education in Japan, information about NI competencies are scarce.

In 2000, the Nursing Division of the JAMI was established and is managed by a team of clinical nurses and academic researchers. In March 2004, the first standard textbook for medical informatics and nursing informatics was published. Some nursing schools offer Nursing Informatics courses or content and lecturers with researchers of health informatics and NI. However, the accreditation program of the Japan Nursing Association does not recognize the training for the informatics nurse specialist. As in India, most nurses have their NI knowledge and skills from training "on the job" in hospital settings. [49]

5. Competencies related to informatics and information management for nurses in Korea

The term nursing informatics was first introduced when the Korean Society of Medical Informatics (KOSMI) was founded in 1987. In 1993, the Nursing Informatics Special Interest Group was organized under the umbrella of KOSMI to serve as a platform for scientists in nursing informatics to disseminate knowledge and exchange ideas. [50, 51] Content related to nursing informatics was introduced into nursing programs in universities in 1994. In the late 1990s, 25% of the graduate programs surveyed in Korea provided their students with nursing informatics courses, but only computer courses (no NI courses) were offered in 77% of the associate degree or undergraduate programs surveyed at that time.[50, 52] A more recent survey which was finished in 2016 reveals a growing trend in offering nursing informatics courses among entry-to-practice nursing education programs, with 57% of the undergraduate programs and 36% of diploma programs offering nursing informatics courses, and more than half of these programs introducing NI courses within less than 5 years. Nine out of the 32 (28%) graduate programs surveyed offered NI courses, among them, one school had programs at both master's and PhD level focusing on nursing informatics. Content analysis of 27 syllabi of NI related courses revealed that computer technology was included in all syllabi. Information systems, telehealth, informatics, and informatics ethics were included in 93%, 89%, 85%, and 77% of the syllabi, respectively. [53]

Based on NI competencies required of nurses in Taiwan, Chung and Staggers [54] developed a modified 112 item questionnaire in measuring NI competencies among beginning and experienced nurses in Korea. Factor analysis revealed a 3-factor structure which explained 45% of total variance. According to their study, three domains of NI competencies for both beginning level and experienced nurses were identified. The three domains are information knowledge, information skills, and computer skills. However, the expectation of NI competencies for beginning level nurses differed greatly from experienced nurses. The levels of NI competencies for beginning nurses were mostly on the knowledge level, while for experienced nurses, the expectation of NI competences were more skill-oriented.

6. Competencies related to informatics and information management for nurses in Singapore

The Electronic Health Records for Nursing Education (EHRNE) software program was recently developed and integrated into the nursing curriculum at National University of Singapore.[33] The aim of this curriculum change is to increase nursing students' awareness of how health information technology (HIT) and electronic health records (EHRs) can improve the quality of their documentation, reduce medical errors, and increase the quality of patient care.[55] However, there is no information indicating that well defined competency of informatics and information management for entry-to-practice or advanced practice nurses are available in Singapore.

7. Conclusion

With rapid advancement of ICT and its extensive use in the healthcare system, acquiring competency related to informatics and information management among practical nurses is essential in delivering holistic and individual-centered care in this world of connected health. Nursing professionals in China and other Asian regions are still in the process of developing and standardizing competencies that are relevant to entry-to-practice nurses who are involved in the daily work within a hospital using a health information system. Meanwhile, although there are institutions and universities in some Asian countries that have incorporated components related to information science into nursing curriculum, the level and extent vary greatly. There is a growing need to adopt more comprehensive curriculum both at entry-to-practice and the advanced level, as well as offering continuing education to help future nurses in developing the knowledge, skills, and attitude related to nursing informatics and information management in order to provide more effective, efficient, and safer healthcare in this connected world.

8. Acknowledgement

This work is supported by faculty members (Lili Ma, Lisha Shi, Liu Sun, Qian Xiao, Shuqin Xiao, Yahong Xu, Peng Yue, Yan Zhang) at the School of Nursing, Capital Medical University, who contributed greatly to the extensive literature review and research required to write the section on "Nursing Informatics Competency for Nurses and Informatics Nurses in Mainland China". We also would like to extend our special thanks to members of CMIA Nursing Informatics Committee and nurses who worked in hospitals in Mainland China for their contributions to the competency research project. We also acknowledge the contributions we received from Ellen Tong, Zuoying Li, I-Ching Hou, Medha Piplani, and Hyeoun-Ae Park, for providing information related to this topic in Hong Kong, Taiwan, India, and Korea, respectively, because much of this information was not available through a traditional literature search.

References

[1]   Zhang, Q. Use of computer systems in nursing management system (in Chinese). Journal of Chinese Nursing, 1992. 27(2): p. 84-86.
[2]   Guo, C. Experience of using No. 1 Military Medical Project in nursing work station (in Chinese). Medical Information, 2000. 13(8): p. 445-446.
[3]   Li, B.L., Ma L. and Xu Y. The application of nursing informatics and communication technology (in Chinese). Chinese Nursing Management, 2009. 9(3): p. 76-78.
[4]   Wang, G. and Zhang J. Application of computer software in analyzing nursing errors. Chinese Journal of Nursing, 1993. 28(5): p. 262-264.

[5]   Wang, G.J. Experiences of involving the development of computer software. Chinese Journal of Nursing, 1994. 29(9): p. 544-546.
[6]   China E. Commerce, Current status of the Hospital Information Systems development in China. 2000. 14: p. 18-19.
[7]   Qi, L.F. et al. The use of 'Military Health No1' in nursing case management in a holistic approach through informatization. Medical Information, 2000. 13(9): p. 499-500.
[8]   Liu, J. et al. Developing an electronic nursing record system. Chinese Journal of Nursing, 2002. 37(8): p. 595-598.
[9]   Ji, H. Wireless mobile nursing cart actualizing the extention of information system to patient's bedside (Chinese). China Information Field: eMedicine, 2012(3): p. 48-49.
[10] Zhang, B. et al. Application of mobile nursing information system in clinical settings. Chinese Nursing Management, 2014(z1): p. 88-89.
[11] Zeng, F. et al. Development and application of mobile nursing information system. China Medical Equipment, 2015. 12(4): p. 18-22.
[12] Jiang, A. and Shen J. Study on the concept and compositions of information literacy of nursing undergraduates. Chinese Journal of Nursing, 2004. 39(2): p. 84-86.
[13] Huang, H. et al. A survey on the information literacy of head nurses in the wards of "high quality nursing service demonstration project". Journal of Nursing Administration, 2012. 12(2): p. 99-100.
[14] Wang, T. and He S. On the evaluation criteria of information literacy of higher vocational student nurses (in Chinese). China Medical Education Technology, 2008. 22(5): p. 419-421.
[15] Chen, Y., Xu X. and Yang H. Analysis of nurses' information ability and influencing factors in Age of Big Data. Chinese Journal of Modern Nursing, 2015. 21(20).
[16] Liu, L., et al. The ability of nursing undergraduates in acquiring nursing informaiton (in Chinese). Journal of Nursing, 2010. 17(3A): p. 24-26.
[17] Shi, F., et al., Current status of information competency of nursing undergraduate students (in Chinese). General Nursing, 2011. 9(9): p. 2525-2526.
[18] Yang, F. et al. A core competency model for Chinese baccalaureate nursing graduates: A descriptive correlational study in Beijing. Nurse Education Today, 2013. 33: p. 1465-1470.
[19] Xu, R. Study on framework of nursing information competencies for undergraduate students (in Chinese), in Department of Nursing. 2012, Hongzou Normal University: Hangzhou. p. 127.
[20] The American Nurses Association, The scope of nursing informatics practice, in Nursing Informatics: Scope and Standards of Practice, The American Nurses Association, Editor. 2015, American Nurses Association Silver Spring: Maryland. p. 1-2.
[21] The American Nursing Association, The Scope of Nursing Informatics Practice: Informatics Competencies Requisite for All Registered Nurses, in Nursing Informatics: Scope and Standards of Practice, The American Nursing Association, Editor. 2015, American Nurses Association Silver Spring: Maryland. p. 37-38.
[22] Technology Informatics Guiding Education Reform, TIGER initiatives, informatics competencies for every practicing nurse: Recommendations from the TIGER Collaborative. Unclear: file:///Users/meihuaji/Downloads/tiger-report-informatics-competencies%20(2).pdf.
[23] Tong, E. Assistance in acquiring info on NI competences. 2016.
[24] The Hong Kong Polytechnic University and H.K.S.o.M.I. Ltd, Course Syllabus: Applied Clinical Informatics. 2015, The Hong Kong Polytechnic University: http://www.polyu.edu.hk/hti/images/pdf_ProfessionalDevelopment/NBM5_leaflet.pdf. p. 1-2.
[25] Liu, CY., Kuo HS., and Wang DW. Health Information Network in Taiwan -- Now and Future in International Nursing Informatics Conference 2009. 2009. Amsterdam: IOS Press.
[26] Li, YCJ. The Health Smart Cards and the National Health Informatics Project in Taiwan. in APAMI 2006 in Conjunction with MIST 2006. 2006.
[27] Feng, RC. and Yeh YT. A new vision of nursing: the evolution and development of nursing informatics. The Journal of Nursing, 2014. 61(4 Suppl): p. 78-84.
[28] Fang, YW., et al. The development of competencies for informatics nurse: Survey of nursing dducators' perception. in 7th International Conference on Computing and Convergence Technology (Iccct2012). 2012.
[29] Feng, RC. and Yeh YT. A new vision of nursing: the evolution and development of nursing informatics (Article in Chinese). Hu LI Za Zhi, 2014. 61(4 Suppl): p. 78-84.
[30] Liu, CH., Lee TT. and Mills ME. The experience of informatics nurses in Taiwan. Journal of Professional Nursing, 2015. 31(2): p. 158-164.
[31] Li, Z. Need help for NI in Taiwan, Y. Wu, Editor. 2016: Beijing.
[32] YangMing, U. <護理學系碩士在職專班簡介.pdf>. 2016.
[33] Kowitlawakul, Y. et al. Factors influencing nursing students' acceptance of electronic health records for nursing education (EHRNE) software program. Nurse Education Today, 2015. 35(1): p. 189-194.

[34] National Yang Ming University School of Nursing, Curriculum of Registered Nurse Master Program Unclear, National Yang Ming University School of Nursing: http://son-e.web.ym.edu.tw/files/15-1186-16465,c66-1.php.

[35] Chang, J., et al. Nursing informatics competencies required of nurses in Taiwan. International Journal of Medical Informatics, 2011. 80(5): p. 332-340.

[36] Staggers, N., Gassert CA., and Curran C. A Delphi study to determine informatics competencies for nurses at four levels of practice. Nursing Research, 2002. 51(6): p. 383-390.

[37] Indian Association for Medical Informatics, Indian Association for Medical Informatics IAMI: Its history, formation, objectives & activities. Unclear, Indian Association for Medical Informatics: http://www.iami.org.in/IAMI%20history/Brief_history_of_IAMI.pdf.

[38] Piplani, M. Nursing informatics in India. 2016.

[39] Sarbadhikari, SN. and Gogia SB., An overview of education and training of medical informatics in India, in IMIA Yearbook of Medical Informatics 2010. 2010, IMIA. p. 106-108.

[40] Kumar, S. and Mahajan P., Computer literacy and student demographics a study of select Indian universities library. Hi Tech News, 2013. 10: p. 21-27.

[41] Shahi, M., Knowledge, attitude and application of computer by bachelor level nursing students. Journal of Institute of Medicine, 2012. 34(2): p. 21-27.

[42] All India Institute of Medical Sciences, Syllabus B Sc at the AIIMS (Hons / Post Certificate) Nursing. 2003, All India Institute of Medical Sciences: http://www.aiims.edu/aiims/academic/aiims-syllabus/Syllabus%20Nursing_Hons-Post%20Certificate.pdf. p. 42.

[43] All India Institute of Medical Sciences, Syllabus: M Sc (Nursing) at the AIIMS. 2004, All India Institute of Medical Sciences: http://www.aiims.edu/aiims/academic/aiims-syllabus/Syllabus%20-%20M%20Sc%20(Nursing).pdf. p. 7.

[44] Indian Nursing Council, PhD Curriculum Unclear, Indian Nursing Council: http://www.indiannursingcouncil.org/pdf/phd-curriculum.pdf. p. 3.

[45] All India Institute Of Medical Sciences, Nurse Informatics Specialists (NIS). 2016, All India Institute Of Medical Sciences: http://www.aiims.edu/en/nurse-informatics-specialists-nis-_menu_28.html.

[46] Abad, J. et al. Chapter 40: Nursing Informatics in Asia, in Nursing Informatics. 2016 updated: http://nursinginformaticspunp.tripod.com/chapter-40.html.

[47] Yamanouchi, K. and Ota K. Education for Japanese informatics nurses. in Internation Nursing Informatics Conference. 2009. Amsterdam: IOS Press.

[48] Okada, M., Yamamoto K., and Kawamura T. Health and medical informatics education in Japan, in IMIA Yearbook of Medical Informatics 2005, R. Haux and C. Kulikowski, Editors. 2005, IOS Press: Amsterdam.

[49] Lacson, JJ. Nursing Informatics In Japan, in Nursing Informatics in Pacific Rim,Asia and South America. 2015: http://glendaletokim.blogspot.com/2015/04/nursing-informatics-in-asia.html.

[50] Park, HA. Nursing Informatics in Korea. Computers, Informatics, Nursing, 2002. 20(3): p. 101-107.

[51] Korean Society of Medical Infromatics, History of Korean Society of Medical Infromatics. Unclear, Korean Society of Medical Infromatics: http://www.kosmi.org/eng/main/main.html#.

[52] Park, HA., Yang YH., and Hyun SK. A survey study of nursing informatics education in Korea. Journal of Korean Society of Medical Informatics, 1999. 5(1): p. 11-25.

[53] Jeon, E. et al., Current status of nursing informatics education in South Korea. Healthcare Informatics Research, 2016. 22(2): p. 142-150.

[54] Chung, SY. and Staggers N. Measuring Nursing Informatics Competencies of Practicing Nurses in Korea: Nursing Informatics Competencies Questionnaire. Computers, Informatics, Nursing, 2014. 32(12): p. 596-605.

[55] Kowitlawakul, Y., et al., Exploring faculty perceptions towards electronic health records for nursing education. International Nursing Review, 2014. 61(1): p. 499-506.

Forecasting Informatics Competencies for Nurses in the Future of Connected Health
J. Murphy et al. (Eds.)
© *2017 IMIA and IOS Press.*
doi:10.3233/978-1-61499-738-2-97

The Roles and Functions of Informatics Nurse Specialists in Taiwan

Tso Ying LEE [a,1]

a Nursing Department, Cheng Hsin General Hospital, Taipei, Taiwan

Abstract. During the modernization process in hospitals, information technology is an important indicator. "Informatics nurses" play a critical role in hospitals and clinics. In Taiwan, the certification system of informatics nurses just recently began in 2016. The development of certificated personnel results from students who have graduated with a university degree in nursing and have taken classes in informatics, as well as nurses who have been trained in informatics at clinics and hospitals, and the establishment of a national nursing informatics association. Clinically, the main responsibilities of Informatics Nurse Specialists are system analysis, training, problem solving, data analysis, and communication. In Taiwan, as of September 2016, only 48 informatics nurses have been certified. They are working either in hospitals or at universities.

Keywords. nursing informatics, informatics nurse specialist, certification of informatics nurse specialist

1. Introduction

The development of information technology has changed the world and allowed the innovation of nursing care services. In recent years, the development of nursing informatics in Taiwan has been catching up with international trends and has been regarded positively by the international nursing informatics community. The integration of information technology into the medical care system has created the new nursing role of "informatics nurse." Although the certification system and job description for these nurses have become increasingly comprehensive in many countries, Taiwan remains in an early developmental stage in these regards [1]. The Taiwan Nursing Informatics Association (TNIA) clearly articulates the role, responsibilities, and job descriptions and defines the training requirements and certification system.

This paper introduces the functions and professional growth of informatics nurses and introduces the framework for a certification system, which gives medical and paramedical staff a better understanding of informatics nursing and helps them to recognize the important role played by informatics nurses in the healthcare industry.

---

[1] Corresponding author: Tso Ying Lee, R.N., Ph.D., Associate Director of Nursing Department, Cheng Hsin General Hospital, Taipei, Taiwan. E-mail : ch4006@chgh.org.tw

2. Evolution of the roles and functions of informatics nurses

The roles and functions of informatics nurses have become increasingly more important in the modernization of hospitals. The evolution of nursing informatics in Taiwan has led to both independent roles and coordinating roles for informatics nurses.

The functions of the independent role are:
- a.　Conducting system and workflow analysis
- b.　Operating system implementation and system evaluation
- c.　Planning of user education and training
- d.　Compiling work manuals
- e.　Updating relevant knowledge and skills
- f.　Solving problems
- g.　Applying information technology to nursing
- h.　Conducting data analysis and information analysis
- i.　Message processing and information integration
- j.　Facilitating communication and coordination
- k.　Providing user support and consulting

The functions of the coordinating role are:
- a.　Nursing care quality control. This includes evaluating system functions, evaluating problem-solving ability and efficacy, improving patient safety and care quality, and monitoring the legality and integrity of patient information.
- b.　Education, training, and consulting. This refers to assisting clinicians in maintaining or improving job readiness.
- c.　Improving the professional ability of nurses and providing education through analysis, planning, or continuing education.
- d.　Communication and coordination. This refers to linking the individual networks of the units in a healthcare team to achieve coordination and integration of professional work content.
- e.　Innovation and development, particularly research in the areas of clinical care guidelines and informatics nursing [2].

3. Nursing informatics education and training

As for the education and training of informatics nurses in Taiwan, some universities offer courses which introduce concepts in nursing informatics within their general nursing programs. With the growing importance of the role of information technology, some universities now require these courses to be taken so that nursing students can fully understand nursing informatics prior to graduation. Some two-year community colleges also offer nursing informatics programs. These courses comply with the two-year community college nursing program curriculum set forth by the Taiwan Ministry of Education. These programs comprise 72 credits in general education and nursing, including 20 credits in required nursing informatics courses such as computer hardware, computer software, database applications, nursing informatics development and status, project design, information ethics and safety, healthcare information, and practicum in nursing informatics. The programs provide students with the necessary knowledge and skills required by informatics nurses [3].

Some universities have established graduate programs in nursing informatics, which provide a platform for nursing professionals who are interested in this career path. In addition, some schools offer nursing informatics courses through their in-service and continuing education departments, providing currently employed nurses with continued training to improve their skills in informatics. [1]

Lastly, professional associations such as the Taiwan Association for Medical Informatics (TAMI) and Taiwan Nursing Informatics Association (TNIA) annually offer courses in practical or applied nursing informatics to assist in the education and training of healthcare informatics professionals in Taiwan.

Currently, most medium-size and large Taiwanese hospitals have established nursing informatics committees to promote and develop work in this field. Some hospitals employ one to three full-time or dedicated informatics nurses to assist in promoting nursing that integrates information technology. Hospitals that value nursing informatics development also generally have both nurses and committees to promote clinical care information systems.

4. Certification of Informatics Nurses

According to a 2010 survey compiled by the Taiwan Nursing Informatics Association (TNIA), 3.1% of clinical healthcare workers expect informatics nurses to have a degree from a community college, 56.8% expect nurses to have a bachelor's degree, and 38.7% expect a master's degree. The same survey showed that 6.2% of respondents expect informatics nurses to have less than three years of clinical experience, 50.6% expect four to six years of clinical experience, and 37.5% expect more than seven years of clinical experience. Regarding the professional training received by informatics nurses, 15.6% of respondents felt that it should be provided by bachelor's degree programs, 20.6% felt that it should be provided by master's degree programs, and 25.8% felt that it should be offered by professional nursing associations, such as the TNIA [2].

Based on the survey results, in 2014, TNIA undertook drafting the certification pre-requisites and qualifications for informatics nurses and informatics nurse specialists [4]. Informatics nurses must be licensed registered nurses and members of TNIA, they must have a bachelor's degree in nursing, they must have two or more years of clinical nursing experience and at least one year of practical experience in informatics, and they must have taken at least 30 hours of informatics courses during the past three years, including least 15 hours in courses which are offered by TNIA.

Certifications are awarded after a review of qualifications or after passing a written exam. Certified informatics nurses who receive an additional 10 hours of informatics training within two years may receive certification as informatics nurse specialists after a review of qualifications or after passing a written exam. The informatics nurse specialist certification is valid for a period of five years, and 60 hours of continuing education in informatics is required to renew the certification [5]. 〔Table 1〕

The Taiwan Nursing Informatics Association began accepting certification applications in February 2015 [5]. As of September 2016, 48 certifications have been awarded, signaling a new milestone in the evolution of the role of informatics nurses in Taiwan.

Table 1 The basic requirements for Informatics Nurses and Specialists t in Taiwan, 2015[5]

Requirements	Informatics Nurses (IN)	Informatics Nurse Specialist (INS)
Certification organization	TNIA	TNIA
Academic degree	Bachelor degree	Bachelor degree
Training hours	at least 30 hours during the last three years	at least 10 hours during the last two years
Clinical nursing experience	at least three years	at least three years
Practical experience	at least one year	at least one year
Method of certification	Paper-based exam & qualification	Paper-based exam & qualification
Period of validity	----	five years

Note : Each applicant must be a registered nurse and a member of TNIA.
Also, in order to be an informatics nurse specialist, a nurse must already be certified in informatics nursing.

5. Conclusion

The development of nursing informatics is a current trend. Over the last 5 years, information technology has made rapid progress in Taiwan. The Taiwan government strongly encourages innovation of medical information. The hospital accreditation committee emphasizes the application of medical information more and more. Thus, hospitals of all sizes are eager to develop medical information systems. As a result, informatics nurses have to continuously learn about information technology as well as nursing knowledge and skills to help hospitals and nursing professionals be ready for the new era of medical information technology in the 21st century.

References

[1] A reflection on nursing education in Taiwan from the perspective of introducing information technology into clinical nursing. Taiwan Association of Nursing Education Newsletter, 9. [cited 20th May 2016]. Available from http://www.tane.org.tw/newsletter_show.php?news_no=104 .
[2] Feng, RC., Liu, JT., Chang, ML., and Wang, MH.: Assessing the feasibility of expanding the roles and functions of nurses: the roles and functions of informatics nurses. Research Project Number DOH099-TD-M-113-099005. Taipei: Taiwan Nursing Informatics Association. ;2010.
[3] Informatics nursing curriculum. [Internet]. ; [cited 2th July 2016]. Available from http://ens.fy.edu.tw/files/11-1031-6344.php?Lang=zh-tw
[4] Certification process for informatics nurses. [internet]; [cited 6th August 2016]. Available from http://www.ni.org.tw/
[5] Feng, RC., Lee, LY., and Lee, TY. (2015). The role development of informatics nurse specialists in Taiwan. J Nurs Res. 2014; 62(3): 23–29.

Forecasting Informatics Competencies for Nurses in the Future of Connected Health
J. Murphy et al. (Eds.)
101
© 2017 IMIA and IOS Press.
This article is published online with Open Access by IOS Press and distributed under the terms
of the Creative Commons Attribution Non-Commercial License 4.0 (CC BY-NC 4.0).
doi:10.3233/978-1-61499-738-2-101

Technology-Based Healthcare for Nursing Education Within The Netherlands: Past, Present and Future

Ybranda KOSTER MSc,[a] and Cornelis T.M. van HOUWELINGEN MSc, RN[b]

[a] Faculty of Nursing, University of Applied Sciences Inholland Amsterdam, The Netherlands
[b] Research Center for Innovations in Health Care, Faculty of Health Care, Utrecht University of Applied Sciences, The Netherlands

Abstract. At the present time, nearly all Dutch nursing schools are searching for suitable ways to implement technology-based healthcare in their curriculum. Some Universities chose elective education, others a mandatory solution. Several studies were executed to determine competencies needed by nurses in order to work with technology-based healthcare. In 2016 a nationwide new curriculum for nurses has been published. Providing technology-based healthcare is included under the core competencies of this new curriculum. All baccalaureate nursing educational institutes must implement this new curriculum at the start of 2016 which will have a huge impact on the implementation of technology-based healthcare in the education programs. In the future, technology centers from Universities will collaborate and specialize, partner with technology companies and crossovers between information and communication technology and healthcare education will be expanded.

Keywords. Technology-based healthcare, curriculum, education, mandatory education, elective education, ICT, information, communication, technology

1. Introduction

Beginning in the fall of 2016, all nursing schools will offer education about technology-based healthcare. This chapter describes the history of how it got to where it is today. It begins by exploring the past education of technology-based healthcare in The Netherlands based on several examples of projects and programs.

Afterward we will elaborate on the present implementation of technology-based healthcare within the Dutch education system. Examples from the Universities of Applied Science of Nursing, the Master Advanced Health Informatics Practice, the platform of Nursing and Healthcare Informatics (VZI) of the Dutch Professional Association of Nurses and Carers (V&VN) will be explored. The role of technology-based healthcare in the new nationwide curriculum of "Bachelor Nursing 2020" will also be discussed.

The chapter will end with a view on the future of technology-based healthcare within the Dutch education system. This will include the future plans on Nursing Informatics from multiple Colleges of Nursing and the ambitions of VZI will be elaborated.

In this chapter the abbreviation ICT will be used. ICT stand for Information and Communication Technology. This term is used for the branch of Information Technology related to digital devices that are used to communicate or interact with digital information. The Dutch national institute for technology in healthcare is NICTIZ (National ICT Institute Healthcare). Since ICT is used in the name of the national institute and is commonly used in Dutch healthcare, the abbreviation ICT will be used in this article.

2. The Past: 1983-2013

The importance of attention for technology-based healthcare within the Dutch education system started early. One of the first publications about technology-based healthcare in the Netherlands is the article of Pluyter (1983) [1] in which early experiences in using a digitally integrated Hospital Information System are discussed. Pluyter indicates that it is important for the nurses who are involved in the construction of computer programs to orientate in the field of informatics, as well as the need for those involved in informatics to orientate in the field of nursing. This laid the groundwork for nursing education to implement technology content in the curriculum. The article ends with the statement: "To all appearances it is not the question whether nurses will use computer facilities, but the manner and extent to which this should be done. Obviously, it is the job of the nurses themselves to give to the desired result and the line of march."

2.1   Local initiatives

Since 1983 there have been several local projects on technology-based healthcare in education. For example, in 1989 at the Noordelijke Hogeschool Leeuwarden, University of Applied Sciences, the development and implementation of Nursing Informatics courses started. A structured approach was used to develop Nurses Informatics education in four different courses. A modified framework was used, based on the framework of Ronald and Skiba (1987) [2]. With the use of this framework courses were developed for the Nurse Teacher program of the Noordelijke Hogeschool Leeuwarden, baccalaureate program of the Noordelijke Hogeschool Leeuwarden and the Nurse Scientist Program of Groningen University. This included one module on how to use the framework and one on education of Nursing Informatics. Learning contents were based on learning objectives and content was based on IMIA guidelines and existing courses [3].

Seven years later, in 1996, the courses had changed. In the course for nursing instructors the focus became more and more on the specialized nursing informatics skills, since the computer knowledge of the students appeared to be sufficient in most cases. Instead new topics were included about integrated electronic patient records, information management and processing, classification and terminology issues, nursing minimum data sets, innovation of care and use of technology to support this. In the baccalaureate program, Nursing Informatics was integrated in the program [4]. But this remained a local development.

The University of Applied Sciences Inholland started with a course in 1991: "Hogere Opleiding voor Verpleegkundige Informatica" (Higher Education of Nursing Informatics), HOVIF for short. This course focused on promoting user-friendly use of health informatics in primary care processes and in organizational levels. Since this was an open course, professionals from all over the country attended and spread the knowledge. Graduates from this course have contributed, in several ways, to the innovative use of ICT in several domains and activities in healthcare. The developments of this course have been intertwined with the developments in Dutch healthcare [5]. Yet it still remained a local initiative.

Dutch nurses can graduate at one of three levels: intermediate vocational education, bachelor's degree level education and master's level education. Nurses can graduate at the intermediate vocational education level at ROC's (Regional Education Centers). ROC's were also searching how to implement technology into their nursing education. In Twente (a province in the eastern part of the Netherlands) one of the ROC's started with a course "Care and Technology" in 2006. In this course nursing students and students of the application developers program of the same ROC worked together. The module included "special learning objects" such as the development of a Care Information Model (reusable building blocks for an EHR) and the development of functional requirements for EHR systems for continuity of care. [6]. Again, this was a local initiative of only one ROC.

2.2   National initiatives

In an attempt to nationalize the use of technology-based healthcare within the education system, the Dutch Association of Higher Healthcare Education (HGZO) started with an ICT project in 2002. Due to changes in the profession, a greater need emerged to develop specific ICT competencies and educational material for non-ICT courses, like nursing. The focus on this project was on Electronic Health Records. Three goals were established: identifying the professional competencies related to information processing and ICT, the development of educational tools to obtain those competencies and the support of the implementation of ICT related education.

The project used key issues and results from previous work, including (among others) the Nightingale Project and Project Eductra, to determine the competencies needed. A start was made with competencies on five levels of skill: recognizing, using, evaluating, applying and integrating. For these levels a proposal for educational tools was made. The competencies that were developed ended up being less about ICT and more about healthcare than anticipated. Attempts to establish an Electronic Health Record for education failed due to high costs. An alternative was found by making simulations using screens of existing systems [7]. Though this initiative was national, it was free for the educational institutes to implement these competencies into their education. However, only a few Universities of Applied Sciences used these recommendations in their curriculum.

In 2012 another push for a national curriculum for nurses was given by the V&VN, who published an advisory for the professional profile of the nurses in 2020 [8]. In the advisory the V&VN stated that ICT can mean a valuable step forward for direct care and in administrative tasks. The nurses of the future should be aware of technological developments like Electronic Health Records, screen-to-screen care and electronic monitoring. One of the important issues is standardization of both language and practice. In an increasing dependency of technology, the V&VN claimed, it is important that nurses (and their professional organization) have a clear role in the development. The advisory also laid the foundation for the "Bachelor Nursing 2020" profile, published in 2016, which will be described in the next section.

3. The Present: 2014-2016

For many Dutch Universities of Applied Science in Nursing and other healthcare educational institutes the advisory from V&VN was a wakeup call to start technology in their educational program. As a result, more nationwide and local initiatives on technology-based healthcare emerged. Several institutes explored the required competencies on technology-based healthcare for nurses. Educational institutes still had different approaches to technology implementation in their curriculum. Some institutes choose for elective education while others integrate the technology into their core curriculum, thus making technology a mandatory element of the nurses' education.

3.1   Exploring required competencies for technology-based healthcare

On December 10th 2014 a symposium was held on healthcare technology within the Dutch healthcare education system. This symposium was necessary because the current education taught too little on technology. Even more, there seemed to be an anti-technology attitude within the Dutch healthcare education system. Traditional healthcare was often described as "warm care" while healthcare technology was described as "cold care". Nurses tended to fill in the needs of their patients with comments such as "my patient isn't capable of using technology, that is too difficult". Important in the education was to learn about developments and possibilities of technology, learning ethical, social and social issues concerning technology. Change in the educational environment needed to start with a change in the teachers. Students had to develop an innovative attitude as well as a critical attitude, not every change is an improvement. Therefore an international minor "care and technology" was developed at Hogeschool Zuyd for bachelor-prepared individuals with at least two years of working experience to train them to become leaders in the use of technology in healthcare [9].

The symposium in December started with a view on the changes health education had to make on behalf of the report on health professions in 2030. During interactive sessions the participants were asked to reflect on which level a healthcare professional should master the competencies as were developed by Hogeschool Zuyd (completed with competencies from several publications). Most participants reflected soft skills concerning healthcare ICT where missing in the list of competencies. The symposium did manage to achieve that healthcare educators needed to start thinking about how they could implement ICT in their education together [10]. The "letter of inspiration, Technology in Healthcare" of the HGZO, a publication of this symposium, stated that 22 competencies were defined as generic after at least 2/3 of the (120) participants stated these were the competencies every healthcare professional should achieve [11]. This showed that the question on how to implement technology into healthcare education is not just an issue for the nursing education but is a topic for every level of health education. This letter of inspiration intended to give a boost to the implementation of technology within the Dutch healthcare education.

Meanwhile Utrecht University of Applied Science investigated which professional activities nurses can perform using telemonitoring devices, video conferencing and personal alarming and what competencies nurses need to possess in order to perform these activities effectively. In this research a panel of experts discussed the activities on relevance for nurses and discussed which competencies would be needed to execute these activities. Fourteen activities were identified and fifty-two competencies were considered to be required for nurses to be able to execute these activities. Of the fifty-two competencies, thirty-two were specifically for telehealth and were new competencies. Home care organizations and healthcare educational institutes benefit from this research by using the activities and the corresponding competencies as a starting point for their curriculum and education [12].

3.2   Elective courses about technology-based healthcare

Some Universities of Applied Science chose to develop a minor or a separate course on technology-based healthcare instead of making it a mandatory part of their curriculum. The Fontys University of Applied Science of nursing founded an Expert Centre Health and Technology (EGT) in order to embed the technology in the education. In this center, students from different educational directions work together in a minor to design and develop solutions that improve the quality of life for people with health limitations or problems. In the third year of the education, students from nursing, ICT, design and other courses participate in a project. Usable prototypes are developed like a special click-lock brake system on walkers of hemiplegic patients or a robot dog with a ball to motivate elderly people to move [13].

Another development in the elective programs is the HOVIF, discussed in the previous section. It evolved into a Master of Science program. The new program, Master of Advanced Health Informatics Practice (MAHIP), covers the professional roles of the Health Care Informatics: the information analyst, the designer, the adviser, the implementation manager and the project manager [14].   Students come from various settings of healthcare and welfare. Some are already working on the area of ICT and want to expand their knowledge others have interest or ambitions to work the area of health, welfare and technology. During the two years, the master's students work on projects related to their own setting, so employers already see and benefit from the effects of the master during the program. One of the assignments is to develop an eHealth application in a patient centred design. In 2015 a pilot started where the eHealth applications designed, on paper, by students of the MAHIP were used in an assignment for the Informatics students of Hogeschool Inholland. The students made a working prototype of the application. One of these designs was so successful, it is now implemented in the intensive care unit where the MAHIP student who designed the application works. The implementation and evaluation of this application will be the theme of his thesis. After this success, more collaboration between the two educational directions will be explored.

Nursing students from the Hogeschool Inholland have been working on a project to create a structured overview of available eHealth interventions organized by health problems which resulted in a table with brief information on the intervention, the name of the eHealth product and a document with further information on the eHealth intervention. A student from the MAHIP is making a database design which will be developed by informatics students. When the database is available, more project assignments will be given to nursing students to generate more input for the database. The plan is to publish this database online so that it can be used by healthcare professionals, patients, students and teachers.

Most Dutch nursing schools have integrated nursing informatics in their existing curriculum, to a lesser or greater extent, by a minor or integrated in the curriculum. Saxion Hogeschool decided on another, creative approach. They started with a combined bachelor degree. The 4 year course of Health and Technology (Gezondheid en Technologie) matches for 60% with the curriculum of the bachelor of nursing while the remaining 40% focuses on technology and innovation. A graduate receives a bachelor of nursing with expertise on health technology. In the curriculum health technology in the home environment, online aid and other technology use in healthcare are discussed. The students that graduate from this program are professionals that use modern technology and are able to contribute to the innovation of healthcare [15].

At Hogeschool Zuyd a special day "Technology in Healthcare" has been held for several years now. In this day all students of the faculty of Healthcare: occupational therapy, speech therapy, physical therapy, nursing and midwifery participate. The day is opened by a lecturer and after that all students start working on assignments in mixed study groups. A market with participation of several vendors is held where the newest technology is shown and the students can try everything.

3.3   Mandatory courses about technology-based healthcare

At Utrecht University of Applied Science, lessons that were learned from a course on home telehealth for care professionals were applied to the curriculum of the nursing education. One of the lessons was that nurses are most interested in the question: "what does this technology add to the care of my patient?" In the lectures on technology-based healthcare, this has become the leading question. Students are motivated by examples told by a patient or a nurse. During the curriculum, lectures on technology-based healthcare are provided in courses on psychiatry, youth healthcare and chronic illness. In each lecture an aspect of technology-based healthcare is covered in class, such as privacy, self-management, laws and regulations and the influence of the role of the nurses. Learning to work with remote healthcare is also integrated in the curriculum in the form of a practicum and during their internship [16].

Research on Assisted Living Technology (ALT: telecare, digital participation services and wellness services) showed not all Universities of Applied science pay attention to this technology. ALT could support healthcare for (especially) elderly people in order for them to be able to stay in their own environment for a longer period. In a study by van Houwelingen [17] a conclusion is drawn that lack of education could have caused the insufficient motivation of healthcare professionals to deploy ALT. The study has focused on two elements of ALT: personal alarming and telecare (screen-to-screen care). Nursing universities from four countries in Europe (Spain, The Netherlands, Germany and The United Kingdom) where questioned on the education of personal alarming and screen-to-screen care in their educational program. Education on social alarming was first offered in 2013. Education on screen-to-screen care started a few years earlier, in 2011. In this short period a lot has happened, since today respectively 30% and 16% of the Dutch nursing schools are offering social alarming and/or screen-to-screen care. For the near future 40% of Dutch nursing schools are planning to offer education on social alarming. 33% of the Dutch nursing schools have plans to offer screen-to-screen care education in the near future. These amounts are very promising for the future of Nursing Technology within the Dutch education system.

One of the institutes that uses ALT in their curriculum is the University of Applied Science Windesheim. Windesheim is one of the Dutch nursing schools who have incorporated screen- to-screen care in their curriculum; a skills lab is used for education on screen-to-screen care. In cooperation with the lectureship "ICT innovation in Healthcare" two classrooms have been designed to create the skills lab. One of these classrooms is fitted with a one-way mirror and is used for observation. The other room is used as a technology care centre. Further on the campus another room is furnished as a living room. Both rooms are equipped with cameras and microphones to record sound and visual for analysis and evaluation. Also both rooms have iPads equipped with an app that can accomplish a save connection between the two settings, the same app is used in home care settings. The use of this skills lab has been intertwined in the curriculum along with practicums on Electronic Health Record and sensor technology [18].

In 2016 the complete edition of the educational profile has been published. This profile is named "Bachelor Nursing 2020, a future ready educational profile" or BN2020 for short. This profile has been developed by LOOV in cooperation with all of the 17 Dutch Universities of applied sciences that offer nursing education. This profile creates the outline of the educational profile and is a firm base for the future. It prepares for the changes in healthcare that are already happening and the changes yet to come. This curriculum ensures that technology-based healthcare will become a mandatory part of the curriculum of all bachelor's of nursing educational institutes. The universities themselves create their own curriculum based on these outlines.

The new profile is based on the CanMEDS (Canadian Medical Education Directions for Specialists) roles: caregiver, communicator, collaborator, reflective EBP-professional, health advocate, organizer and professional and quality enhancer. The CanMEDS is a framework to deepen and describe the complex competencies. For every CanMEDS role, the concerning competencies and key concepts are described. These competencies and key concepts form the core of the profile. The knowledge and skills that operationalize these key concepts and competencies are described in a Body of Knowledge and Skills (BoKS). Even though eHealth can be integrated in (almost) every aspect of the profession in the BN202, the role of communicator specifically focuses on the use of technology with the key concept "the use of information and communication technology". The knowledge that is necessary for this key concept is divided into knowledge, skills and attitude and are:

Knowledge:
- Knows the latest ICT applications aimed at improving and supporting communication in healthcare
- Knows the latest information and communication technologies to organize and execute healthcare

Skills:
- Can use digital skills and available ICT applications to support the professional and personalized communication
- Can adequately use ICT tools and e-health such as remote care
- Can handle and use electronic nurse and multidisciplinary patient records (EHR)
- Can find information on the internet and in professional nursing databases (national and international) fast and competent
- Can use social media and eHealth programs

Attitude:
- Uses the potential of ICT in an integer and professional manner

- Shows an open attitude towards ICT innovations in healthcare [19].

Every university of applied science in the Netherlands will have to use the BN2020 curriculum guidelines to create their curriculum; and all nursing graduates after 2020 should have the knowledge, skills and attitude as described. It is up to the universities as to how they make sure their students reach these competencies at school and/or during their internship.

4. The Future 2017-…

In the years to come, the University of Applied Sciences of Inholland will start with the "Inholland Health and Technology Centre" (IHTC), a collaboration between the domain of the education for Technology, Design and Informatics and the domain of the education for Health, Sports and Welfare. The IHTC creates synergy in the triangle of education between the Education – Research – Professional fields, due to its central position. There is much to learn and research in the field of eHealth. Most knowledge still has to be placed in education. In the field there are many questions on acceptance, implementation and ethics. The IHTC want to link the field of healthcare and technology to the education of healthcare and technology and provide expertise to enhance a crossover of health and technology both in education and field. They will intermediate between field and students to execute projects form which will produce knowledge from which all involved will benefit. In this collaboration a minor eHealth will be developed, it will start out as an eHealth minor for the informatics students but the other educational directions will start to participate later on [20]. The IHTC will cooperate with the Vrije Universiteit Amsterdam (University of Amsterdam) and the technology centre of Hogeschool Zuyd to ensure progress in technology based healthcare. More cooperation and collaboration with other organizations are expected.

Another development at Inholland is that the MAHIP course has attracted attention from professionals who work in the ICT business with a focus on healthcare. Therefore a special pre master's program is being developed to familiarize the ICT-trained professionals with the ins and outs of healthcare so that they are able to follow the same programme as the students who already work in the health or welfare sector. This will further integrate the knowledge of both healthcare and ICT professionals.

A thesis for the MAHIP research will be conducted to explore the expectations of the home care organization concerning eHealth competencies of graduate nursing students. With this information and an analysis of the current curriculum an advisory will be given to the education of nurses of the Hogeschool Inholland. Also, based on the advisory, an innovation project will be started to implement an eHealth application in the curriculum that will help students obtain these competencies.

In 2017 the University of Applied Science Hogeschool Zuyd will set up an app café at their "Technology in Healthcare" day. There will be a challenge for the students to find the best app for a special target audience. Clarification of the criteria of quality will play an important role in this process.

To give nursing the possibility to practice real life scenarios, the University of Applied Science of Utrecht started a collaboration with Verklizan, a European company offering telecare/telehealth services. Together they started with the creation of a simulated alarm and monitoring center and simulated home environment. In these settings several scenarios can be trained and healthcare technology can be tested and experienced by the students (e.g. Google Glass, devices for self-measurement, videoconferencing, and personal alarming). The benefits for the company are publication and testing of their technology. The University benefits from this collaboration because the company supplies their newest technology for both settings and will replace this technology when new systems are available. Collaborations like these can make it possible for Universities to have up to date technology without having to purchase new equipment regularly.

5. Conclusion

Due to Bachelor Nursing 2020, the new Dutch nursing standard, all nursing Universities of Applied Science will have education on technology based healthcare in their curriculum beginning in the fall of 2016. Some universities will start with the first year students and evolve the curriculum for senior students during that year; others will start with a completely changed curriculum. This means that technology based healthcare will be part of every nursing school providing bachelor's degree education. In the cooperation of knowledge centers, lectureships, healthcare practices and technology companies, technology-based healthcare will play an even bigger role in nursing education in the future.

References

[1] Pluyter-Wenting ESP., Nieman HBJ., Computers melden zich aan bij de verpleging, Tijdschrift voor Ziekenverpleging 36(14) (1983), 430-436.
[2] Goossen WTF., Jeuring G., Dassen TWN. Education in Nursing Informatics: seven years of Experience Part 1. The Development, Information Technology in Nursing 8 (1996).
[3] Goossen WTF., Jeuring G., Dassen TWN. Education in Nursing Informatics: seven years of Experience Part 2. The Courses, Information Technology in Nursing 8 (1996).
[4] Goossen WTF., Jeuring G. Dassen TWN. Education in Nursing Informatics: seven years of Experience Part 3. Changes over the years, Information Technology in Nursing 9 (1997).
[5] Doms R. Opleidingsplan Professionel masteropleiding Advanced Health Informa-tics Practice, Domein Gezondheid, Sport en Welzijn Hogeschool Inholland, Amsterdam, 2012.
[6] Goossen WTF., Goossen-Baremans ATM, Hofte L., de Krey B., ROC van Twente: Nursing Education in Care and Technology, Studies in Health Technology and Informatics 129 (2007), 1396-1400.
[7] Hoger Gezondheidszorg Onderwijs (HGZO), Informatievaardigheden binnen de HGZO Beroepscompetenties, eindrapportage HGZO-ICT project, HGZO, Koudekerk aan den Rijn, 2003.
[8] Verpleegkundigen & Verzorgenden Nederland (VenVN), V&V 2020 Deel 3 Beroepsprofiel verpleegkundige, VenVN, Utrecht, 2012.
[9] Verwey R., Onderwijs voor Verpleegkundigen op het terrein van Technologie en Zorg, Nieuwsbrief VZI VenVN December 2014 (2014), 4-5.
[10] Y. Koster, Congres Technologie en Zorgonderwijs, Nieuwsbrief VZI VenVN December 2014 (2014), 15-16.
[11] Hoger Gezondheidszorg Onderwijs (HGZO), Informatiebrief Technologie in de Zorg, HGZO, Koudekerk aan den Rijn, 2015.
[12] van Houwelingen CTM., Moerman AH., Ettema RGA., Kort HSM., ten Cate O., Competencies required for nursing telehealth activities: A delphi-study, Nurse Education Today 39 (2016) 50-62.
[13] van Gorkom P., Harder C., van Lieshout F., van der Zijp T. Community of Practice, Nieuwsbrief VZI VenVN December 2014 (2014), 10.
[14] de Boer U., Doms R. Master Advanced Health Informatics Practice, Nieuwsbrief VZI VenVN December 2014 (2014), 6-7.
[15] Gezondheid &Technologie [Internet]. Saxion Hogeschool, 28 April 2016, Available from: http://saxion.nl/studeren/kiezen_en_kennismaken/Studiekiezer/agz/gt/gezondheid-en-technologie

[16] van Houwelingen CTM., Kort HSM. Verpleegkundigen opleiden voor het verlenen van zorg op afstand, Onderwijs en Gezondheidszorg 37 (2013), 24-27.
[17] van Houwelingen CTM., Assistive Living technology education in Western Europe. In H.Müller, Groot M., Schut D., Awang D., Kort H., de la Cruz IP., Pumpe D., Roelofsma H., Valero MA., van Zandwijk R., Acceptance of assisted living technologies in Europe: Analysis of major differences in the adoption rates of assisted living technologies in Europe, Verklizan, Sliedrecht, 2014.
[18] van Hout A., Prins H.. Nauta J., Hettinga M. eHealth begint in het verpleegkundig onderwijs, Onderwijs en Gezondheidszorg 37 (2013), 19-23.
[19] Lambregts J., Grotendorst A., van Merwijk C., Bachelor of nursing 2020, een toekomstbestendig opleidingsprofiel 4.0, Bohn Stafleu van Loghum, Houten, 2016.
[20] Inholland Health & Technology Centre [Internet]. Inholland Hogeschool, 11 May 2016, Available from: https://www.inholland.nl/ihtc/home/

Forecasting Informatics Competencies for Nurses in the Future of Connected Health
J. Murphy et al. (Eds.)
© *2017 IMIA and IOS Press.*
doi:10.3233/978-1-61499-738-2-111

From Entry to Practice to Advanced Nurse Practitioner – The Progression of Competencies and How They Assist in Delivery of eHealth Programs for Healthy Ageing

Daragh RODGER[a] and Pamela HUSSEY[b]
[a]St Mary's Campus, Phoenix Park, Dublin 20
[b]School of Nursing and Human Science, Dublin City University, Dublin 9

Abstract Most of the health issues encountered in persons of older age are the result of one or more chronic diseases. The evidence base reports that chronic diseases can be prevented or delayed by engaging in healthy behaviors. Education provides a cost effective intervention on both economic grounds in addition to delivery of optimal patient outcomes. Information and Communication Technology (ICT) increasingly is viewed as a critical utility in eHealth delivery, providing scope for expanding online education facilities for older persons. Developing nursing competencies in the delivery of eHealth solutions to deliver user education programs therefore makes sense. This chapter discusses nursing competencies on the development of targeted eHealth programs for healthy ageing. The role of Advanced Nurse Practitioner in Ireland and its associated competency set identifies how a strong action learning model can be designed to deliver eHealth educational programs for effective delivery of healthy ageing in place.

Keywords: eLearning, Competencies, Advanced Nurse Practitioner, Healthy ageing

1. Introduction

The proportion of the world's population over 65 years is expected to rise dramatically in the next 30 years and will account for over 25% of the adult population in some countries. Recent World Health Organization (WHO) projections report a rise from 12% in 2015 to 22% in 2050 of the world population being over 60 years of age – this equates to a rise from 900 million to 2 billion people in this age category [1]. Problems therefore arise with an ageing population to provide and match societal demands for care. Most of the health issues encountered in persons of older age are the result of one or more chronic diseases [2]. In addition to chronic disease is the effect of ageing, which has been widely documented in the literature and referred to as the "Giants of Geriatric Medicine" [3]. The Geriatric Giants include – Instability, Incontinence, Immobility, Intellectual impairment and Iatrogenics. The Giants of Geriatric Medicine are of particular concern in older adults as they impact on the ability to function for those who are over 65 years with associated disabilities and multimorbidity. The evidence base presents exciting opportunities reporting that chronic diseases can be prevented or delayed by engaging in healthy behaviors [1]. Core to the role of the Advanced Nurse Practitioner (ANP) is a need to maintain or support clients in health seeking behavior to maintain optimal health and independence [4].

In Ireland, advanced practice refers to registered nurses who engage in continuing professional development and clinical supervision to practice as expert practitioners and demonstrate exemplary clinical leadership. It is a recognized registration – Registered Advanced Nurse Practitioner – where nurses work within an agreed scope of practice and meet established criteria set out by Nursing and Midwifery Board of Ireland (NMBI) [5]. All ANP's practice under four core concepts:-

- Autonomy in clinical practice
- Expert practice
- Professional and clinical leadership
- Research

Each of the core concepts has specific competencies that the ANP attain.

To operationalise this role effectively, the ANP provides significant time in educational interventions and related research activity. Education provides a cost effective intervention on both economic grounds and on the delivery of prospective patient outcomes [6]. Traditionally nurses have engaged with patients providing most of the education in the management and prevention of disease across all ages and all care settings. Nurses have also historically played a pivotal role in educational initiatives relating to chronic disease management [7, 8]. Recent policy agendas in regard to development of the Clinical Nurse Specialist and Advanced Nurse Practitioner role demonstrate an increase in patient learning, knowledge, and understanding leveraging in improved adherence to treatment, increased wellness and ultimately better management of chronic diseases and associated disabilities [4].

The advancement of Information and Communication Technology (ICT) in healthcare and the development of nursing informatics over the past decade progresses the notion that the use of technology can be considered as a critical utility in health service delivery [9, 10]. In tandem with an ageing population this provides the framework for developing online education programmes to promote action learning models for healthy active ageing, better disease prevention and management and thus supporting the theory that health promotion needs to be delivered through education across all ages.

Competencies are a key requisite to the professional development of all registered nurses and are outlined in scope of practice documents for nurses internationally [11,12,13]. To be safe and effective practitioners, nurses must demonstrate evidence of these competencies, and over time with experience, competency requirements can evolve within practice. Developing nursing competencies in delivery of eHealth solutions on service user education programmes therefore is timely and in line with global policy agendas as outlined by WHO [14]

2. Competencies for development of eHealth programs for healthy ageing

Use of a framework underpinned by evidence to clarify the role of nursing is necessary in competency development. According to Uys, competence is the ability to deliver a specified professional service and nursing provides a framework to clarify the role with sound evidence of safe care through education and regulation [15]. The International Council of Nurses, Competence for ANP defines competency as the effective application of a combination of knowledge, skill and judgement demonstrated by an individual in daily practice or job performance [16, 17]. It is reflected in practice as:

- Knowledge, understanding and judgement
- Skills: cognitive, technical or psychomotor and interpersonal
- A range of personal attributes and attitudes.

Mapping the above principles for the development of eHealth programs for healthy ageing with one of the Giants of Geriatric Medicine – instability, as an example demonstrates the role of how an ANP can provide a specific nursing service, and have an impact on patient safety. Here we provide a summary overview of this mapping process and the associated outcomes as developed by an ANP of older persons in Ireland.

2.1   Knowledge, understanding, judgement

The ANP has extensive experience in older person care to identify the impact of falls on older adults and recognition of the need to provide education on the following facts:

- Falls cause a lot of pain, discomfort and disability to older adults resulting in additional healthcare needs and additional costs to healthcare providers
- Falls cause additional psychological trauma to older people resulting in social isolation, loneliness, anxiety and fear.
- Falls are preventable and measures are required to reduce the risk of falls for older adults.

In Figure 1, this particular message is conveyed as competency 1 impact.

2.2   Skill: cognitive, technical or psychomotor and interpersonal

The ANP through experience recognizes the need for an education program:

- To create an awareness of the potential for falls in older adults and reduce the risk of falls in an ageing population.
- To identify the medium to present the education in order to reach a wide audience as falls is a global phenomenon.
- To identify the need to engage with an educational technologist to develop the online education material.

Competency 2 is illustrated in Figure 1 as definition of scope and aims

2.3   A range of personal attributes and attitudes

- The ANP through working with this client group recognizes that a tailored individualized approach is important as clients may have a varied intellectual background. Education is pitched at a level understandable to all.
- Education is easily accessible and underpinned by action learning.
- Differing formats were developed to meet individual needs.

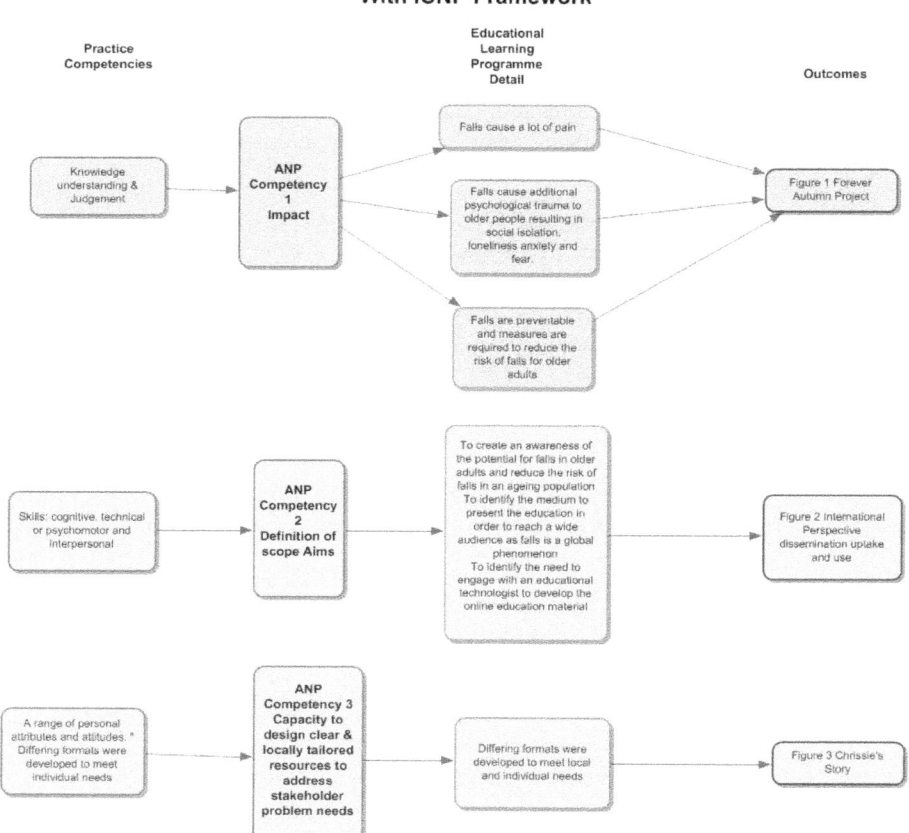

Figure 1: Mapping ANP Competency with ICNP Framework

Identification by the ANP of the education requirements is portrayed as Competency 3 in Figure 1

Such an approach was used to develop a programme on creating awareness of falls and falls risk reduction – Forever Autumn© as an online resource. Also, by adopting an action learning model and engaging with an Educational Technologist to develop the eLearning component with a view to reaching a larger audience within and beyond the organisation has proved most effective. [18] Initial evaluation and professional response to this program not only demonstrates its effectiveness but also exhibits how the skills and competence in nurses to enhance their practice is achieved through targeted educational programs. The competency framework therefore can provide the required elements for nurses to develop both personally and professionally to enhance quality of life of the patients in their care.

This work, completed in Ireland in accordance with national and international healthcare strategy and policy agendas, has recently been recognized as a best practice initiative receiving a national award for best in health service delivery. It provided a case example on how the participatory process of learning is achieved using Web 2.0 technologies as alluded to by Spencer and Hussey [19] to teach, learn collaborate and create knowledge. Using a case study to assist individuals to learn about healthy ageing, the eBonehealth© and Forever Autumn© Falls Prevention Projects [20] portray core competencies acquired by an Advanced Nurse Practitioner (ANP) to design, lead out and deliver on an eHealth patient educational activity. Collaboration with other healthcare professionals is evident in the development of Forever Autumn Community of Practice© (FACOP) which promotes the sharing of knowledge through an online platform [21]. This once again demonstrates the use of competencies to recognize the need for and use of skills required to develop essential education resources for intellectual disabilities community on bone health and falls prevention – (Figure 2) Happy Bones© [22]. Figure 2 provides screenshots of the outcomes from Figure 1 Mapping Framework. This paper concludes with figures 3 and 4 which offer summary detail of the access and dissemination of this programme internationally. To date the combined access to these sites = 3750 views.

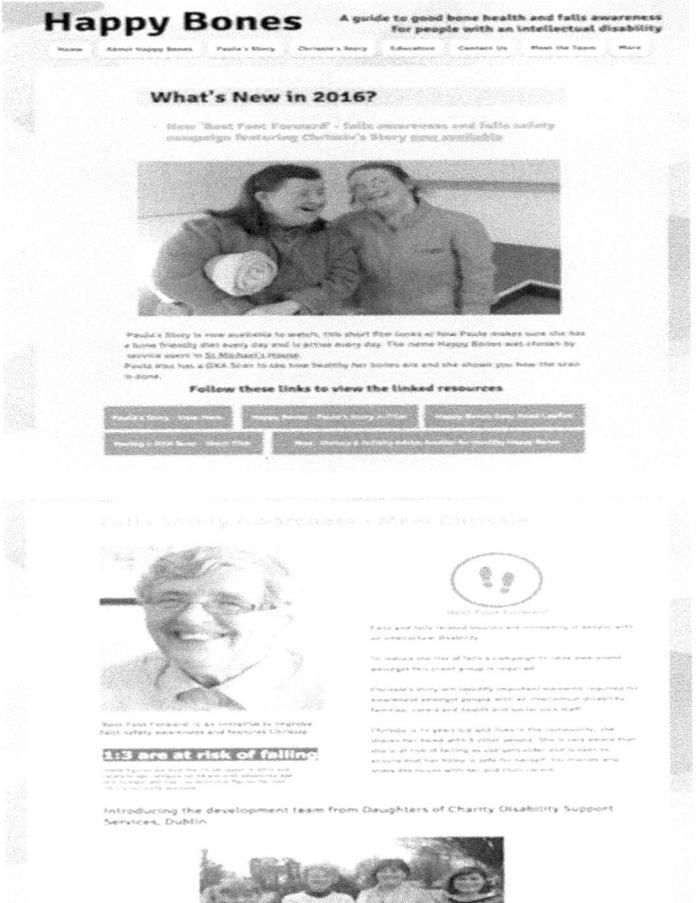

Figure 2: Happy Bones education resource to promote bone health and falls awareness in Intellectual Disabilities

3. Conclusion

In addition to access and dissemination of the program, since its deployment in 2012, Forever Autumn as an educational programme has been implemented in more than twenty four Residential Care Settings across Ireland. It has also has been nominated and awarded a National Irish Healthcare Centre Award as a Department Initiative on Fall Prevention. The FACOP© has a membership of 75 healthcare professionals from eight disciplines and national and international website visits as seen in Figure 3 while Figure 4 highlights the visits to the more recently developed Happy Bones© website.

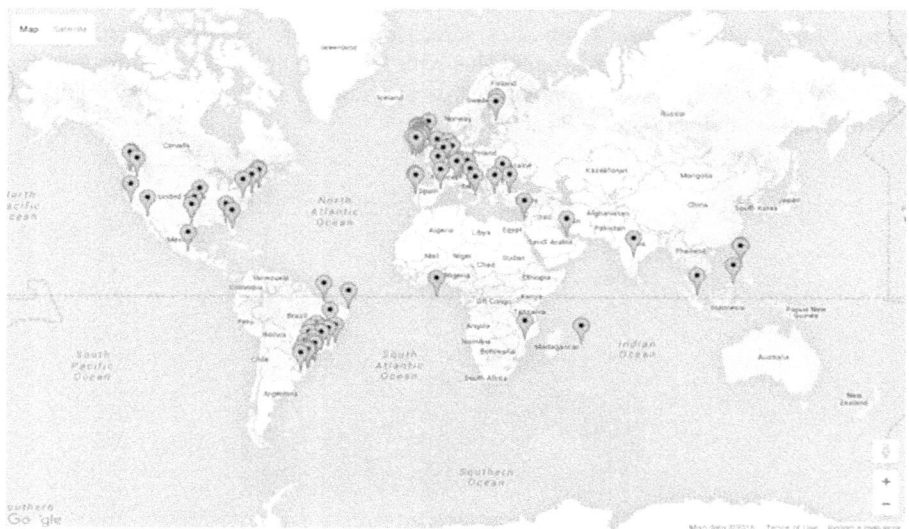

Figure 3 International Perspectives – Forever Autumn Community of Practice Web Site 2015/2016

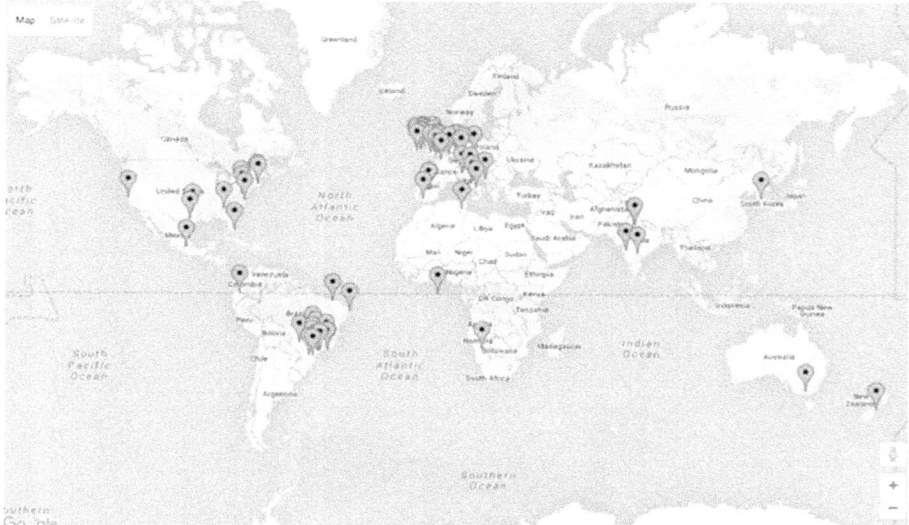

Figure 4: International Perspective – Happy Bones Web Site 2015/2016

The knowledge skills and attributes framework as defined by ICN and NMBI for ANP provides a clear structure to advance knowledge with experience to innovate and create educational programs for other similar eHealth initiatives. Additional evidence of this approach using a second Giant of Geriatric Medicine – incontinence, has produced an effective eLearning programme - Implementing and Supporting Holistic Continence Awareness [23].

The role of the ANP and its associated competency set as explained in this paper can provide a strong action learning strategy to organize and deliver eHealth educational programmes for effective healthy ageing in place. Future research includes creating additional eHealth educational programs to tackle the remaining Giants of Geriatric Medicine and also revising existing design templates for healthy ageing across all age groups in the life span.

References

[1] World Health Organisation World Report on Ageing and Health (2015)
     http://apps.who.int/iris/bitstream/10665/186463/1/9789240694811_eng.pdf?ua=1
[2] McEvoy P. (2014) Chronic Disease Management. Radcliffe, London.
[3] Isaacs B. 1992. *The challenge of geriatric medicine*. Oxford. Oxford University Press.
[4] Nursing & Midwifery Board of Ireland. Evaluation of Clinical Nurse and Midwife Specialist and Advanced Nurse and Midwife Practitioner Roles in Ireland (SCAPE) FINAL REPORT (2010) Available at https://nursingmidwifery.tcd.ie/assets/research/pdf/SCAPE_Final_Report_13th_May.pdf
[5] Nursing & Midwifery Board of Ireland (2016) http://www.nmbi.ie/Registration/Advanced-Practice#sthash.ycLe92uK.dpuf
[6] National Health Service (2014) Using Data and Technology to Transform Outcomes for Patients and Citizens. A Framework for Action. Retrieved from https://www.gov.uk/government/publications/personalised-health-and-care-2020 on 13 January 2015
[7] Corbin J. and Strauss A. A Nursing Model for Chronic Illness Management upon the Trajectory Framework. Scholarly Inquiry for Nursing Practice, 1991, 5, 155-174
[8] Hussey P., Kennedy MA. eHealth A Global Priority, pp35-53, In An Introduction to Nursing Informatics, 4th edn (Hannah K., Hussey P., Kennedy MA. & Ball M. eds), Springer, London, (2014)
[9] Pearce C., MacDougall C., Bainbridge M. & Davidson J. (Ensuring Clinical Utility and Function in a Large Scale National Project in Australia by Embedding Clinical Informatics into Design Pages 28 – 32
[10] Hussey PA. and Kennedy MA. (2016) Instantiating informatics in nursing practice for integrated patient centred holistic models of care: a discussion paper (pages 1030–1041) http://onlinelibrary.wiley.com/doi/10.1111/jan.2016.72.issue5/issuetoc;jsessionid=A4051608C539E5E DE06CD709087D8A15.f02t02
[11] Nursing & Midwifery Board of Ireland Scope of Nursing and Midwifery Practice Framework Practice 2015 Available at http://www.nmbi.ie/Standards-Guidance/Scope-of-Practice
[12] Canadian Nurses Association Framework for the Practice of Registered Nurses in Canada https://www.cna-aiic.ca/en/becoming-an-rn/the-practice-of-nursing
[13] Standards for competence for registered nurses Nursing and Midwifery Council https://www.nmc.org.uk/globalassets/sitedocuments/standards/nmc-standards-for-competence-for-registered-nurses.pdf
[14] World Health Organisation National eHealth Strategy Toolkit 2012 Available at http://www.who.int/ehealth/publications/overview.pdf
[15] Uys L. (2003) COMPETENCY in nursing. WHO Collaborating Centre for Education of Nurses and Midwives in Community Problem Solving School of Nursing University of Natal Durban, South Africa World Health Organization Geneva. Available on line http://reprolineplus.org/system/files/resources/WHOCompetency_in_Nursing.pdf
[16] Styles MM. & Affara FA. (**1997**). International Council of Nurses on regulation: Towards a 21st century model. Geneva, Switzerland
[17] Schober M., Affara F. International Council of Nurses: Advanced Nursing Practice Blackwell Publishing 2006
[18] Instruction Design Models and Theories: Action Learning Model https://elearningindustry.com/action-learning-model

[19] Spencer A. & Hussey P. Knowledge Networks in Nursing, pg. 427- 438 In An Introduction to Nursing Informatics, 4th edn (K. Hannah, P. Hussey, M.A. Kennedy, & M. Ball eds), Springer, London, (2014)
[20] Bone health in the park website www.bonehealth.co
[21] Forever Autumn Community of Practice website www.foreverautumn.co
[22] Happy Bones website www.happybones.ie
[23] Implementing and Supporting Holistic Continence Awareness website www.ishca.net

© 2017 IMIA and IOS Press.
This article is published online with Open Access by IOS Press and distributed under the terms
of the Creative Commons Attribution Non-Commercial License 4.0 (CC BY-NC 4.0).
doi:10.3233/978-1-61499-738-2-119

Competency Recommendations for Advancing Nursing Informatics in the Next Decade: International Survey Results

Charlene RONQUILLO[a], Maxim TOPAZ[b], Lisiane PRUINELLI[c],
Laura-Maria PELTONEN[d], and Raji NIBBER[a]

[a] *School of Nursing, University of British Columbia, Canada*
[b] *Harvard Medical School and Brigham Women's Health Hospital, Boston MA, USA*
[c] *School of Nursing, University of Minnesota, MN, USA*
[d] *Nursing Science, University of Turku and Turku University Hospital, Finland*

Abstract. The IMIA-NIstudents' and emerging professionals' working group conducted a large international survey in 2015 regarding research trends in nursing informatics. The survey was translated into half-a-dozen languages and distributed through 18 international research collaborators' professional connections. The survey focused on the perspectives of nurse informaticians. A total of 272 participants responded to an open ended question concerning recommendations to advance nursing informatics. Five key areas for action were identified through our thematic content analysis: education, research, practice, visibility and collaboration. This chapter discusses these results with implications for nursing competency development. We propose how components of various competency lists might support the key areas for action. We also identify room to further develop existing competency guidelines to support in-service education for practicing nurses, promote nursing informatics visibility, or improve and facilitate collaboration and integration with other professions.

Keywords. Nursing informatics, future trends, informatics competencies

1. Introduction

Following the 11th International Congress on Nursing Informatics (NI2012) in Montreal, Canada, the International Medical Informatics Association – Nursing Informatics (IMIA-NI) Student and Emerging Professionals (SEP) Working Group was founded. To date, the SEP has been successful in bringing together students in nursing informatics (NI) from around the world to engage in collaborative activities, including research.

The SEP members engaged in 2015 in discussions about the future development of NI as a specialty field. Group members were interested in learning more about the current state of NI and how to best facilitate the advancement of the field. This led to a collaborative international study conducted by the SEP in the Autumn of 2015, which aimed to gather the perspectives of nurse informaticians from around the globe on current trends and future priorities for NI.

In this chapter, we present an overview of the nursing informatics (NI) international trends survey that was focused on the thematic analysis of the question:

"What should be done (at a country or organizational level) to advance nursing informatics in the next 5-10 years?" In our previous study, we identified five key areas for action including research, practice, education, collaboration, and visibility [1]. This chapter discusses these results with implications for nursing competency development. The potential overlap and support for these key areas for action provided by existing national and international NI competency recommendations are also explored. Finally, we offer recommendations on how to achieve the best results in the five key areas for action, supported by various national and international NI competency and education initiatives.

2. Nursing Informatics: a survey of current and future trends

2.1. Study methods

The SEP developed and distributed an international survey, which focused on current and future trends in NI. The questionnaire was created based on contemporary NI literature [2, 3] and recommendations from NI experts in the field. The questionnaire was translated from English into Arabic, Korean, Mandarin, Portuguese, Spanish, and Swedish. The translations were conducted by native speaking nurses with a background in NI. The translations were validated by at least two other NI professionals. The questionnaire had the following demographic questions: city, country, highest degree received, position (clinical or academic), professional background and years of NI experience, and a set of 18 questions regarding the current or future state of NI. This chapter focuses on the open-ended question: "What should be done (at a country or organizational level) to advance nursing informatics in the next 5-10 years?"

The study received a supportive ethical statement from the ethics committee of the University of Turku in Finland, where it was coordinated. The survey was distributed online through Google forms. Any nurse or other allied health professional with experience in NI in the clinical setting or in academia was eligible to respond. We used snowball sampling and 18 SEP members from fourteen countries distributed the survey through their networks. The nurses who translated the original survey question translated the responses to the open-ended question into English for analysis. Data were collected from August to October in 2015.

2.2. Thematic analysis

All responses were saved into an Excel® spreadsheet and each answer was independently analyzed with thematic content analysis by two of the authors (CR, MT). This qualitative descriptive approach was used to identify, analyze, and report themes in qualitative data [4]. Each answer was examined independently by both authors and assigned one or more initial theme. These themes were then discussed by the two authors and a consensus of five major themes was reached. Thereafter, both authors re-examined their analyses based on these identified major themes and they reached agreement regarding each answer [4]. The results were reviewed by two other authors (LP, LMP) for validation.

3. Survey respondents

Out of 402 total survey participants, 272 (67.7%) responded to the question regarding recommendations on the advancement of NI. Responders were from 31 different countries in Asia, Africa, North and Central America, South America, Europe, and Australia. The majority of respondents were nurses (87.8%) with Bachelors (28.25%), Masters (39.75%), and PhD (28.75%) degrees. Clinical roles ranged from staff (33%), middle management (25.8%), upper management (16.4%), or other (24.8%). Training in NI varied: 57.8% of respondents did not receive formal education in NI, 32.9% received formal NI education, and 9.3% were current students or received education in another informatics field. Those identifying with academic roles included students (22.9%), teachers/instructors (16.9%), and professors (36.4%).

4. Study results

Five key themes for action were identified through the thematic analysis: 1) Education and training; 2) Research; 3) Practice; 4) Visibility; and 5) Collaboration and Integration. Figure 1 presents a word cloud of the most common words that appear in responses to the open-ended question on the next steps to advance nursing informatics. A brief summary of the key themes for action is provided in the following sections. For a more detailed discussion of these key themes, please refer to the original paper [1].

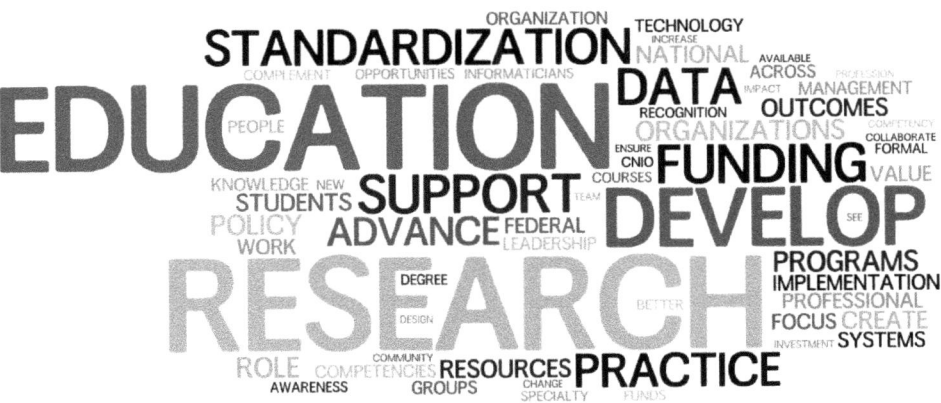

Figure 1. Word cloud of the most common words that appear in responses to open-ended question on the next steps to advance nursing informatics.

4.1. Education and training

Survey participants frequently mentioned the need for better training and specialized NI education. There are many strong advocates for incorporating NI education into all levels of nursing learning (Bachelors-Masters-PhD level programs) and professional development training. Inclusion of informatics content was recommended as a required component of undergraduate nursing curriculums, staff nurses' training and continuous education, and for nurses in leadership and administrative roles. Others further highlighted the need for further development of specialized NI education in nursing for those who wish to pursue advanced NI specializations.

4.2. Research

Participants suggested that further investments should be made to advance NI research as this can generate more evidence on the benefits of NI approaches, e.g., improved patient safety or providing more efficient care. Participants identified significant topic areas as priorities for the future including big data science, standardized terminologies, education and competencies, clinical decision support, mobile health, usability, patient safety, data exchange and interoperability, patient engagement, and clinical quality measures [5]. Participants also recommended increasing NI specific research funding to advance the discipline.

4.3. Practice

Participants suggested that better health care quality and an increased availability of nursing-specific information systems are critically needed across the board, regardless of high or low adoption of health information systems. Participants also emphasized the importance of thinking beyond acute care and keeping patient outcomes at the center, rather than focusing on profession-specific terminology and issues. Usability was another key area identified as needing advancement. Another sub-theme was the need to establish and support specialist health informatics roles across multiple levels within organizations. For instance, the importance of having leadership roles in nursing informatics such as Chief Nursing Information Officers (CNIO) was highlighted as a way of ensuring the inclusion of nursing practice perspectives and considerations in the design and implementation of health information technologies.

4.4. Visibility

Participants pointed to the need to increase the awareness and knowledge of what NI is across practice, organizational, and policy levels, as well as to the public. Responses suggested that an important aspect of improving the understanding and perceptions of NI is demystifying it within the field of nursing as well as other disciplines. The ability to articulate the relevance and advantages provided by NI in health systems is an area for further development, identified by respondents. Many also pointed to the increased efforts that should be invested to ensure NI representation and leadership in high-level decision-making.

4.5. Collaboration and Integration

Participant recommendations centered on establishing a common voice across the field of nursing, with the aim of placing patient outcomes at the center. Others have advocated an integrated approach across all health informatics fields, where nursing informatics is harmonized with medical and other informatics sub-specialties. Overall, these thoughts reflected two key sub-themes around: 1) the integration and inclusion of all health professions as integral components of health information systems; and 2) the need for collaboration across health informatics disciplines in high-level strategic planning, design, development, implementation, and evaluation of health information systems. Participants also pointed to opportunities for national and international collaboration and facilitating the exchange of expertise, knowledge, and resources across nursing organizations, clinical practice, and academia, as additional key areas for action.

5. Nursing informatics competency recommendations to support the survey results

5.1. Recommendations for NI education

There are numerous historical and recently developed efforts that aim to address the survey recommendations on promoting NI education. So far, the focus on NI capacity building through entry-level nursing education programs seems to be a dominant approach. For example, the Technology Informatics Guiding Educational Reform (TIGER) led to the TIGER Informatics Competencies Collaborative (TICC) model in 2010. The TICC was developed to function as informatics recommendations for all nurses and comprised of basic computer competencies, information literacy and information management (see section B chapter 3 for a more detailed discussion of the TIGER competencies). In agreement with our survey results, TIGER suggests that NI education should span across all levels of nursing learning, from baccalaureate to doctoral level. The TICC model focuses primarily on the competency needs of nursing students, practicing nurses, and advanced and expert skill levels relating primarily to practice. However, we suggest that the development of competency requirements for advanced and highly specialized NI education levels (i.e., doctoral level competencies) are areas for future development, as these are not currently well addressed in established competencies.

Beyond TIGER, there are several other attempts at developing country-level NI education recommendations both for entry-level nursing practice and as continuing education efforts for experienced nurses. For example, the Canadian Association of Schools of Nursing (CASN) Entry to Practice Nursing Informatics Competencies' recommendations target both students and faculty needs related to the use of information technologies [6]. CASN developed the entry-to-practice nursing informatics competencies so that faculty can have a better understanding of what would be expected of the nursing students upon graduation. CASN also developed resources and a toolkit for faculty to support integrating informatics competencies into current nursing education curriculums [7]. The CASN focus on education and knowledge needs not just at the nursing student level but also of nursing faculty (i.e., those who are responsible for ensuring these competencies are met by student nurses) addresses the survey recommendation of incorporating NI as a required component of undergraduate nursing curriculums. Specifically, addressing the needs of faculty ensures that infrastructure is built in order to deliver NI education to students in a way that can be sustainable. Similarly, one goal of the TIGER education and faculty development collaborative [8] is to encourage foundational investment in NI research, curriculum development, NI practice, and IT adoption. Detailed discussions of country-level NI education efforts in Brazil and South America, China and Asia-Pacific, Taiwan, the Netherlands can be found in section B, and in section B chapter 1 for New Zealand, the United States of America, England, Australia, Finland, and Canada.

The final recommendation from the survey relates to the further development of specialized NI education at advanced education and leadership levels, and for those who wish to pursue advanced NI specializations. An initiative led by the AMIA task force on the Knowledge, Education, and Skillset Requirements of Chief Clinical Informatics Officers, addressed this through provision of recommendations for skillsets needed in informatics and different education and training requirements for CNIO roles [9]. The report pointed to the need of a doctorate level training with leadership focus for CNIO positions. Specifically, the report highlighted that doctorate level education should prepare nurses for leadership roles spanning beyond the substantive aspects of NI, such as development and evaluation of programs, advocacy, conducting research, and understanding the financial aspects of NI. An important group that have been identified are nurse leaders and executives, who may not necessarily have NI substantive expertise but are responsible for making decisions around NI infrastructure, technology procurement, and the like. Existing competency recommendations suggest that nurse leaders should ideally have sufficient substantive informatics knowledge to thoughtfully inform decision-making about information systems in institutions. However, they do not necessarily need to be NI specialists themselves (see section D chapter 1 for a detailed discussion of Informatics Competencies for Nurse Leaders). Recognizing this important group, an instrument to assess NI competencies of nurse executives and leaders have been recently developed and is shown to be valid and reliable (see section D chapter 2).

Students at the Masters level are envisioned to become experts in informatics lingo and foundational concepts delineated by the ANA's Nursing Informatics Scope and Standards of Practice [10]. Masters level training can be a foundational first step developing advanced NI leaders, as graduates will be well-positioned to serve as nurse informaticians in clinical analytics, system configuration, IT training, and other tasks around the system development lifecycle, with the potential to build on this expertise towards higher level decision-making positions. Ideally, such educational preparation will initiate the continued development of competencies and capabilities for both CNIO-type roles and other nurse executive roles that oversee information systems decisions to serve on corporate tables and participate in high-level decision-making.

5.2. Recommendations for NI research

To address the survey recommendation of conducting more NI research, continued development of NI researchers with sufficient research skills is a foundational requirement. The research priorities identified by participants highlight the need for continued development in "traditional" quantitative and qualitative research methods, but also point to the need for researchers' development and training in emergent methods. For instance, big data analytics has seen substantial emergence as a key research priority in future years and requires innovative research methodologies and approaches. Specifically, clinical knowledge and multidisciplinary skills on data management and research methods are needed to develop cutting-edge research models where big data science can be incorporated into nursing research (see section C chapter 3 for a more detailed discussion of big data analytics). Another example is natural language processing, which requires the development of new sets of skills and expertise to best make use of narrative nursing data. Development of these methodological skills can also facilitate making use of standardized nursing terminologies in EHRs that can be mined to gain important insights into nursing care and nursing-specific outcomes. As demonstrated by a recent systematic review, this type of NI research is limited, to date, with only ten of forty-five studies identified to have used of standardized nursing data from EHRs in research and those limited to only two countries (USA and South Korea) [11].

A proposed research agenda for NI in 2008-18 highlight genomic healthcare and the role of environmental factors in health, data visualization, predictive modeling, and development of middle-range NI theories, among other topics as areas where priorities should be focused [12]. Similarly, the most recent international survey examining priorities for research in NI identified two highly ranked areas of importance for research: 1) development of systems to provide real time feedback to nurses; and 2) assessment of the impact of HIT on nursing care and patient outcomes [14]. The diversity and complexity of the topic areas mentioned above further underscore the importance of the development of skills in NI research. The importance of competencies in analytic and research methods appears to be an enduring aspect of NI research, as highlighted in earlier work [13].

The need for skills in NI research is supported by the work of Staggers et al. [14], who divide nurses into four levels: beginning nurses, experienced nurses, informatics specialists, and informatics innovators. They derived a research-based list of 281 competencies for entry-level and experienced informatics nurse specialists. The competencies of experienced nurses, informatics specialists and informatics innovators all include some knowledge of nursing research from using computer applications for nursing research to advanced responsibilities such as developing conceptual frameworks and techniques in NI research. Finally, it is suggested that the highest levels of expertise (i.e. informatics specialists and informatics innovators), should have the skills in obtaining research funding [14]. We did not identify competencies aimed specifically at developing skills that will highlight the benefits of NI approaches and increase NI specific research funding. Further competency development work should examine the necessary skills such as advocating for NI specific research funding and knowledge mobilization or translation science.

5.3. Recommendations for NI practice

The survey findings highlighted the need for better inclusion of nursing practice perspectives in the design and implementation of health information technologies. This finding is underpinned by two key assumptions: 1) that nurses have opportunities to participate; and 2) that nurses will have sufficient understanding of health information systems in order to participate. Staggers et al.'s [14] competency list supports the second assumption related to the need for a foundational understanding of NI in order to participate – it includes nurses' knowledge and skills to take part of system development and implementation processes.

Addressing the second assumption is critical as specific skillsets are needed to implement and adopt evidence based information systems, educate other nurses on clinical technology, transform health care through the use of information technology, and translate policy into practice and delivery towards the aim of improving clinical outcomes. Indeed, this importance is illustrated by the various efforts towards providing continuing education and specialized NI training geared towards practicing nurses, including in Brazil the United States, Finland, Australia, New Zealand, China, and Taiwan (see section B chapters 1 and section B for detailed descriptions). However, it is important to highlight that the goal of increasing practicing nurses' foundational understanding of NI is only possible by addressing the first assumption that it is reliant on – ensuring nurses' have opportunities to participate and engage with NI in practice. Further, efforts to establish a baseline understanding of NI for all nurses is arguably only possible through advocacy for the need of these specialized efforts and commitment to investment of resources by nurse leaders in health care organizations. One way this can be ensured is through the establishment of specialist health informatics roles across multiple levels in organizations (e.g., CNIO, NI specialists, etc.).

The remaining survey findings around the need to increase nursing-specific information systems, thinking beyond acute care, broadening the focus beyond profession-specific terminology and issues, and issues related to usability of systems appear to have limited overlap with existing competency recommendations. Increasing the development and availability of nursing-specific information systems can arguably benefit from competencies related to advocacy and leadership development among NI professionals, in order to voice the importance of including such systems in health regions. Competency guidelines around working as part of multidisciplinary teams with various perspectives and expertise is another area of development that should be considered, perhaps in future iterations of existing competency recommendations. Finally, skills and knowledge related to NI in the context of public and community health are additional areas that can benefit from further focus and investigation. For instance, initial efforts can be focused on identifying public and community-health specific NI competencies across multiple levels of education and nursing experience, similar to what has been outlined in acute care (e.g., from baccalaureate nursing level to continuing professional nursing education) and identifying unique needs and requirements of nurses in these contexts related to usability.

5.4. Recommendations for increasing NI visibility

As NI visibility varies significantly across institutions and countries, advancing visibility and articulating the value of NI in health care systems relies on competencies related to leadership development and advocacy. Approaches to developing these competencies can, for example, include formal training in well-designed programs, board examinations and certifications, and the development of specialized NI roles [9]. A more detailed discussion of some these approaches in various countries can be found in section B chapter 1 and section B. In line with our survey finding, the need to invest in efforts to promote NI visibility has been acknowledged in the TIGER Leadership Collaborative report [15]. They recommend the development of programs for nurse executives that emphasize the importance of IT and empowers the user of health IT [15].

An important step in demystifying NI and increasing its visibility within nursing can involve targeting nursing students at early stages of education, which is what many of the competency recommendations focused on. Beyond targeting basic nursing education, CASN entry-to-practice competencies touch on the notion of visibility and inclusion of the nursing voice in health IT development, design, and implementation. For example, a CASN competency indicates that users of health information systems should "recognize the importance of nurses' involvement in the design, selection, implementation, and evaluation of applications and systems in health care" [6].

5.5. Recommendations to promote and facilitate collaboration and integration

A clear understanding that the nurse informaticians role is imperative for collaborative work, both inside institutions and across settings and countries. Nurse informaticians collaborate with interdisciplinary teams to promote all aspects of health and develop better models of care for better outcomes. The need for specific competencies at the organizational level exists as nurses' knowledge and skills in NI vary between setting and countries. There are numerous efforts to address NI competency needs through the development of country specific competency guidelines in connection with the TIGER initiative, for example in Germany, Austria, Switzerland [16], Ireland [17], Australia [18], New Zealand [19] and Portugal [20]. Efforts like that, supported by TIGER, are undoubtedly important first steps. However, the focus of TIGER and other competency recommendation efforts focus primarily on NI competencies as related to the acute setting, and more specifically, as related to the use of EHRs. Therefore, there is room for the development of broad, high-level general guidelines to steer NI education and practice at the (inter)national level that could support the development of standardized NI competencies across countries in contexts that are broader than acute care. In terms of broader efforts to promote collaborative working, perhaps one approach is to look at recommendations not limited to NI. For instance, this may include looking to the Interprofessional Education Collaborative Practice (IPEC) [21] competencies, as described in section A chapter 1.

Recommendations to promote cross-organizational collaboration are mentioned by some existing competency recommendations. For example, The TIGER Leadership Collaborative report promotes the sharing of best practices through health IT and promotes alignment of health organizations with the American Nurses Credentialing Centre Magnet Recognition Program®, as a way to demonstrate excellence [15]. However, the skills needed by NI professionals in order to do so are not well described. Identification of these competencies, likely related to multidisciplinary collaboration and organizational dynamics, are areas requiring further development and should be considered in future NI competency recommendations. This can then provide the foundation to address the key recommendations made by the survey participants, namely, enabling the possibility for developing integrated approaches across nursing and the health informatics fields and have a unified voice in high-level strategic planning, design, development, implementation, and evaluation of health information technologies. Perhaps one possibility is drawing from recent efforts toward broadening of the work of TIGER to increase the focus on interprofessional and international issues, with the TIGER International Competency Synthesis Project, currently underway (see section B chapter 3).

6. Limitations

Our study has several limitations. First, the generalizability of our survey results is limited due to small numbers of participants from certain geographic regions (e.g. from African countries). The snowball sampling approach was also limited by the reach of our respective networks and only reached certain organizations and practitioners while others were not included. In addition, we only reviewed some NI competency recommendations and might have missed others.

7. Conclusions

We conducted one of the largest international surveys to identify key areas for action in order to advance the field of NI. Qualitative analysis of the survey themes identified five specific key areas: education and training; research; practice; visibility; and collaboration and integration. In this chapter we suggested how components of various national and international guidelines and competency lists (e.g., TIGER, CASN, etc.) might support the key areas for action. We also identified room for further development of existing competency guidelines to support advancement of several key areas. For example, although several competencies exist to guide the education of nursing students, in-service education for practicing nurses and their competencies remain largely unaddressed. In comparison to efforts aimed at addressing NI education and practice, our search identified the need for further development to identify competencies necessary to promote NI research, NI visibility, or ability to collaborate and integrate with other professions and across institutions and countries. Although our survey results have limitations, we believe that the key areas and our suggestions can be used to evaluate and further develop NI competency efforts.

References

[1]   Topaz M, Ronquillo C, Peltonen LM, Pruinelli L, Sarmiento RF, Badger MK, et al. Advancing nursing informatics in the next decade: recommendations from an international survey.   13th International Congress in Nursing Informatics: NI2016; June 25-29, 2016; Geneva, Switzerland2016.
[2]   Saba VK, McCormick KA. Essentials of Nursing Informatics. 6th Edition ed: McGraw-Hill Medical; 2015.
[3]   Topaz M, Ronquillo C, Pruinelli L, Ramos R, Peltonen LM, Siirala E, et al. Central Trends in Nursing Informatics: Students' Reflections From International Congress on Nursing Informatics 2014 (Taipei, Taiwan). CIN: Computers, Informatics, Nursing. 2015;33(3):85-9.
[4]   Vaismoradi M, Turunen H, Bondas T. Content analysis and thematic analysis: Implications for conducting a qualitative descriptive study. Nursing & health sciences. 2013;15(3):398-405.
[5]   Peltonen LM, Topaz M, Ronquillo C, Pruinelli L, Sarmiento RF, Badger MK, et al. Nursing informatics research priorities for the future: recommendations from an international survey. 13th International Congress in Nursing Informatics: NI2016; June 25-29, 2016; Geneva, Switzerland2016.
[6]   Nagle L, Borycki E, Donelle L, Frisch N, Hannah K, Harris A, et al. Nursing informatics: Entry to practice competencies for registered nurses. Ottawa, Canada; 2012.
[7]   Nagle LM, Crosby K, Frisch N, Borycki EM, Donelle L, Hannah KJ, et al., editors. Developing entry-to-practice nursing informatics competencies for registered nurses. Nursing Informatics; 2014.
[8]   TIGER Initiative. Transforming education for an informatics agenda: TIGER Education and Faculty Development Collaborative. 2009. 2012.
[9]   Kannry J, Fridsma D. The Chief Clinical Informatics Officer (CCIO). Journal of the American Medical Informatics Association. 2016;23(2):435-.
[10. American Nurses Association. Nursing informatics: Scope and standards of practice. 2nd Edition ed. Maryland, USA: American Nurses Association; 2014.
[11] Park JI, Pruinelli L, Westra BL, Delaney C, editors. Applied nursing informatics research-state-of-the-art methodologies using electronic health record data. Nursing Informatics; 2014.
[12] Bakken S, Stone PW, Larson EL. A nursing informatics research agenda for 2008–18: Contextual influences and key components. Nursing Outlook. 2008;56(5):206-14. e3.
[13] Goossen W. Nursing informatics research. Nurse Researcher. 2001;8(2):42-54.
[14] Staggers N, Gassert CA, Curran C. A Delphi study to determine informatics competencies for nurses at four levels of practice. Nursing research. 2002;51(6):383-90.
[15] TIGER Initiative. The TIGER Initiative Foundation The Leadership Imperative: TIGER's Recommendations for Integrating Technology to Transform Practice and Education 2009.
[16] Hübner UH. Towards defining nursing informatics competencies in Austria, Germany, and Switzerland. 2015.

[17] Hussey P. Healthcare Informatics Society of Ireland: Response to TIGER international group on the creation of informatics competencies relating to nursing and midwifery. 2015.
[18] Australian Nursing & Midwifery Federation. National informatics standards for nurses and midwives. 2015.
[19] Day K, Honey M. Country specific competencies for New Zealand. 2015.
[20] Cardoso A, Souza P. Nursing informatics core competencies for Portugal. 2015.
[21] Interprofessional Education Collaborative Expert Panel. Interprofessional Education Collaborative Expert Panel. Washington, DC: Interprofessional Education Collaborative; 2011.

Section C

Trends in Health and Nursing Informatics

Forecasting Informatics Competencies for Nurses in the Future of Connected Health
J. Murphy et al. (Eds.)

doi:10.3233/978-1-61499-738-2-133

Semanticification in Connected Health

Anneke GOOSSEN-BAREMANS [a] , Sarah COLLINS[b] and Hyeoun-Ae PARK[c]
[a] *Results 4 Care, Amersfoort, The Netherlands*
[b] *Partners Healthcare System, Wellesley, MA United States*
[c] *Seoul National University, Seoul, Republic of Korea*

Abstract. The purpose of the implementation of nursing terminologies is to capture and process meaningful health data wherein facts about patients and nursing care can be recorded and inferences for nursing care, patient outcomes and associations with all care delivered by the interprofessional team can be made. This paper describes the clinical information landscape, implementation of semantic content, and competencies required for nurses. Health data can be outlined in a high level clinical information ecosystem where nursing terminologies can be represented for implementation. This ecosystem consists of both the structural and dynamic aspects of the support of care.

Keywords. Semantics, Terminology, Data Models, Ontology, Competencies.

1. Introduction

Nursing has traditionally been using words to describe patients' problems and nursing care and developing nursing terminologies to support their documentation. Today, approximately a dozen nursing and health terminologies are being used to support nursing practice documentation. During the 1990s, nursing focused on the development and application of these terminologies. Until recently, the adoption of Electronic Health Records (EHR) has been slow so there remain many paper-based patient records. Therefore, application of these nursing terminologies was not consistent in the EHR systems. The initial applications of nursing terminologies primarily focused on recording and classification of nursing data. However, since the adoption of EHRs is reaching a critical mass and the application of nursing terminologies becomes matured, the need for interoperability, in particular semantic interoperability of nursing data and patient outcomes, has increased. Semantic interoperability is the ability for systems to exchange data and perform automated processing to interpret that data based on unambiguous and shared meanings. Semantic interoperability is essential for an EHR to be considered "meaningful", in that the system can process, analyze, interpret, and exchange data based on the shared and pre-defined meaning of the data.

The Nursing Terminology summits taught us that there could not be one "best" terminology solution [1]. In order to achieve semantic interoperability, it is important to use a standardized terminology. However, also the underlying information model of the EHR system is critical to assure unambiguous meanings of shared data. Current information model initiatives include Health Level 7 (HL7) v3 Reference Information Model based messages and templates, ISO 13606 and OpenEHR Archetypes from European standards (EN) and International Standards Organization (ISO), and EN ISO TS 13972 Detailed Clinical Models (DCM) [2]. HL7 Terminfo project is a project dealing with how to use the information model in relationship with terminologies. This Terminfo project will be described in this contribution.

However, as health IT is evolving, nurses need to learn how to deal with not only meaningful EHRs, but also with medical devices connected to the EHR, Patient Portals or Personal Health Records (PHRs), and apps that can be connected to either an EHR or PHR system. In the near future, the Clinical Information Ecosystem is going to be much broader than that of today's EHR and PHR. It is going to be a fully connected health landscape, including mobile devices and connected Health Apps. In this context, we refer in this chapter to these systems broadly as Clinical Information Ecosystems.

To effectively leverage electronic patient data for automated processing, analytics, and information exchange based on the defined meaning of the data for nursing practice, a minimum level of competency related to semantic interoperability is needed for nurses. According to COACH [3] competencies are the knowledge, skills, attitudes, and judgments required to perform activities safely and effectively in a broad range of environments and practice settings.

2. Background

Health information can be outlined in a high level clinical information ecosystem in which nursing terminologies can be represented for EHR implementation. This ecosystem consists of both the structural and dynamic aspects of the support of care. The structural aspect of the ecosystem (including devices, apps and systems) consists of data entry, services, databases, linkage to knowledge, communication and secondary use of data from a data warehouse. The dynamic aspect supports the workflow and decision support, among others.

The purpose of the implementation of nursing terminologies is to have a meaningful ecosystem wherein data about patients and nursing care can be documented so inferences for nursing care and patient outcomes can be made. In the next section, each component of the ecosystem wherein a terminology can be implemented is described with the value, advantages and disadvantages of such an implementation.

A terminology by itself has limited impact, however, the implementation of a terminology within an EHR system adds value to the ecosystem. One implementation approach is to bind a terminology to clinical information models, such as archetypes, detailed clinical models and HL7 templates.

3. The Clinical Information Ecosystem

To achieve semantic interoperability and enable the exploitation of clinical/ health data, it is important to use terminology in EHR systems consistently [4]. Unfortunately, it is common that independent healthcare systems use different EHR systems or terminology systems or that the local configurations of the same EHR system and terminology implementation are not aligned. During the SNOMED CT Implementation Showcase in 2014 the SemanticHealthNet proposed a semantic infrastructure consisting of an ontology framework and a set of ontology patterns (semantic patterns) that use the proposed framework as reference [4]. A more detailed discussion of ontologies and their relationship with terminologies is included in section 4.3.

With the addition of PHRs, devices and apps to the clinical information ecosystem, one can imagine that the problem of semantic interoperability dramatically increases. If we want to connect medical devices, apps, and the PHR with the EHR system, having a semantic framework for only an EHR system will not solve the problems of semantic interoperability.

A terminology is not effective on its own. However, when it is appropriately implemented as an essential part of an EHR system, it delivers value as part of that system [5]. To meet user requirements, a terminology needs to be connected to an EHR system for data capture and retrieval in ways that maximize the power of the terminology. To realize the value, a terminology used in an EHR system must be fit for the purpose it intends to serve (e.g. representing clinical information, retrieving data, carrying out analytics and statistics etc.). However, implementation of a terminology in only the EHR system will not be enough to meet future requirements of the Clinical Information Ecosystem.

Within the Clinical Information Ecosystem, identified purposes for implementation of a terminology include [6]:

1. Data entry: capturing and displaying clinical information in EHRs, PHRs, medical devices and apps (terminology used as an interface terminology);
2. Storing (clinical) information (terminology used as a code system);
3. Retrieving clinical information (terminology used as an indexing system);
4. Communicating in a meaningful way (terminology facilitating data exchange);
5. Integrating heterogeneous data (terminology used as a common terminology);
6. Secondary use of data for querying, analyzing and reporting data (terminology used as an indexing system);
7. Linking systems, devices and apps to knowledge resources (terminology used as a dictionary); and
8. Representing new types of clinical data (terminology used to extend knowledge) [5].

Figure 1 illustrates the implementation of terminology services in a clinical information ecosystem.

During the delivery of nursing care, data are captured in EHRs to record assessments and interventions, and support planning and decision making for the patient. These data are stored in a database and may be displayed to the interprofessional care team and patient through various user interfaces and patient-facing portals. The stored data, either saved directly in the EHR database or sent to the data warehouse, can be used for reporting and analytics as well as quality improvement and research. Increasingly, PHR technologies, such as Patient Portals operated and managed by a health system, allow patients to enter and send wellness and health data for integration into the EHR. Expanded efforts are underway to integrate these data with the broader health ecosystem. Patients use devices and apps to monitor their wellness and these data will increasingly be transferred to and stored in PHR and EHR data bases. These types of personal device data can be displayed to the patient through the device, app, or PHR system.

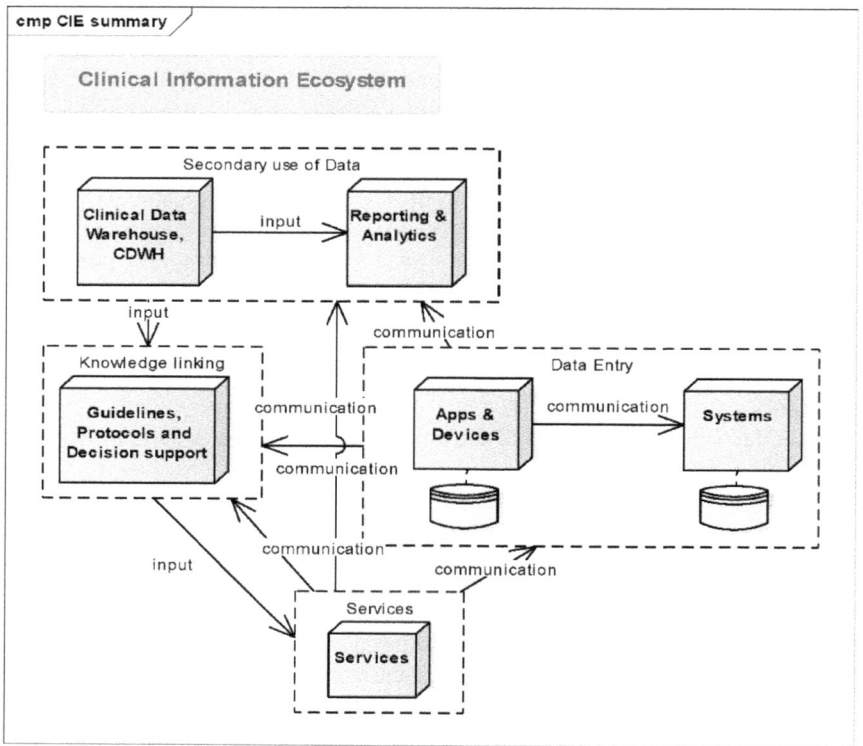

Figure 1. Clinical Information Ecosystem, an abstract.

Patient data can also be sent to different systems for the purpose of communication to maintain continuity of care. These models of information exchange are continuously expanding and include communication between EHRs and between PHRs and EHRs. Emerging models of information exchange use Apps to support continuity of care for specific use cases. These information exchange capabilities are bi-directional typically leveraging Application Programming Interfaces (APIs) from the EHR, PHR, or Apps to send or receive patient data externally. External data received into any clinical information system should have adequate metadata (i.e., data about the data such as its provenance) to ensure that data displayed to clinical end-users and patients, and any inferences made for analytics or clinical decision support can be validated and tracked.

Clinical content in a clinical information system (stored as clinical data elements) can be linked to knowledge assets via terminology and standards such as Infobutton services to support the implementation of evidence based nursing care and to provide context-specific knowledge to the nurses at the point of care [7].

Data in clinical information systems can lead to development of new knowledge through reporting, research and analytical processes. Data-driven new knowledge can be used to refine data definitions for unambiguous data capture, optimize user interface visualizations and data entry displays, and evaluate and design clinically relevant decision support systems.

Terminology services are needed to support the functionality described above and displayed in Figure 1. The use of standardized terminology in clinical information systems is critical to communicate nursing practice activities with the multidisciplinary team and capture the impact of those activities on patient outcomes. The representation of nursing knowledge in a meaningful way across disciplines and care settings is needed to meet the requirement to deliver quality patient care, and achieve efficacy, efficiency and cost containment. Recording nursing care within EHR systems enables data-driven demonstration of the impact of nursing care on patient outcomes and validates the significance of nursing practice [8].

The key challenge in demonstrating the impact of nursing care on the patient outcomes is to identify specific concepts of nursing activities within a vast set of clinical documentation, capture those data in a structured coded way, and link those data with other relevant concepts of coded clinical activities and outcomes. A clinically validated, semantically rich, controlled terminology enables identification of concepts for clinical assessments, activities and outcomes within documentation.[5] Linking those concepts to terminologies supports meaningful use of EHR data [5]. SNOMED CT is one of the concept oriented clinical terminologies that enables identification of clinical concepts for both continuity of care and the secondary use of patient data.

4. Semantic content

4.1. Terminology

The core process for nursing information management consists of the following components [9].

- assessment: the systematic and dynamic collection and analysis of data about a client;
- diagnosis: the clinical judgment of a nurse about the client's response to actual or potential health conditions or needs;
- outcomes and planning: together with the client the nurse sets measurable and achievable short- and long-term goals (based on the assessment and diagnosis) for this client;
- implementation: nursing care or interventions are provided for the purpose of continuity of care, and documented in the client's EHR;
- evaluation: the client's status and the effectiveness of the nursing care is continuously evaluated, the care plan modified as needed.

To document the elements of this process with sufficient detail, standardized data elements with bindings to terminologies, as well as free text capabilities to capture unique data descriptions that were not anticipated or modeled in advance are required. Significant efforts to capture nursing process data have focused on nursing terminologies, which will briefly be described.

Currently there are at least 12 terminologies that support nursing practice. These include: NANDA (North American Nursing Diagnosis Association- Nursing Diagnoses), NIC (Nursing Interventions Classification), NOC (Nursing Outcomes Classification), Nursing Management Minimum Data Set (NMMDS), (Systematized Nomenclature of Medicine Clinical Terms) (SNOMED CT), Nursing Minimum Data Set (NMDS), ABC Codes, Logical Observation Identifiers Names and Codes

(LOINC®), Omaha System, Clinical Care Classification, Preoperative Nursing Data Set (PNDS), and the International Classification for Nursing Practice (ICNP) [10]. With the development of more advanced Natural Language Processing (NLP) tools the meaning (also known as semantics) from free text data entry can be extracted [11]. However, use of NLP also requires the use of terminologies to assign the proper semantics. The choice of a terminology depends on several factors, such as breadth and depth of coverage for the intended content domain, licensing costs, and local expertise. Other considerations include availability of electronic versions for a terminology service and proper coding in the terminology.

While the choice of a particular terminology can be made at a local level to meet the particular needs of an organization, to enable data exchange and semantic interoperability across systems and meaningful associations with patient data documented by other clinical professions, the terminology selected should be mapped to reference terminologies such as SNOMED CT, ICNP or LOINC. SNOMED CT is a well-recognized standard clinical reference terminology owned and distributed around the world by the International Health Terminology Standards Development Organization (IHTSDO). ICNP is an integral part of the global information infrastructure that informs health care practice and policy to improve patient care internationally [12]. LOINC is a database and standard coding system for tests, measurements, and observations. Data exchange standards such as HL7 use LOINC to electronically transfer diagnostic test results between different electronic health systems. Concepts from some nursing terminologies are mapped to SNOMED CT and LOINC. These mappings include concepts for nursing observations and assessments, nursing problems/diagnosis, nursing interventions, and patient outcomes.

Nursing observations are a type of nursing assessment. The assessment concepts include two components: 1) questions and 2) answers. Each component is handled with a unique approach for terminology mapping. An example of a nursing assessment question is: "What is the patient's pain location?" and may be included as a data element name on an EHR form or flowsheet. A nursing assessment answer for this example question may be: "upper right abdominal quadrant" and can be referred to as the value, which may be part of a coded value set for anatomical location. Nursing assessment questions can be coded using LOINC and nursing assessment answers can be represented as values using SNOMED CT. Therefore, in this example the question "What is the patient's pain location?" can be coded using LOINC and the answer value "upper right abdominal quadrant" can be coded using SNOMED CT. This approach can be recommended for all nursing assessment concepts with one exception: this is not done when a validated instrument is included in LOINC in its entirety (e.g., questions and answer values are included and coded). More work is needed to identify and standardize recommended value sets for representing assessment "answers" in SNOMED CT for a particular clinical assessment and this work should leverage Nursing Terminologies that are mapped to SNOMED CT.

SNOMED CT includes a Nursing Problem List Subset and nursing terminologies, such as ICNP, that are already mapped to SNOMED CT and follow the existing SNOMED CT process for adding additional problem concepts to this subset to drive consistency of use [13]. Nursing interventions can be modeled with SNOMED CT. This model is consistent with ISO 18104 and ICNP both of which separates out activities by type of action (e.g., assess, teach).

There is varied level of adoption in the use of both LOINC and SNOMED CT for outcomes. If a patient outcome is a measurement, this can be coded using LOINC as a LOINC observation. If it is an observed assessment that a patient state has improved, this can be coded using SNOMED CT. Many validated instruments that are proprietary cannot be put into standard terminologies that are freely available, such as LOINC. This is a barrier to interoperability and subsequently, has downstream impacts. Further work is needed to identify best approaches for using these proprietary instruments in conjunction with/mapped to standard terminologies, particularly LOINC.

According to the ICN [14] ICNP can also be used for the documentation of nursing care based on the nursing process. ICNP provides a dictionary of terms and expressive relationships that can be used to describe and report nursing practice in a systematic way. Data collected using ICNP can be mapped to SNOMED CT[15, 16]. The ICN [14] states that the resulting information is used reliably to support care and effective decision-making, and inform nursing education, research and health policy. It is intended for the nursing domain and thus it is difficult to share with other domains. However, the potential benefits of a consistent approach to capture nursing data can be used to deliver the value of nursing care.

4.2. Clinical Information models

Various examples of clinical modeling initiatives exist. Clinical modeling work started with the two level modeling approach for EHRs by Rector et al [17]. Rector et al split the basic EHR system functions and the specification of medical content into two levels, each handling parts of the EHR functionality. Level one describes the basic system functions and level two specifies the required clinical content. Examples are described below.

4.2.1. HL7 v3 Reference Information Model

Health Level Seven (HL7) is an international standards development organization. The mission of HL7 is to provide standards for the exchange, management, and integration of data that support clinical patient care, including nursing care, and the management, delivery, and evaluation of healthcare services [18]. The Reference Information Model of HL7 (HL7 RIM) version 3 is a comprehensive, non-discipline-specific, object-oriented information model of patient care and of the providers, institutions, and activities involved [19]. The HL7 RIM represents health care concepts for which information needs to be available, processed, and exchanged [19]. The HL7 RIM uses an object oriented approach, the Unified Modeling Language (UML) [20]. The HL7 RIM has six core classes and their relationships: "Entity" (e.g., any person, institution, material), "Role" (a role the entity normally has, such as "Patient" or "Physician"), "Role Link" (a feature to relate different roles to each other, such as patient to nurse), "Participation" (the actual behavior of an entity in a specific act) and "Act" (any health related activity). The "Act" class also has an "Act_Relationship" class, which allows combining and relating Activities as necessary. The Act_Relationship class allows instances of Act to be "collected" in sections such as: 1) *container* (vital signs contains heart rate, blood pressure, etc.), 2) *rules* (care plans, protocols, etc.), and 3) *judgments* (such as medical or nursing diagnoses). Several RIM classes also have subclasses. The

RIM classes have specific characteristics such as the attributes as time, codes and values. Typical UML features as Relationships between classes, Specialization (adding characteristics) and Cloning (duplicating of classes and their characteristics) make it possible to create representations that are meaningful for healthcare. To ensure overall consistency of the standard, these features must be handled carefully, in order to allow interoperability of data within and between different information systems [19]. Further, the classes have behaviors, allowing the dynamics of care to be expressed. Integrating nursing data standards with the HL7 RIM helps to apply information modeling in the nursing domain [21]. For instance, the representation of the nursing process as a dynamic series of phases includes the following [21]:

- Data collection or assessment
- Diagnosis
- Identification of goals or desired outcomes
- Planning of interventions
- Implementation of treatment and care
- Evaluation.

Another initiative is the Fast Health Interoperable Resources (FHIR) ® from HL7 [22]. Unlike HL7 RIM v3 approach, FIHR does not require all content to be specified according the standard, but allows extensions. The assumption is that FIHR standardizes 80% of the use cases and clinical data. FIHR uses technology supporting apps and devices, such as Restful interfaces and JSON. A caveat is that FIHR allows non standardized content, this might be a risk for interoperability [22].

4.2.2. CEN ISO 13606 and OpenEHR Archetypes

The group of EN ISO 13606 standards (consisting of 5 parts) developed within CEN and approved by ISO, are designed to achieve semantic interoperability in the EHR communication [23]. Its overall goal is to define a rigorous and stable information architecture for the communication of a part or all of the EHR about a single subject of care (patient) between EHR systems, or between EHR systems and a centralized EHR data repository [23].

The Dual Model architecture defines through a Reference Model a separation between the core system functions and basic, and specific clinical knowledge based on archetypes.

The development of archetypes is carried out since the approval of the EN ISO 13606 standard. Archetypes are both 'computable definitions of single, discrete clinical concepts' and 'computable expressions of a domain content model in the form of structured constraint statements [24]. Archetypes are based on a Reference Model, either the EN ISO 13606 Reference Model or the OpenEHR Reference Model [25,26], and created using Archetype Definition Language, an abstract human-readable and computer-processable syntax [24].

The clinical concept definitions in an archetype are described in an artifact that allows operations in compliant EHR systems [27]. Each archetype is designed to be inclusive of all attributes about a given concept. The openEHR Clinical Knowledge Manager [28] is an online resource to develop and store archetypes and on which a formal content review process can be initiated and carried out. There are minor differences between the 13606 and OpenEHR archetypes. These differences are preliminary based on the fact that EN13606 is a few years old and stable, and OpenEHR has moved further based on experiences in projects. However, the EN13606 Association has recently worked on implementations of the 13606 archetypes.

4.2.3. EN ISO TS 13972 Detailed Clinical Models (DCM)

Currently there are several initiatives around detailed clinical modeling. These will be described briefly. Intermountain Health Care creates and deploys Clinical Element Models (CEM) in their electronic patient records. The University of Minnesota Big Data Science Conference is focused on detailed clinical modeling for nursing flow sheet data [29]. The ISO 13606 archetypes/ OpenEHR archetypes are described in the paragraph above, however it is important to mention their large collection of available archetypes, which are a kind of clinical models. HL7 creates various v3 RIM compliant templates for use in for example the Care Record message and Clinical Document Architecture (CDA). Researchers in Korea developed and published a large set of Clinical Contents Models (CCM), and clinical models on nursing assessments/observations and nursing actions/interventions. Korea uses these DCMs with nursing content to generate structured nursing narratives using natural language generating systems. These structured nursing narratives are imported into electronic nursing records system so nurses can use nursing documentation [30,31]. Unfortunately, they are developed in Korean and not available on the web. The Netherlands created about 300 DCMs based on Unified Modeling Language (UML).

The ISO Technical Specification 13972 on Detailed Clinical Models expresses the requirements for clinical models independent of the logical modeling approach or the technical implementation formalism of choice [32]. It is beyond this contribution to discuss all of the TS 13972, but the core will be presented here. The core requirements for clinical models are: name for each data element in the model, definition of the date element, unique binding of the data element to a unique code from a standardized terminology, data type, if data type is a physical quantity then the unit must be added, if data type is a coded element with a value set, then the value set must have an identifier and each value must have an unique code. Hence, several examples of clinical modeling mentioned above qualify as DCM.

4.2.4. CIMI models

The Clinical Information Modeling Initiative (CIMI) is currently an HL7 work group providing a common format for detailed specifications for the representation of health information content [33]. The goal of CIMI is to achieve semantically interoperable information that is created and shared in health records, messages, and documents.

The CIMI approach takes into account a basic meta model in UML (BMM) to define clinical models. CIMI further uses the archetype definition language (ADL) from ISO 13606 / openEHR, but upgraded this to version 2.0 which overcomes many of the limitations of older archetypes. For instance, ADL 2.0 now includes code bindings to terminologies.

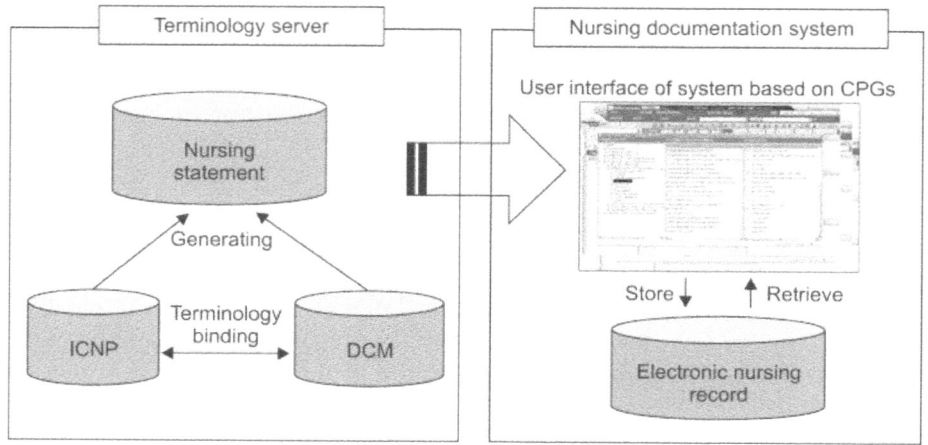

Figure 2. Relationship between Terminology and Detailed Clinical Models (Park et al, 2012).

4.3. Why do we need ontologies in healthcare applications?

An ontology is an explicit formal specification of the terms in the domain and relations among them [34]. It includes explicit description of concepts in a domain of interest (classes), properties of each concept describing various features and attributes of the concept (slots), and restrictions on slots (facets) [35]. Classes are the focus of ontologies. We develop ontologies to separate domain knowledge from the operational knowledge, to analyze domain knowledge, to share common understanding of the structure of information, and to reuse domain knowledge.

Healthcare ontologies define concepts that are represented in healthcare – patients, their symptoms, their diseases, treatment and so on. An ontology is a comprehensive representation of relevant concepts, whether or not the data for each concept are always known to the clinician. For example, all patients have a diagnosis; however, the diagnosis may not be known or recorded. Standardized and structured vocabularies such as SNOMED CT and the semantic network of the Unified Medical Language System are examples of healthcare ontologies.

Ontology is different from coding systems and information models. Rector, Qamar, and Marley [36] described the relationship between ontologies, coding systems, and information models in their paper titled "Binding Ontologies & Coding systems to Electronic Health Records and Messages". Ontology is our understanding and conceptualization of the world. A conceptualization is an abstract, simplified view of the world that we wish to represent. Ontologies are based on an "Open World Assumption" (which means essentially that Anyone can say Anything about Any topic).

Information models of data structures describe and constrain how the data is stored in database and transmitted in messages. Information models of data structures are based on a Closed World Assumption (CWA). This means that any statement that is not known to the message or database are considered false as opposed to unknown. If an information model has a field for diagnosis, that field cannot be missing for any given patient, but it can be empty, that is there is no value inserted.

Codes are symbols to be used in data structures. Although coding systems are derived from ontologies, coding systems in contrast contain an enumerated list of codes to choose from. Rector, Qamar, and Marley [36] propose a code binding interface between the models of meaning (i.e., the ontology), the model of codes (i.e., the terminology) and the information model.

Thus, based on the relationship between ontologies, coding systems and information models proposed by Rector, Qamar, and Marley [36]: We first need to create an ontology to describe our conceptualization (or understanding) of the world. Second, we derive an enumerated list of codes called code system from the ontology. Third, we use the codes in healthcare applications databases and messages which are data structures. Last, we validate the binding between the ontology, the information model, and the code.

Creating an ontology includes: defining classes in the domain, arranging the classes in a taxonomic (subclass–superclass) hierarchy, defining slots and describing allowed values for these slots, and filling in the values for slots for instances. A knowledge base can be created by defining individual instances of these classes and by filling in specific slot value information and additional slot restrictions.

Given the complexity and scale of healthcare knowledge today, the use of ontology-based reasoning will become essential in applications such as health terminologies, clinical knowledge management for clinical decision support, and big data analytics. See for instance section C chapter 3. Ontologies are being used for health terminology development, integration and evaluation. Schuster and Stuckenschmidt used ontologies for terminology integration [37], Rector, Brandt, and Schneider [38] used an OWL representation of SNOMED CT to unearth errors in SNOMED CT hierarchies. ICD-11 is being developed using OWL to allow consistency checking and linking to other biomedical terminologies and ontologies.

Ontologies are being used for modeling the medical knowledge contained in Clinical Practice Guidelines (CPGs) and Care Pathways (CPs). Zheng et al.[39] introduced guideline representation ontologies for evidence-based healthcare practice. An ontology in this context is a specification of conceptualizations that constitutes evidence-based clinical practice guidelines. A guideline representation ontology would define a set of medical decisions and actions (concepts), as well as a set of rules (relationships) that relate the evaluation of a decision criterion to further reasoning steps or to its associated actions. Several ontology-based approaches to modeling CPGs and CPs have been proposed in the past including PROforma, HELEN, EON, GLIF, and SAGE. Peace and Brennen [40] used ontology design methods to create a nursing representation of family health history.

An ontology can be used to address the semantic challenges presented by big data sets created from diverse sources in healthcare [41]. The availability of big data in healthcare has introduced complexities that we must address, not only in terms of semantics and analytics but also in terms of data management, storage, and distribution. Currently, the capabilities to analyze, and manage big data sets have underscored the limitations of our analytics capabilities supported by relational database management systems. An ontology-based approach to data analytics provides a practical framework to address the semantic challenges presented by big data sets.

4.4. Interdependencies between Terminology and Clinical Information Models

There is a dependency between terminology and clinical information models. The way the terminology is used in, for instance an EHR system, is depending on the information model and the structure of that EHR system. Park and Hardiker [42] describe in their article that attempts to standardize the capture, representation and communication of clinical data rely upon three layers of artifacts to represent the meaning of clinical data. They describe that semantic interoperability solutions include generic reference models, data models and terminologies. These three layers for representing clinical data include reference models such as HL7 Reference Information Model (RIM), and the EHR Reference Model; agreed clinical data structure definitions such as openEHR archetypes, HL7 v3 templates, and DCMs; and clinical terminology systems, e.g LOINC, ICNP and SNOMED CT.

Semantic interoperability is the exchange of information in such a way that the receiving application is able to retrieve and process the communicated information in the same way as that information is managed in its original application. The meaning of the information must be represented in an agreed upon, consistent and adequate format to meet this requirement [43].

The IHTSDO is representing the interdependencies between SNOMED CT and structural EHR models, like ISO 13606, OpenEHR and HL7 v3, as pieces of the puzzle that fit together because of the use of terminology binding, see Figure 3.

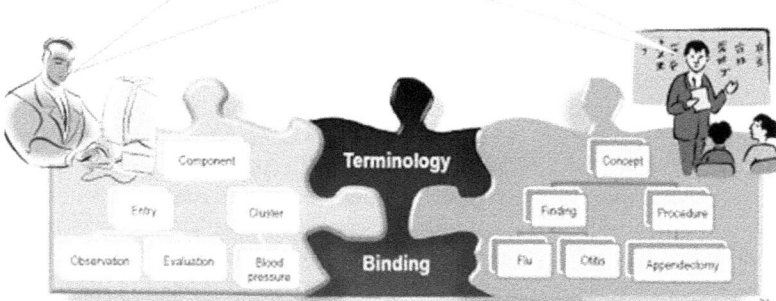

Figure 3. Interdependencies between SNOMED CT and structured EHR models [44] (used with permission).

Terminfo focuses on a specification of an approach to resolve issues related to the interface between HL7 information models and various terminologies or code systems. This example is often used in other information modeling approaches such as archetypes and DCMs. The terminology binding is the focus of the HL7 Terminfo project, because similar information can be represented in varied and potentially complex ways (Figure 3). The HL7 Terminfo project develops specific guidance on the use of SNOMED Clinical Terms (SNOMED CT) concepts in the HL7 Version 3 communication standards [45].

Since an ontology is a model of a domain describing objects that inhabit it, all described data models can be thought of as ontologies. Hence, ontologies range from the most expressive one that describes business concepts and processes (the conceptual model) to less expressive and progressively moving from describing business semantics to describing physical structures of the data as it is stored in the databases (the logical and physical data model). A physical model can be thought of as an ontology of a particular database. Thus, in clinical modeling, a collection of different ontologies is usually required.

5. Integration of clinical knowledge, information models and terminology

5.1. Application in connected health

Nursing care, as part of healthcare, can be seen as knowledge intensive and information is a key factor within, and enabler of, the nursing care system. To place accurate, complete information at the hands of nurses when and where it can best support quality patient care, and to enable sharing and use information in a meaningful way throughout the healthcare system is the purpose of an EHR system. The objective is better outcomes for patients, populations and the healthcare system as a whole [46].

An example of implementation of nursing relevant terminology in HL7 version 3 consists of perinatal data that are exchanged for both clinical and reporting purposes [47]. Use cases from perinatology were modeled using the Health Level 7 version 3 Reference Information Model (HL7 RIM). The results of this project include descriptions of care processes and communication of information. Several domain information models for perinatology were drawn up. These models allow healthcare professionals to recognize their communication, content and work. Examples include the referral from a midwife to a gynecologist as a process, the obstetric assessment as a large structure, the Apgar score as an assessment scale, and birth weight as an individual observation. These examples represent data models from the business level to the most detailed level.

Another example is presented by Hübner et all [48] who created the eNursing summary, based on the HL7 version 3 Clinical Document Architecture (CDA). The eNursing Summary was developed on the basis of several internationally accepted concepts, such as various nursing data sets, the nursing process, and the ISO 18104 Reference Terminology Model for Nursing [49]. Examples of the content include nursing assessments, diagnosis, goals, procedures and outcomes. Further, it includes the HL7 version 3 representation of a patient biography, references to legal documents, the homecare status and medical information as the medical diagnosis and medication. The eNursing Summary project standardized the content during several phases in which nursing experts were involved to validate the structure and content of the summary. Finally the eNursing Summary was evaluated within a large network of healthcare organizations.

The integration of clinical knowledge, information models and terminology enables the implementation of evidence based care represented in clinical guidelines, specified in information models and bound to terminology. Park et al [50] tested the feasibility of an electronic nursing record (ENR) system for perinatal care that was based on detailed clinical models (DCMs) and clinical practice guidelines (CPGs). Also in this work, components of DCM were mapped to ICNP. This study was carried out in five steps: 1) generation of nursing statements using DCMs, 2) identification of the relevant evidence, 3) linkage of nursing statements with the evidence, 4) development of a prototype ENR system based on DCMs and CPGs, and 5) evaluation of the ENR prototype system, including decision support. Figure 4 shows the elements of the ENR prototype system plotted in the overall EHR system design.

Standardization of elements in clinical guidelines enables the implementation of decision support [51]. In their SNOMED CT Showcase presentation, Lee & Cornet showed the elements in the clinical guideline which must be standardized, examples are Problem List and Encounter Diagnoses, Medications, Laboratory tests, and Laboratory test result values. This approach is another one than described by Park et al [50]. Park et al used the knowledge in clinical guidelines to develop DCMs from nursing statements derived from these guidelines. In the DCMs ICNP was used to bind the concepts in the DCM to terminology.

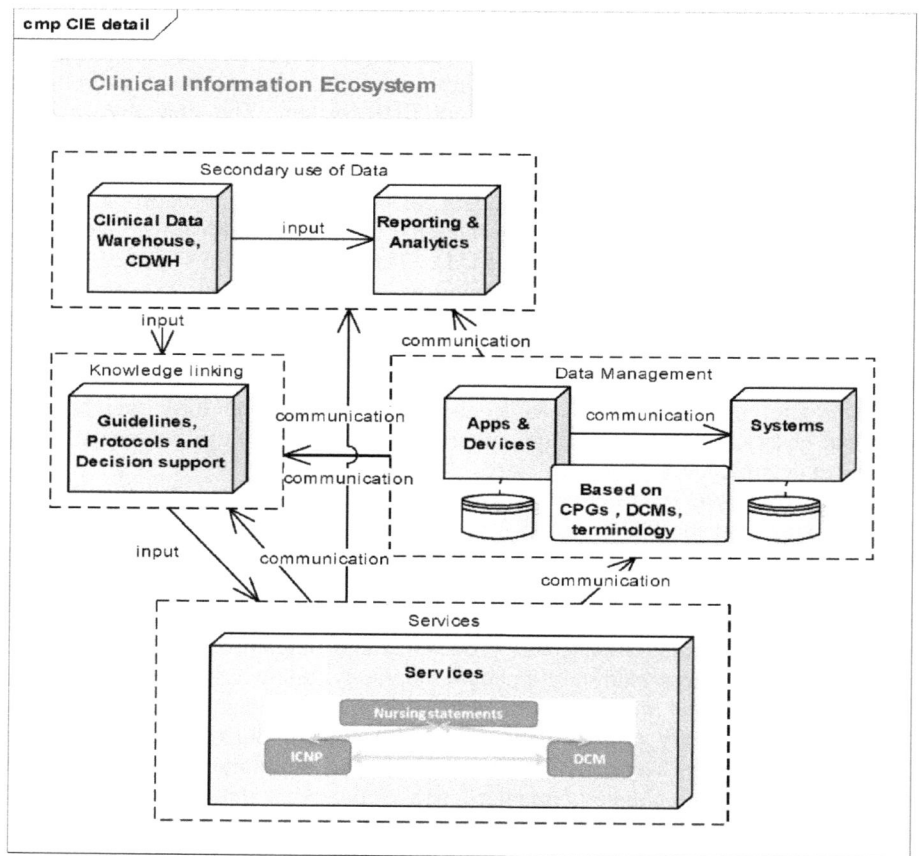

Figure 4. Clinical Information Ecosystem & Elements of use to the ENR.

5.2. Application in quality indicators for nursing care

In order to obtain quality indicators, data from different sources need to be combined. The relationship between quality indicators and terminologies, information models and ontologies concentrates on the semantics. If the meaning is not clear or imprecise it is not possible to calculate a quality indicator.

Dykes and Collins [52] described the prerequisites and challenges to measuring quality indicators for nursing care. A key challenge to measuring quality indicators for nursing is the ability to aggregate data across organizations for benchmarking and comparisons overtime. The number of resources that were required for measuring quality indicators when clinical data were captured on paper records was high; however, barriers still remain to process and analyze electronic data for nursing quality indicators. eMeasures are defined as the secondary use of electronic data to populate standardized performance measures [53] and can greatly facilitate this work. However, successful eMeasurement for comparisons within and across organizations overtime requires four components: 1) standardized, electronic performance measures; 2) the capture of structured, coded data in an EHR; 3) administrative and clinical workflows that facilitate consistent documentation or capture of the data needed to populate the electronic measures, and 4) standard approach to data capture and quality measurement across organizations for benchmarking [54].

Fowles et al, [55] with funding from the Commonwealth Fund, developed a typology for categorizing five broad types of eMeasures within increasing technical sophistication and scalability. While some nursing data may remain in narrative form in an EHR, nursing quality indicators can guide the types of nursing data that should be structured and coded using, for instance SNOMED CT and LOINC, and integrated into the nurses' workflow for consistent and reliable data capture.

6. Competencies

In order to participate in a professional manner in this challenging world, nurses on all levels do need to acquire the knowledge and skills essential for working in a connected health environment. The topic discussed in this paper, semantification of connected health, implies very specific competencies for nurses on all levels.

Nursing has a tradition in the development and use of nursing terminologies. However, connected health does require additional knowledge and skills about clinical system architectures and information modeling. This implies that education needs to go beyond nursing terminologies.

Nurses should be able to understand the architecture of connected health, the concepts used in such an architecture and their role towards making this architecture patient friendly and supportive for nursing care. In addition, the need for and importance of information modeling should become part of their knowledge and skills. However, being able to read such a model would be sufficient, unless nurses actually engage in EHR development.

The skills needed for semantics, information modeling, and ontology building are different from the skills needed for computer programming and systems administration. They include abstract thinking, conceptual design, user liaison, and communication compared to concrete thinking, hardware and software knowledge, and systems integration experience needed for the programming and systems administration.

While clinical modeling and ontology building are creative processes, and one's understanding and view of the domain will affect models and ontologies built; there are basic requirements for modeling and ontology building. These requirements include combination of domain knowledge and the ability to think abstractly and conceptually, to extract a domain's terms from vague and often conflicting natural language text, to demonstrate logical thought processes, and to communicate these concepts well, including through visual presentation.

The recommended competencies are summarized in Table 1. It is emphasized that as technology advances these competencies will too.

Table 1. Current State Competencies for nurses on semantics for connected health.

Level for competencies / Competencies	Entry level nurse	Advanced level nurse	NI specialists	Nurse leadership & informatics
Health terminology in general				
can discuss the Clinical Information Ecosystem	X	X	X	X
can compare the Clinical Information Ecosystem with the current situation on Health IT	X	X	X	X
can explain the importance of health information exchange between stakeholders (e.g professionals, consumers) systems and countries.	X	X	X	X
can explain the importance of standardized terminology in health information exchange	X	X	X	X
can verbalize the purposes for implementing a standard terminology	X	X	X	X
Nursing terminologies				
can record clinical/patient information in practice with the use of standard nursing terminology	X	X	X	
can explain the relationship of nursing concepts to quality, patient safety, nursing value and research	X	X	X	X
can describe the semantics of nursing data and the consequences of ambiguous data definitions	X	X	X	X
Data Modeling and ontology in general				
can explain the re-use or secondary use of stored clinical/patient data	X	X	X	X
can describe the different types of data, e.g unstructured data (free text), structured data (code list, physical quantity, interger)	X	X	X	X
can discuss the importance of clinical models and ontology in health information exchange.	X	X	X	X
can participate in the communication with stakeholders on a clinical model and the terminology binding in the clinical model		X	X	
can explain the need for add semantics of visualizations of clinical models.	X	X	X	X
can create the semantics and visualizations of clinical models.			X	
can explain the need for a conceptual design of clinical information system	X	X	X	X
can create a conceptual design for clinical information systems			X	
Use and application of terminology				
can discuss the differences in standarized terminologies according to their purposes		X	X	X
can describe the components of the clinical term (conceptualization), including its structure and its concepts, e.g Pulmonary cancer		X	X	X
can operate Natural Language processing to map recorded terms to terminology concepts		X	X	
Management of terminologies				
can explain the management lifecycle of terminology		X	X	X
can develop new terminology content in a given terminology		X	X	
can discuss the significance of data provenance for interoperability	X	X	X	X
can operate Natural Language processing to identify and validate terminology concepts		X	X	

7. Conclusion

The purpose of this chapter was to explore semantification of connected health content by describing the clinical information ecosystem and the semantic content as the relationship between clinical guidelines, information models, terminology and ontologies. It is important for nursing education to be aware of and have knowledge of this semantification of connected health. A distinction can be made between nurses, both on entry and advanced level, leadership and nurse informaticians. The competencies described in this chapter can be used to determine this distinction. If nurses want to be prepared for the future with connected health, they should strive to acquire these competencies.

References

[1] Ozbolt J. Terminology standards for nursing: collaboration at the summit. J Am Med Inform Assoc. 2000 Nov-Dec;7(6):517-22.

[2] Goossen W, Goossen-Baremans A, van der Zel M, (2010). Detailed Clinical Models: A Review. Healthc Inform Res. 2010 December;16(4):201-214. doi: 10.4258/hir.2010.16.4.201.

[3] Canada's Health Informatics Association, COACH (2012). Health Informatics Professional Core Competencies, COACH, Toronto, Canada.

[4] Martínez-Costa C., Schulz S. and Kalra D., (2014). A Semantic Infrastructure Towards Semantic Interoperability. SNOMED CT Implementation Showcase 2014 Presentation or Poster Abstract SemanticHealthNet.   Available   from: http://ihtsdo.org/fileadmin/user_upload/doc/showcase/show14/SnomedCtShowcase2014_Abstract_140 33.pdf

[5] SNOMED CT – Adding Value to Electronic Health Records. Available from: http://www.ihtsdo.org/resource/resource/248

[6] Bird L., SNOMED CT Implementation Approaches, IHTSDO, Copenhagen, 2016.

[7] HL7 Infobutton Standard. Available from: http://www.openinfobutton.org/hl7-infobutton-standard

[8] Lundberg C., Warren J., Brokel J., Bulechek G., Butcher H., McCloskey Dochterman J., Johnson M., Mass M., Martin K., Moorhead S., Spisla C., Swanson E. & Giarrizzo-Wilson S. (June, 2008). Selecting a Standardized Terminology for the Electronic Health Record that Reveals the Impact of Nursing on Patient Care. Online Journal of Nursing Informatics (OJNI), 12, (2). Available at http:ojni.org/12_2/lundberg.pdf

[9] American Nurses Association The Nursing Process. Available from: http://www.nursingworld.org/EspeciallyforYou/StudentNurses/Thenursingprocess.aspx

[10] American Nurses Association. Recognized Terminologies that Support Nursing Practice. Available from: http://www.nursingworld.org/MainMenuCategories/Tools/Recognized-Nursing-Practice-Terminologies.pdf

[11] Nadkarni PM, Ohno-Machado L, Chapman WW. Natural language processing: an introduction. Journal of the American Medical Informatics Association : JAMIA. 2011;18(5):544-551. doi:10.1136/amiajnl-2011-000464.

[12] International Council of Nurses (ICN) About ICNP. Available from: http://www.icn.ch/what-we-do/vision-goals-a-benefits-of-icnpr/

[13] Matney SA., Warren JJ., Evans JL., Kim TY., Coenen A., Auld VA., (2012). Development of the nursing problem list subset of SNOMED CT®. J Biomed Inform. 2012 Aug;45(4):683-8. doi: 10.1016/j.jbi.2011.12.003. Epub 2011 Dec 20.

[14] International Council of Nurses (ICN) ICNP® Definition. Available from: http://www.icn.ch/what-we-do/definition-a-elements-of-icnpr/

[15] Hardiker N. (ICN), Millar j. (IHTSDO. Using ICNP to enhance SNOMED CT®. Available from: http://www.icn.ch/images/stories/documents/pillars/Practice/icnp/Benefits_of_ICNP-SNOMED_CT.pdf

[16] International Health Terminology Standards Development Organisation (IHTSDO) ICN. Available from: http://www.ihtsdo.org/about-ihtsdo/partnerships/icn

[17] Rector AL, Nowlan WA, Kay S, Goble CA, Howkins TJ. A framework for modelling the electronic medical record. Methods Inf Med. 1993 Apr;32(2):109-19.

[18] Health Level 7 (HL7). Health Level 7 Web site: Mission statement. Available from: http://www.hl7.org/
[19] Health Level 7 (HL7). HL7 Version 3: Reference Information Model (RIM), Available from: http://www.hl7.org/implement/standards/product_brief.cfm?product_id=77
[20] Booch G, Rumbaugh J, Jacobsen I. The Unified Modeling Language User Guide. Boston, etc. Addison-Wesley, 1999.
[21] Goossen W., Ozbolt J., Coenen A., Park HA., Mead C., Ehnfors M., Marin H.. (2004). Development of a provisional domain model for the nursing process for use within the Health Level 7 RIM. J Am Med Inform Assoc., 11 (3): 186-194. http://www.jamia.org/cgi/content/short/M1085v1
[22] FHIR. Fast Healthcare Interoperability Resources. Available from: https://www.hl7.org/fhir/
[23] EN ISO 13606. Health informatics - Electronic Health Record Communication. Geneva, ISO, Brussels, CEN.
[24] OpenEHR Foundation, (2015). The open EHR Archetype Model. Archetype Definition Language ADL 2. Available from: http://www.openehr.org/releases/trunk/architecture/am/adl2.pdf.
[25] Beale T. Archetypes Constraint-based Domain Models for Futureproof Information Systems. Web documents 2000. http://www.openehr.org/publications/archetypes/archetypes_beale_web_2000.pdf Accessed 22 November 2010
[26] Beale T. (2003). Archetypes and the EHR. Stud Health Technol Inform.;96 (2003) 238-244.
[27] Hovenga E., Garde S., Heard S. (2005). Nursing constraint models for electronic health records: a vision for domain knowledge governance. Int J Med Inform. 2005 Dec;74(11-12):886-98.
[28] OpenEHR foundation. OpenEHR Clinical Knowledge Manager. Available from: http://www.openehr.org/ckm/
[29] Westra BL., Latimer GE., Matney SA., Park JI., Sensmeier J., Simpson RL., Swanson MJ, Warren JJ., Delaney CW., (2016). A national action plan for sharable and comparable nursing data to support practice and translational research for transforming health care. J Am Med Inform Assoc. 2015 May;22(3):600-7. doi: 10.1093/jamia/ocu011. Epub 2015 Feb 10.
[30] Park HA., Min YH, Kim Y, Lee MK, Lee Y, Development of detailed clinical models for nursing assessments and nursing interventions. Healthcare Informatics Research 17 (2011), 244–252.
[31] Min YH, Park HA, Lee JY, Jo SJ, Jeon E, Byeon N, Choi SY, Chung E. Automatic generation of nursing narratives from entity-attribute-value triplet for electronic nursing records system. Stud Health Technol Inform. 2014;201:452-60.
[32] ISO/TS 13972:2015 Health informatics -- Detailed clinical models, characteristics and processes. Available   from: http://www.iso.org/iso/home/store/catalogue_tc/catalogue_detail.htm?csnumber=62416
[33] Clinical Information Modeling Initiative (CIMI). Introduction to CIMI, Available from: http://opencimi.org/about_cimi and http://www.hl7.org/Special/Committees/cimi/index.cfm
[34] Gruber, T.R. (1993). A translation approach to portable ontology specification. Knowledge Acquisition 5: 199-220.
[35] Noy NF., Mcguinness DL.(2001), Ontology development 101: A guide to creating your first ontology. Available from: http://protege.stanford.edu/publications/ontology_development/ontology101.pdf
[36] Rector I.L., Rahil Qamar R. Marley T, Binding ontologies and coding systems to electronic health records and messages. Applied Ontology 4(1): 51-69 (2009)
[37] Schuster G., and Stuckenschmidt H. Building shared ontologies for terminology integration. KI-01 Workshop on Ontologies, Vienna, Austria. 2001.
[38] Rector AL., Brandt S. and Schneider T. "Getting the foot out of the pelvis: modeling problems affecting use of SNOMED CT hierarchies in practical applications." Journal of the American Medical Informatics Association 18.4 (2011): 432-440.
[39] Zheng, Kai, et al. "Guideline representation ontologies for evidence-based medicine practice." Handbook of Research on Advances in Health Informatics and Electronic Healthcare Applications: Global Adoption and Impact of Information Communication Technologies: Global Adoption and Impact of Information Communication Technologies (2009): 234.
[40] Peace J., Brennan PF. (2009) Formalizing nursing knowledge: from theories and models to ontologies. Studies in Health Technology and Informatics. 146: 347-51. PMID 19592863 DOI: 10.3233/978-1-60750-024-7-347
[41] Kuiler EW. (2014). From big data to knowledge: An ontological approach to big data analytics. Review of Policy Research. 31(4). DOI: 10.1111/ropr.12077.
[42] Park HA, Hardiker N, Clinical terminologies: a solution for semantic interoperability. Journal of Korean Society of Medical Informatics 15 (2009),1–11.
[43] Semantic interoperability of clinical information in Using SNOMED CT in HL7 Version 3; Implementation   Guide,   Release   1.5.   Obtained   in   August   2016,   from http://wiki.hl7.org/index.php?title=Background

[44] Markwell D., SNOMED CT as a component of Electronic Health Records (EHR), IHTSDO, Copenhagen, 2011.

[45] HL7 Terminfo project. Available from: http://www.hl7.org/Special/committees/terminfo/overview.cfm

[46] Buchanan R., Koehn M., Building the Business Case for SNOMED CT® Promoting and Realising SNOMED CT®'s value in enabling high-performing health system, 2014, Gevity

[47] Goossen WT, Jonker MJ, Heitmann KU, Jongeneel-de Haas IC, de Jong T, van der Slikke JW, Kabbes BL. Electronic patient records: domain message information model perinatology. Int J Med Inform. 2003 Jul;70(2-3):265-76.

[48] Hübner U, Flemming D, Heitmann KU, Oemig F, Thun S, Dickerson A, Veenstra M. The need for standardised documents in continuity of care: results of standardising the eNursing summary. Stud Health Technol Inform. 2010;160(Pt 2):1169-73.

[49] ISO 18104:2014 Health informatics -- Categorial structures for representation of nursing diagnoses and nursing actions in terminological systems. Available from: http://www.iso.org/iso/home/store/catalogue_ics/catalogue_detail_ics.htm?csnumber=59431

[50] Park HA., Min YH., Jeon E., Chung E.. Integration of Evidence into a Detailed Clinical Model-based Electronic Nursing Record System. Healthc Inform Res. 2012 Jun;18(2):136-44.

[51] Lee D, Cornet R. (2013). A Practical Approach to Meaningful Clinical Records with SNOMED CT. IHTSDO Implementation Showcase Friday, October 11, 2013.

[52] Dykes, P., Collins, S., (September 30, 2013) Building Linkages between Nursing Care and Improved Patient Outcomes: The Role of Health Information Technology. OJIN: The Online Journal of Issues in Nursing Vol. 18, No. 3, Manuscript 4

[53] National Quality Forum. (2013a). Electronic Quality Measures Available from: www.qualityforum.org/Projects/e-g/eMeasures/Electronic_Quality_Measures.aspx

[54] American Hospital Association. Quality Measurement Enabled by Health IT. Response to Agency Healthc Res Qual Req Inf 2012. Available from: http://www.aha.org/advocacy-issues/letter/2012/120919-cl-ahrqhitquality.pdf

[55] Fowles JB, Kind EA, Awwad S, Weiner JP, Chan KS, Coon PJ, et al. Performance measures using electronic health records : five case studies. 2008.

152   *Forecasting Informatics Competencies for Nurses in the Future of Connected Health*
J. Murphy et al. (Eds.)
© 2017 IMIA and IOS Press.
This article is published online with Open Access by IOS Press and distributed under the terms
of the Creative Commons Attribution Non-Commercial License 4.0 (CC BY-NC 4.0).
doi:10.3233/978-1-61499-738-2-152

Genetic and Genomic Competencies for Nursing Informatics Internationally

Kathleen A. MC CORMICK[a] and Kathleen A. CALZONE[b]
[a] *Principal/Owner SciMind, LLC*
[b] *Senior Nurse Specialist, Research, Center for Cancer Research, Genetics Branch,*
National Institutes of Health, National Cancer Institute

Abstract. The majority of health professionals now have genetic and genomic competencies and some are measured by certification standards. Nursing has a proud history of defining roles for nursing in informatics and genetics. In addition, the nursing professional organization, the American Nurses Association, has a Certification Center that has successfully achieved ISO 9001:2008 certification in the design, development, and delivery of global credentialing services which encompasses certification of advanced practice nurses in genetics. ISO 9001:2008 certification is the firmly established global standard for assuring stakeholders of an organization's ability to satisfy quality-related requirements. However, despite the addition of genomics into the Informatics Scope and Standards of Practice, there is a need to define the integration of the genetic, genomics and other omics competencies into the informatics domain, especially the Electronic Health Record. Currently, there are also international and interprofessional activities and organizations that have established or are identifying competencies in genetics and genomics. There remains a need for more international collaborations to build upon the current resources and strategies implemented by several countries, to learn from each other, support each other, and to collaborate to answer questions and reduce duplication of efforts.

Keywords. Competencies in genetics, genomics and omics, Healthcare Professionals, Consumers, Integration into Electronic Health Records, Certifications, International efforts in genetics and genomics, Opportunities for international collaboration

1. Introduction

Nursing has a proud history spanning over a decade in developing competencies for nurses and certification of advanced practice level nurses in genetics. To begin with, two definitions are important: 1) Genetics is the study of individual genes and their impact on relatively rare single gene disorders, and 2) Genomics is the study of all the genes in the human genome together, including their interactions with each other, the environment, and other psychosocial and cultural factors [1]. The impact of genetics and genomics information and technology has the potential to improve the quality of care and result in safer practices at lower costs. These are so important to the future of the nursing profession, that the American Nurses Association included the concept of genetics and genomics in the new Nursing Informatics: Scope and Standards of Practice, 2nd edition. The statement specifies that informatics nurses must be able to: "Incorporate genetic and genomic technologies and informatics into practice." and

"Demonstrate in practice the importance of tailoring genetic and genomic information and services to clients based on their culture, religion, knowledge level, literature, and preferred language" [1].

2. Rapid Advances in Genetics, Genomics, and other Omics

There have been rapid advances over the past 25 years since the sequencing of the human genome [2]. The global community has engaged in the identification of human genetic variation through several projects such as: establishing the Encyclopedia of DNA Elements (ENCODE) to identify genomic functional elements; completed the International HapMap Project to identify genetic variation associated with human diseases, developed The Cancer Genome Atlas (TCGA) to identify genetic variation associated with cancer and cancer sub-types; and established the international 1000 Genomes Project to catalogue human genetic variation. Other United States (US) supported projects include finding Mendalian disease genes and supporting drug discovery and genomic underpinnings to drug metabolism. Because of these advances, we are now witnessing the application of these discoveries in clinical care.

The National Human Genome Research Institute (NHGRI) in the US is placing increased emphasis on validation and implementation of genomics into healthcare, in addition to the biology of genomes [3]. Programs focus on cancer genomics, pharmacogenomics, genomic medicine, newborn genomic analysis, clinical genomics information systems, and rare and/or undiagnosed genetic disease diagnostics. Additionally efforts surrounding genomic translation continue to grow, such as the IGNITE (Implementing GeNomics In PracTicE) initiative aimed at conducting projects designed to translate genomic information into clinical care [4]. Across the healthcare continuum the influences of genetics and genomics can be found in preconception/prenatal care, newborn screening, disease susceptibility, screening/diagnosis, prognosis and therapeutic decision, and monitoring disease burden and recurrence. Several publications in nursing journals and books have identified the major advances relevant to nursing and patient care, achieving outcomes, and improving safety at a reduced cost [5-7].

The prospect of Precision Medicine was greatly accelerated with the launch of the Precision Medicine Initiative [2]. Since then the biology of genes and genomes and the translation to health care and nursing practice applications has continued to expand. In the United States and elsewhere around the globe, Precision Medicine has been identified as a priority with funding secured to conduct vital research including the generation of large scale cohorts that include not just biospecimens but robust clinical and lifestyle data. The US has increased funding to accelerate the use of genomic variation information in healthcare with specific emphasis on cancer treatments and resistance. In addition, over 1 million Americans will be recruited to consent to study their biospecimens, diet, lifestyle, and other health information that is linked to their electronic health record (EHR). Effective implementation, however, has brought attention to the need for appropriate policy and regulation of information, the adequate preparation of the healthcare workforce to understand and use this new evidence, and the informatics infrastructure needed to manage these data.

3. New Advances in Pharmacogenomics are now Impacting the Safety and Quality of Healthcare Outcomes.

There are now several guidelines, workflows, and algorithms for determining the pharmacogenomics effects of several medications, their effectiveness, and the potential for adverse reactions even when the medications are administered at the correct dose [8, 9]. An international database to provide knowledge of the pharmacogenomics findings, called the Pharmacogenomics Knowledge Base (PharmGKB) it contains the evidence from literature, curated by experts, and disseminated on human genomics variation and potential differences in drug metabolism and responses [10]. Building on this evidence, PharmGKB and the Pharmacogenomics Research Network established a collaboration called the Clinical Pharmacogenetics Implementation Consortium (CPIC) to produce guidelines. The goal is to establish evidence based guidelines that are open access, peer reviewed, provide detailed drug and clinical information, and are updatable as the evidence base evolves. CPIC guidelines are amenable to integration into Electronic Health Records using Clinical Decision Support (CDS). To date, 33 CPIC guidelines with sufficient evidence for implementation into clinical practice are available on the website [9].

An important ongoing initiative focuses on workflow and algorithm pathways for the inclusion of the CPIC guidelines into the EHR. Hoffman et al. have developed a model workflow that supports CPIC guidelines, knowledge sources, and clinical decision support for pharmacogenomics integration into the EHR [8].

4. Formal competencies for nursing at all Academic Levels

Initial genetic and genomic competencies for US nursing defined a core of expected knowledge, skills, and attitudes required of all registered nurses regardless of academic preparation or specialties were published in January 2006 [11]. These competencies have since been revised to incorporate changes in technology and the addition of outcome indicators, and more recently competencies were developed for advanced practice [12, 13]. The most recent version of core competencies for all health professionals identified minimum levels of competencies, knowledge, skills, and attitudes from the National Coalition for Health Professional Education in Genetics (NCHPEG) [11]. These have been built upon similar to the nursing efforts by other disciplines including physician assistants, pharmacists, and most recently physicians [14-16]. Building on the work from NCHPEG, the Inter-Society Coordinating Committee for Practitioner Education in Genomics (ISCC) was established in 2013. Aims of the interprofessional ISCC is to help generate evidence and address provider competency gaps [17].

Not surprisingly, across all the disciplines with genomic competencies, there is considerable overlap. Competencies surrounding basic genetic concepts, assessments and indications for a genetic specialist referral, and ethical, legal, and social issues are underpinnings common across all disciplines. These commonalities support some interprofessional core educational activities.

In the international community, genomic based competencies have continued to develop. The United Kingdom (UK) recently updated their 2003 competency framework for nurses [18]. Building on the work in the US and UK, other countries have developed country specific competencies such as Japan and Brazil, or are moving in that direction [19].

5. Examples of Competencies in Nursing in Clinical Practice

Since genetic and genomic competencies have been established for all US registered nurses regardless of academic degree, clinical role, or specialty, implementation into clinical practice is important. A recent study of US Magnet® Recognition Program Hospital integration of genetics and genomics into practice demonstrated what strategies nurse leaders developed to diffuse this important information in order to improve nursing genomic competency thereby impacting quality and safety [20]. The project recruited twenty-one Magnet® hospitals and 2 control hospitals which participated in a one-year education intervention to help them understand the basic concepts sufficient enough to design and implement institutional integration efforts. Each hospital used several on-line and other resources to access information. Hospitals had to complete environmental scans to identify policies that needed to be changed, developed, or extended. Continuing education and staff development activities were found to be effective means to introduce this subject in practice. One of the most popular methods of incentivizing learning was a one-page monthly series called GeneSplash, a single concept learning tool that provided new discoveries and genetics and genomics and facts pertinent to diseases they managed. The Magnet® hospital study participants have partnered with the investigators to develop an online toolkit of all their strategies for use by other educators and administrators to facilitate implementation of these changes in the practice environment [21].

6. Certification of Advanced Practice Nurses in Genetics from the American Nurses Credentialing Center (ANCC) and ISO certified group

The American Nurses Credentialing Center (ANCC) has built on the work of the Genetic Nursing Credentialing Commission and developed a certification in Advanced Genetics Nursing [22]. In the US and worldwide, nurses who demonstrate genomic skills, knowledge and abilities, and who have a minimum of 1,500 practice hours in a genomic area within a 5 year period, and have 30 hours of continuing education credits within a 3 year period, are eligible to submit a portfolio for expert peer review and certification. The ANCC certifications focus on professional development; professional and ethical nursing practice; teamwork and collaboration; and quality and safety. These ANCC certifications are available worldwide since they have successfully achieved ISO 9001:2008 certification in the design, development, and delivery of global credentialing services and support products for nurses and healthcare organizations [22]. ISO 9001:2008 certification is the firmly established global standard for assuring stakeholders of an organization's ability to satisfy quality-related requirements.

7. What are sources of information for Consumers?

One only has to listen to lay or social media through radio, television, internet, and advertising to find that consumers are being bombarded with information on where to test their genome, what they should look for at hospitals testing their genomics and pharmacogenomics, and determining their roots and ancestry through genetics. A reliable source for patients to obtain information on genetics and genomics is genome.gov/patients [23]. There they will find definitions of terms, policies, and resources to follow. Additionally, large private sector alliances continue to develop tools to improve consumers' and patients' knowledge about genetic services (http://geneticalliance.org/programs/geneslife) [24]. Additionally, the Center for Disease Control and Prevention (CDC) Public Health Genomics also offers a number or reliable resources (http://www.cdc.gov/genomics) [25].

8. Effective Integration of Genetics/Genomics, other Omics, and Pharmacogenomics into the Electronic Health Record (EHR)

Several genetic and genomic data and tools are recommended for integration into EHRs. These nursing informatics components for genomic implementation are included in Table 1. They are separated into entry level and advanced level components [4]. The entry level includes more users of the information resources, and the advanced level includes more developers, evaluators, and researchers of the information resources.

Table 1. Nursing Informatics Components for Genomic Implementation Management at the Entry and Advanced levels.

Entry level
1. Facilitate Consumer Engagement in Consent – Signatures and Date
2. Include Pedigree Maps for Family History and Family Values
3. Use and access to Pharmacogenomics Knowledge Bases and other Data Repositories
4. Use Diagnostic and Treatment and Path Report Protocols/Orders
5. Use Evidence Guideline Databases
6. Provide client with interpretive services for genomic tests
Advanced level
1. Develop Data Standards to Ensure Privacy, Security, and Integrity for Big Data Analytics and Data Exchange
2. Incorporate genetic/genomic/adverse reactions into Vocabulary and Terminology Standards to Monitor Quality of Outcomes and the Safety of Care
3. Map to Pharmacogenomics Knowledge Bases and other Data Repositories
4. Link to Advanced Biomarker Discovery Databases, Laboratory findings, Tissue databanks, and Imaging data
5. Include Sequencing and Pathogen Discovery
6. Link to Diagnostic and Treatment and Path Report Protocols/Orders
7. Link to Evidence Guideline Databases
8. De-identify Patients for Data Sharing
9. Enhance EHRs and Mobile Devices to Promote Precision Medicine
10. Develop New Algorithms and Workflows
11. Identify Patients for Genetic/Genomic Services and Consults
12. Develop Point of Care Computerized Clinical Decision Supports
13. Participate on teams developing advanced security and cybersecurity solutions securing genomic data
14. Conduct research data mining on genomic diagnosis, treatment, and symptom management
15. Conduct research on patient access, diversity, and ethnic variation in patient care
16. Identify health services research sites where patient access information on their genetics/genomics
17. Develop new information access sources for clinicians and consumers

A recent National Academy of Medicine Workshop Summary recommended links among genomics, clinical research and a learning health care system (LHCS). In a LCHS, the data from the patient, the genomics data, and other external repositories are integrated into the EHR [26]. They make a significant point that the regulations and policies of individual countries vary, challenging nurses to develop standards across continents to address informed consent and data sharing guidelines that address country specific society and cultural differences.

Several large studies are demonstrating the integration of genetic and genomic data into EHRs. The Electronic Medical Records and Genomics Network (eMERGE) is a project that supports the development of infrastructure for integration of genomic biorepository findings into the EHR to facilitate clinical implementation [26]. Several projects have resulted from eMERGE including: phenotyping algorithms available in an online public repository called Phenotype KnowledgeBase (PheKB) [27]; MyResults, a website where patients and families can learn more about their genetic results; eMERGE SPHINX, to facilitate drug and genomic variation discovery; PheWAS, designed to facilitate understanding of the variation in phenotypes associated with a single genotype [28]; as well as other efforts. eMERGE is also identifying actionable variants and including Clinical Decision Support (CDS) tools in the EHR in the program sites [29].

The Displaying and Integrating Genetic Information Through the EHR Action Collaborative (DIGITizE) working group at the Institute of Medicine (now called National Academy of Medicine- NAM) is developing implementation guides, Logical Observation Identifier Names and Codes (LOINC®) transfer codes, as well as other means to integrate the information into Electronic Health Records. This group includes companies such as Cerner, Epic, and Allscripts working together to implement genetics and genomic workflows into the EHR. SMART (Substitutable Medical Applications and Reusable Technology), the HL7 v3 message on clinical genomics information and family pedigree [30, 31], and FHIR (Fast Healthcare Interoperability Resources) are potentials to connect genomic information into the vendors' EHRs [32, 33].

Another NHGRI supported project is called the Implementing GeNomics In pracTicE (IGNITE) Consortium [24]. The goal of this consortium is to create Genomic Medicine Pilot Demonstration projects that integrate genomics into the EHR and incorporate clinical decision support tools. There are currently multiple IGNITE sites and a coordinating center that focus on: 1) common health conditions including hypertension, kidney disease, and diabetes; 2) the family health history evaluation in diverse care settings applies an implementation science approach to the collection and evaluation of family history and development of implementation guidelines, and 3) the personalized medicine program with a pharmacogenomics focus that aims to include the development of best practices for genomic medicine implementation resulting from pharmacogenomics [4].

The Pharmacogenomics Research Network was established to conduct research on pharmacogenomics and evaluate the impact on clinical care of genetic variants predicting drug metabolism, toxicity and adverse drug effects. An international initiative is call the Pharmacogenomics for Every Nation Initiative (PGENI) which targets countries with good healthcare infrastructure but limited capacity to integrate pharmacogenomics into practice. PGENI is conducting research to ascertain what drugs and genetic variants would be most informative given ethnic variation. The intent is to establish country specific national formulary recommendations informed by genomic variation [34].

Figure 1 identifies the components of a simplified global strategy for moving genetically competent nursing informatics to the integration of genomics translated into precision clinical care. The process components include many subcomponents that detail multiple paths that can be taken by informatics nurses to assure integration into practice. The first building block is education/knowledge of genetics/genomics by all IT nurses because a lack of knowledge is an obstacle to translating genomics into information systems. The second building block is the data standards and vocabulary standards in order to utilize the data to measure quality, safety and for big data analytics. The third building block are the regulatory and policy changes needed nationally, globally, and locally to fulfill the inclusion of nursing with genomics into informatics nursing. The fourth component is nursing IT involvement in Health Information Technology at the stakeholder level, the vendor level, the repository level, and the development of tools integral to decision support. The fifth building block is developing a research agenda. A Genomic Nursing Science Blueprint has been developed by the US based on evidence gaps [35]. The sixth building block is the translation of genetic and genomic content into the EHR, mobile devices, and the Internet of Things for patients and practitioners.

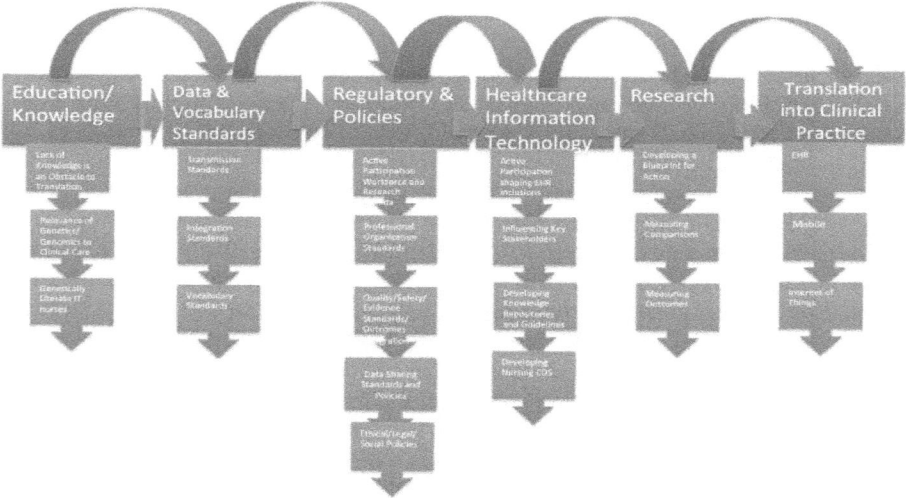

Figure 1. Components of a Global Process for Moving Genetically Competent IT Nurses toward Translation in Precision Clinical Care

9. Identification of Some Global Resources and Country Efforts in Genetics/Genomics

There are several areas where genomic medicine is entering a global environment. One effort, part of the NHGRI larger Genomic Medicine implementation initiative, was global in nature. Genomic Medicine VI (comprised of 50 leaders from 25 countries): Global Leaders in Genomic Medicine, met at the National Academy of Sciences in January 2014 [36]. They defined 4 major objectives:
  1) Identify areas of active translation and implementation of genomic medicine,

2) Frame a policy agenda to advance the field,
3) Highlight nations with unique capabilities, and
4) Discuss opportunities for international collaborations.

Key issues that were identified included: the development of evidence for value of genomics in healthcare, ways to engage both institutional leaders and professionals in genomics, education of professionals and patients, effective integration of genomic results into EHR, and design of financial models that provide cost reductions rather that increases. Building on this work was the establishment of the Global Genomic Medicine Collaborative (G2MC) which is aimed at furthering global collaborations.

In nursing, similar international efforts are underway. The International Society of Nurses in Genetics (ISONG) is a truly international organization whose membership consists predominately of nurses with genetic/genomic expertise. The organizations mission surrounds development of their membership to increase research, clinical, and academic genomic integration as well as genomic information management [37].

A coalition of ISONG members collaborated to secure funding to begin the next steps for establishing a Global Genomics Nursing Alliance (G2NA) to explore strategies for knowledge mobilization and action. The first meeting of this initiative is now funded and nursing leaders globally will be meeting in January 2017 to learn from each other, share resources and expertise. The intent is to establish an Alliance to reduce duplication through sharing and building on work in other countries to accelerate the effective integration of genomics in to nursing practice and education. To facilitate that work the first meeting will include steps to establish a Maturity Matrix to guide and benchmark progress to accelerate integration of genomics into everyday healthcare practice.

There are several other global initiatives that are comprised of several countries and organizations throughout the world. Notable are the following:

The Global Alliance for Genomics and Health (GA4GH) is a network of over 375 institutions internationally that work together to create a common framework of harmonized approaches to enable secure data transfer and data sharing of genomic data linked to clinical data [38]. The International Rare Disease Research Consortium (IRDiRC) is a group of teams of researchers and organizations investing in rare diseases. It is the goal of the group to establish diagnostic tests for all rare diseases and create 200 new rare disease therapies by 2020 [39].

The European Union has identified several initiatives on the continent that seek to develop personalized medicine in the diagnosis and treatment of specific diseases. One initiative called the European Observatory on Personalized Medicine seeks to provide a closer link between research and innovation funding, and policy objectives by funding key initiatives in Personalized Medicine in Europe [40].

A listing of several genomics resources and URLs are provided in Table 2. These include programs, organizations and global initiatives mentioned in this chapter. They also include content about broad genomic programs, education specific programs for clinicians and patients, and detailed repositories and toolkits.

Table 2. Genomics Programs and URLs Mentioned in this Chapter

Global Genomics Programs	URL
Human genomics strategy group: Building on our inheritance—Genomic technology in healthcare	www.gov.uk/government/uploads/system/uploads/attachment_data/file/213705/dh_132382.pdf
European Science Foundation. Forward look: Personalised medicine for the European citizen	www.esf.org/uploads/media/Personalised_Medicine.pdf
Genome Canada: 2012 Large-scale applied research project competition in genomics and personalized health	www.genomecanada.ca/en/portfolio/research/2012-competition.aspx
European Association for Predictive, Preventive, and Personalised Medicine (EPMA)	www.epmanet.eu
European Commission: EuroBioForum observatory	www.eurobioforum.eu/2028/observatory
Genomic Medicine Alliance	www.genomicmedicinealliance.org
International rare diseases research consortium (IRDiRC).	www.irdirc.org
Eurogentest: Harmonizing genetic testing across Europe	www.eurogentest.org
National human genome research institute	www.genome.gov
Genomics England	www.genomicsengland.co.uk
Belgian medical genomics initiative (BeMGI)	www.bemgi.be
Database of genotypes and phenotypes (dbGaP)	www.ncbi.nlm.nih.gov/gap
PharmGKB: The pharmacogenomics knowledgebase	www.pharmgkb.org
Genatak: Pioneering personalized genomic medicine	www.genatak.com
Implementing genomics in practice (IGNITE)	www.ignite-genomics.org/IGNITE_ABOUT.html
Australian New Zealand cLinical trials registry	www.anzctr.org.au
E.U.Clinical TRials register	www.clinicaltrialsregister.eu
U.S. NIH Clinical Trials Registry	https://clinicaltrials.gov
National Health and Medical Research Council of Australia: Principles for the translation of "omics"-based tests from discovery to health care	http://consultations.nhmrc.gov.au/files/consultations/drafts/attaevidentialstandardsdocument.pdf
A guide to the Exome Aggregation Consortium data set, MacArthur lab, Massachusetts General Hospital	http://macarthurlab.org/2014/11/18/a-guide-to-the-exome-aggregation-consortium-exac-data-set
Clinical Genomics Resource (ClinGen)	www.clinicalgenome.org
European translational information and knowledge management services (ETRIKS)	www.etriks.org
National coalition for health professional education in genetics: Core competencies for all health professionals (2007)	http://www.nchpeg.org/index.php?option=com_content&view=article&id=237&Itemid=84
Coursera and University of California, San Francisco. Genomic and precision medicine	www.coursera.org/course/genomicmedicine
The EuroGenTest clinical utility gene cards	www.eurogentest.org/index.php?id=668
Pharmacogenomics knowledge base (PharmGKB): International consortium for antihypertensives pharmacogenomics studies (ICAPS)	www.pharmgkb.org/page/icap
Pharmacogenetics for every nation initiative (PGENI)	www.pgeni.org
Global alliance for genomics and health (GA4GH)	http://genomicsandhealth.org
U.S. National Academy of Medicine (formerly Institute of Medicine): Roundtable on translating genomic-based research for health	www.iom.edu/Activities/Research/GenomicBasedResearch.aspx

10. Future Opportunities and Summary

Informatics remains a cornerstone to the integration of genomics into nursing practice. The ongoing efforts to establish international collaborative networks to build upon the resources and strategies implemented by other countries to learn, support, and collaborate to answer questions and to reduce duplication of effort are vital to realizing the benefits of genomics to health. Informatics experts can play critical roles in adapting successful tools such as Clinical Decision Support for other countries without or with less developed resources. Additionally, efforts to expand the evidence-base and improve the understanding of global genomic variation can facilitate effective genomic implementation.

International collaborative opportunities for IMIA-NI are provided in Table 3. IMIA-NI could expand the International Medical Informatics Association (IMIA) standards activity to engage with other genetic and genomic groups to identify gaps and develop global resources filling those gaps. There are other global needs that include what data to be aggregated for variant/phenotype association, how to define the federated databases for genomic data, and development of a vocabulary to phenotype ontology, standardized phenotype ontology, and inventory of existing phenotype ontologies. Work needs to continue to build on what is already available to disseminate globally, the genomic medicine implementation guidelines, algorithms, CDS, workflows, and pharmacogenomics guidelines.

Table 3. Opportunities for Collaboration in IMIA-NI

• Develop Repositories within ICN and UMLS for Data Standards and Share Data Sharing Policies Integrated with Nursing Classifications
• Share Models for Bioinformatics Integrated into the EHRs
• Share Models for Incorporation of New Algorithms, Workflows, and Evidence into EHRs
• Share New CDS tools
• Promote Collaboration in Pharmacogenomics & Guidelines
• Compare Outcomes with and without Guidelines
• Link Educational content as well as Federated Databases for Variants/Phenotypes/Ethnic Associations
• Identify Global Toolkits of Resources, Link them, and Disseminate to IMIA-NI members
• Identify genetic/genomic resources globally and Collaborate on nursing IT content
• Establish link with ICN and ISONG to collaborate on resources for informatics management of genomic content

There remains a need to collect and disseminate data on different countries on existing nursing workforce prepared in genetics/genomics and/or clinical translation. There is a need to assess the state of genomic competency of the interprofessional workforce and implement strategies to address competency deficits.

There are several opportunities that IMIA NI-WG can engage in educational programs to highlight the importance of genetic and genomic competencies in nursing and other healthcare professionals. IMIA-NI-WG could provide:

- Websites that link nurses in all participating countries with competencies, certification and literature resources in genetics and genomics internationally;
- Conduct international webinars and through telemedicine links, establish regular educational programs;
- Provide links to ongoing educational resources internationally;
- Provide links to studies implementing genetic and genomic education into practice, similar to the Magnet® study in the US;
- Develop and disseminate a repository to compile and conduct studies comparing certifications at the certificate level, baccalaureate level, and advanced practice level internationally;

- Compile and deliver new evidence in pharmacogenomics through the current network of best practice centers developing guidelines throughout the world;
- Collaborate with other global nursing organizations such as ICN and ISONG to provide resources for informatics management of genomic content.

This paper has provided an overview of the journey over the past 25 years of the science of genetics and genomics, and of the nursing profession establishing practice standards, competencies for general and advanced practice nurses, and an internationally ISO accepted certification for advanced practice nurses. In addition, some major discoveries with implications for nursing and the integration into the EHR and nursing informatics were provided. A study implementing genetics and genomics into Magnet® Hospitals and the development of a toolkit were discussed. National efforts from around the world were highlighted. Finally, future opportunities for the IMIA-NI working group were described. Most importantly, this review highlights that there are similar needs across the globe that are amenable to international collaborations that can accelerate the integration of genomics into healthcare world-wide to improve health outcomes.

11. Acknowledgments

The authors acknowledge the contributions of all nurses who have defined the competencies for general nurses, advanced practice nurses, and interprofessional groups. It is only by reaching consensus on common principals that the science of genetics and genomics and the integration into practice to improve quality outcomes and achieve safer care will be provided.

References

[1]   American Nurses Association, Nursing Informatics: Scope & Standards of Practice, 2nd Edition. 2015, American Nurses Association.2.   Collins, F.S. and H. Varmus, A New Initiative on Precision Medicine. N Engl J Med, 2015.
[3]   Green, ED. and Guyer MS. Charting a course for genomic medicine from base pairs to bedside. Nature, 2011. 470(7333): p. 204-13.
[4]   Weitzel KW., et al., The IGNITE network: a model for genomic medicine implementation and research. BMC Med Genomics, 2016. 9: p. 1.
[5]   McCormick KA. and Calzone KA. The impact of genomics on health outcomes, quality, and safety. Nurs Manage, 2016. 47(4): p. 23-6.
[6]   Williams JK., et al., Advanced nursing practice and research contributions to precision medicine. Nurs Outlook, 2016. 64(2): p. 117-23.
[7]   McCormick KA., Calzone KA. , Big Data Initiatives: Genomics and Information Technology for Personalized Health, in Essentials of Nursing informatics, 6th Edition. Saba,VK &. McCormick,KA Editor. 2015, McGraw-Hill: New York. p. 707-725.
[8]   Hoffman JM. et al., Developing knowledge resources to support precision medicine: principles from the Clinical Pharmacogenetics Implementation Consortium (CPIC). J Am Med Inform Assoc, 2016.
[9]   Clinical Phamacogenetics Implementation Constorium. CPIC Guidelines. 2016 [cited 2016 4/2/2016]; Available from: https://www.pharmgkb.org/view/dosing-guidelines.do?source=CPIC#
[10] Relling MV. and. Evans WE, Pharmacogenomics in the clinic. Nature, 2015. 526(7573): p. 343-50.
[11] Consensus Panel on Genetic/Genomic Nursing Competencies, Essential Nursing Competencies and Curricula Guidelines for Genetics and Genomics. 2006, American Nurses Association: Silver Spring.
[12] Consensus Panel on Genetic/Genomic Nursing Competencies, Essentials of Genetic and Genomic Nursing: Competencies, Curricula Guidelines, and Outcome Indicators, 2nd Edition. 2nd ed. 2009, Silver Spring, MD: American Nurses Association.

[13] Greco KE., Tinley S., Seibert D. Essential genetic and genomic competencies for nurses with graduate degrees. 2012 [cited 2013 8/31/2013]; Available from: http://www.nursingworld.org/MainMenuCategories/EthicsStandards/Genetics-1/Essential-Genetic-and-Genomic-Competencies-for-Nurses-With-Graduate-Degrees.pdf.

[14] Korf BR. et al. Framework for development of physician competencies in genomic medicine: report of the Competencies Working Group of the Inter-Society Coordinating Committee for Physician Education in Genomics. Genet Med, 2014. 16(11): p. 804-9.

[15] Consensus Panel on Pharmacist Pharmacogenomic Competencies. Pharmacist Phamacogenomic Competencies 2012 [cited 2016 2/17/2016]; Available from: http://g-2-c-2.org/files/Pharmacist-Comp.pdf.

[16] Rackover M., Goldgar C., Wolpert C., Healy K., Feiger J., Jenkins J., Establishing essential physician assistant clinical competencies guidelines for genetics and genomics. Journal of Physician Assistant Education, 2007. 18(2): p. 48-49.

[17] Manolio TA. and. Murray MF, The growing role of professional societies in educating clinicians in genomics. Genet Med, 2014. 16(8): p. 571-2.

[18] Kirk M., Tonkin E. and Skirton H. An iterative consensus-building approach to revising a genetics/genomics competency framework for nurse education in the UK. J Adv Nurs, 2014. 70(2): p. 405-20.

[19] Kirk M. et al. Genetics-Genomics Competencies and Nursing Regulation. Journal of Nursing Scholarship, 2011. 43(2): p. 107-116.

[20] Calzone KA., et al. Introducing a New Competency Into Nursing Practice. J Nurs Regul, 2014. 5(1): p. 40-47.

[21] Jenkins J. et al. Methods of genomic competency integration in practice. J Nurs Scholarsh, 2015. 47(3): p. 200-10.

[22] American Nurses Credentialing Center (ANCC). Advanced Genetic Nursing. 2016 [cited 2016 3/7/2016]; Available from: http://nursecredentialing.org/AdvancedGenetics.

[23] National Human Genome Research Institute. Genetics/genomics for Patients. 2016 [cited 2016 3/30/2016]; Available from: http://www.Genome.gov/patient.

[24] Genetic Alliance. Genes in Life. 2016 [cited 2016 3/30/2016]; Available from: http://geneticalliance.org/programs/geneslife.

[25] Center for Disease Control and Prevention (CDC). Pubic Health Genomics. 2016 [cited 2016 5/18/2016]; Available from: http://www.cdc.gov/genomics.

[26] Gottesman O. et al. The Electronic Medical Records and Genomics (eMERGE) Network: past, present, and future. Genet Med, 2013. 15(10): p. 761-71.

[27] Pathak J. et al. Mapping clinical phenotype data elements to standardized metadata repositories and controlled terminologies: the eMERGE Network experience. J Am Med Inform Assoc, 2011. 18(4): p. 376-86.

[28] Pendergrass SA. et al. The use of phenome-wide association studies (PheWAS) for exploration of novel genotype-phenotype relationships and pleiotropy discovery. Genet Epidemiol, 2011. 35(5): p. 410-22.

[29] Herr TM. et al. Practical considerations in genomic decision support: The eMERGE experience. J Pathol Inform, 2015. 6: p. 50.

[30] HL7 V3 CG PEDINTEROP, R1 HL7 Version 3 Implementation Guide: Family History/Pedigree Interoperability, Release 1

[31] ANSI/HL7 V3 CGPED, R1-2007 HL7 Version 3 Standard: Clinical Genomics; Pedigree, Release 1 7/5/2007 HL7 International

[32] Warner JL. et al. SMART precision cancer medicine: a FHIR-based app to provide genomic information at the point of care. J Am Med Inform Assoc, 2016.

[33] Mandel JC. et al. SMART on FHIR: a standards-based, interoperable apps platform for electronic health records. J Am Med Inform Assoc, 2016.

[34] Pharmacogenomics for Every Nation Initiative (PGENI). Pharmacogenomics for Every Nation Initiative (PGENI) 2016 [cited 2016 4/1/2016]; Available from: http://www.pgeni.org/.

[35] Genomic Nursing State of the Science Advisory Panel, C., Jenkins KA., Bakos J., Cashion AD., Donaldson AK., Feero N., Feetham WG., Grady S., Hinshaw PA., Knebel AS., Robinson AR., Ropka N., Seibert ME., Stevens D., Tully KR., Webb LA. A Blueprint for Genomic Nursing Science. Journal of Nursing Scholarship, 2013. 45(1): p. 96-104.

[36] Manolio TA., et al. Global implementation of genomic medicine: We are not alone. Sci Transl Med, 2015. 7(290): p. 290ps13.

[37] International Society for Nurses in Genetics. Mission. 2016 [cited 2016 5/21/2016]; Available from: http://www.isong.org/.

[38] Lawler M. et al. All the World's a Stage: Facilitating Discovery Science and Improved Cancer Care through the Global Alliance for Genomics and Health. Cancer Discov, 2015. 5(11): p. 1133-6.

[39] Baxter K. and Terry SF. International Rare Disease Research Consortium commits to aggressive goals. Genet Test Mol Biomarkers, 2011. 15(7-8): p. 465.
[40] European Observatory on Health Systems and Policies. European Observatory on Health Systems and Policies 2016 [cited 2016 3/7/2016]; Available from: http://www.euro.who.int/en/about-us/partners/observatory

Forecasting Informatics Competencies for Nurses in the Future of Connected Health
J. Murphy et al. (Eds.)
© 2017 IMIA and IOS Press.
This article is published online with Open Access by IOS Press and distributed under the terms
of the Creative Commons Attribution Non-Commercial License 4.0 (CC BY-NC 4.0).
doi:10.3233/978-1-61499-738-2-165

Big Data and Nursing: Implications for the Future

Maxim TOPAZ[a] and Lisiane PRUINELLI[b]

[a] *Harvard Medical School & Brigham Women's Health Hospital, Boston, MA, USA*
[b] *School of Nursing, University of Minnesota, Minneapolis, MN, USA*

Abstract. Big data is becoming increasingly more prevalent and it affects the way nurses learn, practice, conduct research and develop policy. The discipline of nursing needs to maximize the benefits of big data to advance the vision of promoting human health and wellbeing. However, current practicing nurses, educators and nurse scientists often lack the required skills and competencies necessary for meaningful use of big data. Some of the key skills for further development include the ability to mine narrative and structured data for new care or outcome patterns, effective data visualization techniques, and further integration of nursing sensitive data into artificial intelligence systems for better clinical decision support. We provide growth-path vision recommendations for big data competencies for practicing nurses, nurse educators, researchers, and policy makers to help prepare the next generation of nurses and improve patient outcomes trough better quality connected health.

Keywords. Big data, Data science, Nursing, Natural language processing, Data mining, Data visualization

1. Introduction

The discipline of nursing is charged with several core missions, including: protecting, promoting and optimizing human health and ability; alleviating suffering by diagnosing and treating the human response; advocating for individuals, families, communities, and populations; and preventing injury and illness [1]. Nursing informatics (NI) incorporates the science of nursing with information, technological, communication and analytical sciences to support the integration of data, information, knowledge, and wisdom into the provision of evidence-based nursing care [1].

The concept of big data became widespread around 2010 [2] and is often defined by the "4Vs": *Volume, Velocity, Variety, and Veracity* [3]. *Volume* refers to the large amount of data, e.g., millions of patients records or detailed genomic data. *Velocity* refers to the rate of high-frequency, real-time generated data, such as data from smartphones and sensors devices. *Variety* refers to the heterogeneity of the data, e.g., structured, semi-structured, and unstructured data, such as electronic health records (EHRs), monitoring devices, genomics, sensors, imaging, claims data, social media, patient generated data, and others real time data. *Veracity* is the uncertainty of the data, either in terms of accuracy of the data for the original purpose for which the data were collected or appropriateness of the data for secondary use. Recently, an additional fifth "V" was suggested for *Value*, representing the value of information extracted from the data leading to knowledge discovery [4, 5].

The scholarship of working with data is known as data science and it draws on knowledge and theories from multiple disciplines, including nursing. Big data science uses a variety of methods for analyzing data from traditional statistics to visualization techniques, data mining, and natural language processing [3]. Use of big data is assuming a critical role in healthcare analytics as the complexity and variety of data available are increasing. In addition, advanced computational methods and tools to analyze big data are increasingly more available. However, nursing relevant big data applications and research are still in their infancy, often because they require a rare combination of multidisciplinary skills in computer science, statistics, mathematics, and health informatics. There is an urgent need in further understanding and recommendations on what nurses need to learn in order to be competent in data science and analytics. Once NI research is able to incorporate data that represent the "5Vs" into research, education and practice, nurses have the potential to achieve better outcomes for populations and individuals.

This chapter aims to identify competencies necessary for big data management and analytics, and provide recommendations concerning policy, educational, research, and practice needs related to big data. We understand that some of the identified competencies might present a challenge for practicing nurses and educators today; nevertheless, we strongly believe that our recommendations will provide a growth-path vision for nurses of the near future practicing in the realm of connected health.

2. Big data types and data processing steps

Health data is the raw and uninterpreted object that contains health attributes or characteristics [6]. In order to manage data effectively, nurses need to understand several basic concepts presented below:

a) *Types of data*: data can be divided in two generic types: qualitative (or categorical) and quantitative (or numeric). Commonly, qualitative data can be represented as nominal/ ordinal/ or free-text values whereas quantitative data can have interval/ratio/dichotomous or discrete values. Health data are often highly heterogeneous, such as electronic health records data that include lab values, narrative notes, diverse time points and large number of medical abbreviations. This data is also often quite messy with missing values, noise, outliers, inconsistencies, duplicate concepts, and might contain other types of human or system errors (e.g., misspellings or erroneously recorded time points). Thus, knowledge domain expertise needed to evaluate the quality of health data.

b) *Data processing steps*: an individual or an organization using health data need to have a clear understanding of the data use goals and the analytic methods they might want to apply. Then, the data needs to be pre-processed and prepared for the analysis. These steps may include: aggregation, sampling, dimensionality reduction, feature selection, feature creation, discretization, binarization, transformation and so on. Another import part is de-identification of data. With big data sets usually containing all health information from a person, additional security measures should be implemented to preserve patient's privacy and confidentiality. For instance, data about rare conditions may be discarded or grouped to prevent potential individual identification. A similar situation can occur if a specific condition is related to a postal code, leading to identification of an individual.

Nursing informaticians expertise, with the domain knowledge of health problems and implications of data for these problems, is crucial in driving more intelligent models where data can be used to improve health of populations through implementation of best evidence-based practices.

3. Common methods and technologies applied for big data with implications for nursing

3.1   Data mining

Data mining refers to a suite of statistical tools that enable knowledge discovery. These techniques help to identify novel patterns that might otherwise remain unknown in large data sets and diverse data types. Data mining techniques help to analyze large multidimensional datasets and identify relationships between different types of data. It is often used for data driven hypothesis generation, for example when novel relationships between diseases to abnormal lab findings are discovered. Data mining tasks are generally divided into two major categories: predictive modeling and descriptive tasks. In addition, data mining tasks can be supervised (e.g., when the outcome is known) or unsupervised (when there is no known outcome). An example of data mining in nursing can be found in Bowles et al. [7] where decision trees were used to identify factors associated with nurses post-acute care referrals. Another example is the Dey et al study [8] where discriminative pattern mining was used to discover patterns associated with improvement in homecare patient mobility.

Data mining is becoming increasingly more prevalent and those techniques are being applied in everyday applications, such as traffic detection, personalized advertisement, fraud detection, and many others. Several existing open access data mining applications, such as Weka [9] and KNIME [10], can be readily utilized by nurses to conduct data mining and knowledge discovery with big data.

3.2   Natural Language Processing

Natural language processing is concerned with creating automated approaches for understanding human language. It is an interdisciplinary field that combines linguistics, computer science and informatics. One of the main goals of health oriented natural language processing is to create computer algorithms capable of understanding different types of free text data. The different types of data include narrative, clinician generated texts from EHRs, social media data (e.g., Twitter, Facebook, online health forums), patient or family generated data, and research literature, among others. The increasing need in natural language processing is based on the fact that about 80% of the data in EHRs, and up to 100% in some other data sources, is stored as free text.

In the past several decades, a few health natural language processing systems were developed, mostly focused on working with texts from the medical domain. For example, an open source system called cTAKES can assist in extracting symptoms from physician narrative notes [11]. Another system called MTERMS can assist with capturing information about medication dosage, route, etc. in physician notes to enable improved medication reconciliation [12].

Although nurses' recorded clinical narratives are similar to data generates by other disciplines, e.g., medicine, there are several unique features that require specific nursing-focused approaches. For example, when nursing narratives are analyzed, nursing interventions or nursing problems should be mapped to nursing standard terminologies (e.g., to the International Classification for Nursing Practice, ICNP). This mapping would allow further use of extracted data for scalable analytics or automated reasoning (e.g., clinical decision support). For example, when a computer algorithm is trained to identify patients with pressure ulcers (ICNP code 10015612) or self-management issues (ICNP code 10022155) in a large pool of clinical notes, the system can generate automated nursing specific treatment recommendations (e.g., facilitate adherence to regime, ICNP code 10036273) or reminders for health promotion (e.g., provide health promotion, ICNP code 10008776). For more information on the role of nursing terminologies please see this book's chapter addressing with semantics.

Unfortunately, there are only a very few natural language processing systems that focus explicitly on nursing data [13]. To analyze nursing-relevant narrative big data, nurses will need the support and close collaboration of other disciplines, such as computational linguistics and computer science and understand machine learning methods.

3.3　Artificial Intelligence

Artificial intelligence is often referred to as the theory and development of information systems able to perform tasks that usually require human intelligence, such as visual or speech recognition, decision-making, and language translation. In health related fields, artificial intelligence systems can be used to assist in data analytics, clinical decision making, and diagnostics, among others. Some examples of artificial intelligence systems in healthcare include esophageal image recognition to enable better intubation [14] or genetics based predictions [15].

In nursing, work on artificial intelligence based systems started in early 1980s when first rule based systems were proposed. For example, Ryan [16] described a development of an interesting system called COMMES (an acronym for Creighton On-line Multiple Medical Expert System). COMMES was an artificial intelligence based expert system simulating a professional consultant designed to assist with nursing decision making about a patient condition. The system had a robust knowledge base and an extensive hierarchy of nursing and medical diagnoses and treatment options. COMMES was envisioned to be used as an educational tool for nurses, capable of generating diagnosis oriented care protocols and testing nurses' knowledge. Similar work on nursing artificial intelligence systems was done by several other groups throughout the years [17-20].

However, most of the systems proposed so far were rule based systems where an expert would pre-define some logical order for the system to follow. This is in contrast to a more probability-based systems that can do reasoning on their own, as envisioned by artificial intelligence pioneers. Also, there is still a wide gap between the developed systems and nursing practice where such systems are not common. To create nursing-sensitive artificial intelligence systems of a new generation, there is a need in thoroughly developed and tested machine learning and natural language processing approaches, which are scarce. Other potential domains that need to be integrated to produce best artificial intelligence results are speech and image recognition. Seeing the trends of increasing use of artificial intelligence systems in healthcare, we expect significant advances in this field for nursing and nurses need to be ready to integrate nursing knowledge into the emerging systems.

3.4   Visualization

Information visualization is the study of visual representations of different data to assist in human cognition and decision making. Big data analytics and applications require appropriate visualizations to enable users to grasp the extent and sometimes the significance of big-data driven inferences. In healthcare, data visualization is often used to present patient specific (e.g., blood pressure levels over time) or population trends (geographical spread of zika virus over time). However, an increasing body of literature indicates that healthcare visualization approaches need better integration within the existing clinical systems. For example, a recent study evaluated the graphical displays of laboratory test results in eight EHRs in the U.S. None of the systems met all 11 quality of visualization criteria and the magnitude of deficiency was significant. One system even presented results in reverse chronological order [21]. Similarly, there were a few recent studies that indicated significant problems with EHR systems used by nurses in terms of visualizations and usability [22]. Traditionally, nurses are used to working with paper charts presenting trends in patient's condition, for example blood pressure, breathing, and heart rate. Big data approaches could potentially offer much insight and help interpret patient's vital signs compared to the population average, for example. To accomplish that, nurses working with big data will need to draw from other disciplines, such as human computer interaction and graphic design, to be able to come up with appropriate visualization approaches.

4. Big data related growth-path competency recommendations for nursing education, practice, research and policy

4.1   Education

Academic and inservice education programs in nursing should teach the concept of big data to students. Students need to be able to discuss big data characteristics and understand the increasing impact of using big data on clinical decision making. Ideally, students in academic nursing programs should understand the limitations and benefits of big data while practicing nurses should learn on how big data is used to shape everyday clinical practice. Nurse educators should also be knowledgeable about big data related concepts and their implications for students.

4.2   Practice

Practicing nurses should understand how to use big data to extract and apply clinically relevant evidence-based information in practice. Also, there is a need to be able to understand how to extract data from different formats and reuse it for quality improvement and better decision making.

4.3   Research

Nurse researchers need to be able to understand the big data characteristics and be able to collaborate effectively with interdisciplinary teams to use big data in their programs of research. They also need to learn about analytic tools and methods (e.g., data mining and natural language processing) that assist in working with big data. More efforts should be spent on data quality validation and merging different data formats/types together for further use in clinical decision making.

4.4   Policy

Nursing policy makers should be able to use big data to visualize the effect of nursing on patient outcomes. Also, there is a need to start building comprehensive national and international data pools that are capable of storing different data types. The large data storages can help design nursing relevant policies that work (e.g., identify the ideal number of patients per nurse during the hospital shift to achieve best outcomes).

Table 1 provides an overall summary of growth-path vision recommendations for entry level and advanced level nurses.

Table 1: Big data growth-path vision competency recommendations for entry and advanced level nurses.

Entry level nursing competencies
Nurses should understand the types and sources of data captured by the information systems, including data quality, type (e.g., structured data, free text narratives, etc.)
Nurses should understand the importance and value of data for nursing care.
Nurses should develop and apply critical thinking when using the data in clinical decision making.
Nurses should be able to communicate with multidisciplinary teams to use data for enhanced clinical decision making.
Advanced level nursing competencies
Nurses should understand the big data characteristics and be able to collaborate effectively with interdisciplinary teams to use big data in their programs of research.
Nurses should learn about analytic tools and methods (e.g., data mining and natural language processing) that assist in working with big data.
Nurses should use data quality validation techniques to merge different data formats/types together for further use in clinical decision making.

5. Conclusion

Big data, with all its complexity, is becoming increasingly more prevalent and it affects the way nurses learn, practice, conduct research and develop policy. The discipline of nursing needs to maximize the benefits of big data to advance the vision of promoting human health and wellbeing. However, current practicing nurses and nurse scientists often lack the required skills and competencies necessary for meaningful use of big data. Some of those key skills for further development include the ability to mine narrative and structured data for new care or outcome patterns, effective data visualization approaches, and further integration of nursing sensitive data into artificial intelligence systems for better clinical decision support. We hope that our big data competencies recommendations' for practicing nurses, nurse educators, researchers, and policy makers will provide a vision for the growth-path and help prepare the next generation of nurses to improve patient outcomes trough better connected health.

References

[1] American Nurses Association. Nursing informatics: Scope and standards of practice. 2nd ed. Silver Spring: MD: Nursesbooks.org; 2014.

[2] Gandomi A, Haider M. Beyond the hype: Big data concepts, methods, and analytics. International Journal of Information Management 35 (2015), 137-144.

[3] Bellazzi R. Big data and biomedical informatics: A challenging opportunity. Yearbook of Medical Informatics 9 (2014) 8-13. doi:10.15265/IY-2014-0024

[4] Kitchin R, McArdle G. What makes big data, big data? Exploring the ontological characteristics of 26 datasets. Big Data and Society 3 (2016),1-10.

[5] Brennan P, Bakken S. Nursing needs big data and big data needs nursing. J Nurs Scholarsh (2015), doi: 10.1111/jnu.12159

[6] McCormick K, & Saba V. Essentials of Nursing Informatics, 6th Edition McGraw-Hill Education, Philadelphia, PA, USA, 2015. Topaz M., Radhakrishnan K., John VL., Zhou L. Mining clinicians' electronic documentation to identify heart failure patients with ineffective self-management: A pilot text-mining study. Stud Health Technol Inform- NI2016 Proceedings (2016).

[7] Bowles KH, Holmes J, Ratcliffe S, Liberatore M, Nydick R, & Naylor MD. Factors identified by experts to support decision making for post acute referral. Nursing research, 58(2009), 115-128.

[8] Dey S, Cooner J, Delaney CW, et al. Mining Patterns Associated With Mobility Outcomes in Home Healthcare. Nurs Res 64(2105), 235-45.

[9] The University of Waikato. Weka 3: Data Mining Software in Java. http://www.cs.waikato.ac.nz/ml/weka/index.html (accessed 27 October 2016).

[10] KNIME.com AG. Open for Innovation. https://www.knime.org/ (accessed 27 October 2016).

[11] Lin C, Karlson E, Dligach D, et al. (2014). Automatic identification of methotrexate-induced liver toxicity in patients with rheumatoid arthritis from the electronic medical record. Journal of the American Medical Informatics Association 22(2105),e151-61.

[12] Zhou L, Plasek J, Mahoney LM, et al. Using Medical Text Extraction, Reasoning and Mapping System (MTERMS) to process medication information in outpatient clinical notes. AMIA Annu Symp Proc (2011), 1639-48.

[13] Topaz M, Lai K, Dowding D, Lei V, Zisberg A, Bowles K, Zhou L. Using natural language processing to automatically identify wound information in narrative clinical notes: application development and testing. Home Healthcare and Hospice Information Technology Conference (H3IT) Proceedings 2 (2015), 3-4.

[14] Carlson JN, Das S, De la Torre F. A Novel Artificial Intelligence System for Endotracheal Intubation. Prehosp Emerg Care 17 (2016), 1-5.

[15] Severin J, Beal K, Vilella K, Fitzgerald S, et al. eHive: an artificial intelligence workflow system for genomic analysis. BMC bioinformatics, 11(2010), 1-7.

[16] Ryan SA. An Expert System for Nursing Practice. Computers in Nursing 3(2)(1985), 77-84.

[17] Bloom KC, Leitner JE, Solano JL. Development of an Expert System Prototype to Generate Nursing Care Plans Based on Nursing Diagnoses. Computers in Nursing 5(2)(1987), 140-5.

[18] Ozbolt JG, Schultz S, Swain MA, Abraham IL. A Proposed Expert System for Nursing Practice: A Springboard to Nursing Science. Journal of Medical Systems 9(1-2)(1985), 57-68.

[19] Ozbolt JG. Developing Decision Support Systems for Nursing. Computers in Nursing 5(3)(1987), 105-11.

[20] Norris J, Cuddigan J, Foyt M, Leak G, Lazure L. Decision Support and Outcomes of Nurses' Care Planning. Computers in Nursing 8(5)(1990), 192-7.

[21] Sittig DF, Murphy DR, Smith MW. Graphical display of diagnostic test results in electronic health records: a comparison of 8 systems. Journal of the American Medical Informatics Association 22(2015), 900-904.

[22] Cho I, Kim E, Choi WH, Staggers N. Comparing usability testing outcomes and functions of six electronic nursing record systems. Int J Med Inform 88 (2016), 78-85.

Forecasting Informatics Competencies for Nurses in the Future of Connected Health
J. Murphy et al. (Eds.)
© *2017 IMIA and IOS Press.*
This article is published online with Open Access by IOS Press and distributed under the terms
of the Creative Commons Attribution Non-Commercial License 4.0 (CC BY-NC 4.0).
doi:10.3233/978-1-61499-738-2-172

Nursing Competencies for Multiple Modalities of Connected Health Technologies

Kaija SARANTO[a], Charlene RONQUILLO[b] and Olivia VELEZ[c]
[a] *University of Eastern Finland, Department of Health and Social Management,*
Finland
[b] *School of Nursing, University of British Columbia, Canada*
[c] *Hudson River HealthCare, Inc. And ICF International, USA*

Abstract. An overview of the rapid and diverse number developments in health information technologies (HIT) in recent years are described in this chapter and the move towards more integrated and connected health is described. The evolution of HIT is described as it has increased in complexity, diversity, connectivity, and more recently, the move towards multiple modalities. Examples of developments in various settings are represented from clinical settings, at home, and in low-resource settings. The implications of the move towards multiple modalities for nursing competencies and the move towards personalized and connected health are discussed, highlighting important areas for consideration and development in the future.

Keywords. eHealth, mHealth, uHealth, integrated care, connected health, IoT

1. Introduction

Connected health as a concept has been integrated into development and change in producing health care services. In recent decades several technologies have been introduced to help the transition in practice from physical to virtual and from manual to digital actions in health care [1]. Thus, connected health is linked not only to technologies, but also to management, and social aspects of providing timely, continuous and high quality care.

Changes in patient profiles, care contexts and costs are challenges for delivery of nursing care globally. The growth in the amount of elderly citizens and complexity of their care needs and services is seen as a driving force to focus on integration at professional, organizational, regional and national level. Early discharge and on the other hand demand for cost-effective services emphasize to provide additional home care beside hospital care [1, 2].

This chapter gives an overview and examples of the diversity of what is considered "connected health" and discuss some of the implications of connected health for nursing competencies. First, the focus will be on providing basic definitions (e.g., eHealth, mHealth, and pHealth) of the diverse terminology related to advanced technologies (e.g., Internet of Things). Next, case examples of connected health will be presented divided by setting (e.g., clinical, home, low-resource settings), with the aim of illustrating the growth towards multiple modalities. Finally, considerations and implications for nursing informatics competencies will be discussed.

2. The evolving field of connected health

Connected health is close to the concept integrated care highlighting the role of patients, collaboration among professionals, and coordination of health care services at multiple levels with advanced technologies. Sharing care information and focusing on the continuum of health care delivery are the key components of integrated care to ensure high quality, safe and efficient care to patients and populations with disabilities or chronic diseases across settings and organizations [1, 3]. Both integrated and connected health are premised on use of advanced technologies with aims on access, sharing, analysis, and use of health data through applications and information systems. Further, the premise of connected health also includes potential cost-effectiveness provided by creative and novel ways of delivering health care, compared with traditional face-to-face care [1].

Technologies that can be seen as encompassed under the broader term of connected health has grown in diversity in recent decades, signaling evolution in the field towards multiple modalities. The adoption of various terms e.g., eHealth, uHealth, mHealth, pHealth, and Internet of Things (IoT) have been connected not only to technologies used in health care but also to describe the practical consequences of advantages as well as disadvantages of the usage. More recent developments are exploring the potentials of wearable electronic devices that can monitor physical and physiological changes in the body and "smart" spaces that incorporate environmental biosensors and facilitate pervasive monitoring [3-5].

Figure 1 illustrates the ecosystem of connected health supported by advanced technology, focusing on continuum of services and service providers. In the ecosystem, mHealth describes the actors of the service system who are connected to services and service providers through mobile technology. One of the main advantages mHealth provides is the independence of location and timing to access and use information and services [1, 6]. In the ecosystem, pHealth represents the continuum of personal health data content/items from disease to wellness which are stored and shared through eHealth applications [1]. It also includes the growing field of personalized health, where treatment of diseases is adjusted to specific personal characteristics [7] Finally, the ecosystem should provide accessible connections with various means and technologies when and where ever needed (uHealth) as well as connect to recent advances in technologies in various formats and be able change and share data and information (IoT).

To aid in providing clarity around terminologies and modalities under the umbrella of connected health, the following sections provide brief definitions of some common terms.

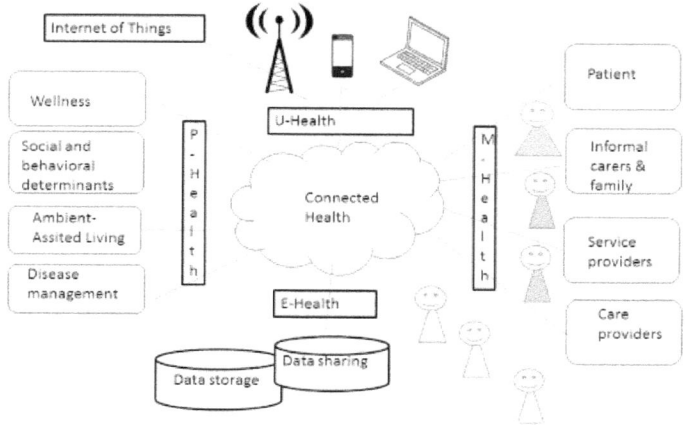

Figure 1. Connected health ecosystem.

2.1   From eHealth to uHealth

The concept of eHealth was introduced in the beginning of 2000's [8] and the number of studies focusing on various aspects of eHealth adoption in health care has grown extensively since then [9]. A remarkable growth of research is especially seen since 2010, based on reviews [1, 4]. The vast amount of eHealth definitions have a lot of commonalities in regard to use of technologies in support health and health-related fields by electronic means and to improve the availability, quality and efficiency of health services [9-10]. eHealth as a concept has been regarded as an umbrella term for the use of Information and Communication Technology (ICT) in healthcare. The outstanding definition by Eysenbach describing the meaning of "e" as not only electronic but far more important aspects of the vowel e.g., education, empowerment, ethics [8]. In terms of connected health eHealth focuses on methods providing safe information management.

Almost parallel to concept eHealth the term uHealth started to appear in the literature in the mid 2000's (e.g., NI2006 proceedings) [11]. Information and communication technology was regarded to have ubiquitous possibilities for use in health care (uHealth). For instance, within the proceeding of the 9th International Congress on Nursing Informatics, a track for submissions focused on ubiquitous computing. Papers and posters presented at this conference described Intranet, Internet, websites, wireless and mobile terminals use in clinical practice and education. On the other hand, Internet and videoconferencing were topics already in the 6th International Congress on Nursing Informatics in 1997. This verifies that nurses, researchers and educators have been early adopters of advanced technology. Overall, uHealth provides wide insights to multiple use of technology in connected health especially highlighting the flexibility of use.

2.2   From telehealth to mHealth

The introduction of the concept mHealth occurred slightly after the concept eHealth. However, mHealth has its origin in telemedicine which has its potential to provide asynchronous communication between care provider and patients. For instance, telemedicine and telehealth can be seen as initial forays into connected health. Telemedicine is described as using electronic communications to facilitate medical information exchange and telehealth can be viewed as a further expansion to include the participation of consumers by providing access to health education resources and support for self-management through the use of the Internet [1, 4].

With advances in technologies came the rise of mobile health that accompanied the rapid proliferation of the use of cellular phones and mobile devices [1]. Within mHealth, we have seen the delivery of health information and facilitating the work of health care providers through short message services on basic cellular phones, to the delivery of sophisticated medical functions and decision support for health providers, given the introduction of smart phones with access to the Internet. mHealth is also regarded more consumer-centered in terms of providing support and information sharing both to patients and professionals. Interestingly, based on previous studies more facilitating than restraining factors were revealed in m-health adoption. However, it seems that external factors for instance human and organizational environment have challenges to overcome [4]. mHealth has advantages to connect citizens, patients, relatives, and care providers with the use of technology to improve especially co-operation in terms of care coordination, information flow and exchange [7].

2.3   From pHealth to IOT

The various definitions focusing on personal health information management highlight the role of an individual and his/her rights on accessing, managing and sharing electronic information in a confidential, secure, and technically sound environment [4]. The number of applications and software developed to maintain personal health information is expanding yearly. The size of devices, connectivity, and mobility enables various groups of citizens and patients to maintain their health data easily, even continuously if needed. pHealth services tend to be highly distributed from virtual environment independent of location and time. Services are individually tailored to diagnose, care, prevent, and provide lifestyle services [12]. The use of sensors and sensor systems have abilities to monitor a variety of activities not only for wellness and lifestyle assessment. With the advances of wearable systems they have a huge potential for clinical use as well as home care based on the patients' signs and symptoms to be monitored and assessed. [4].

The amount of data, diversity of technology in use and multiplicity of actors in health care demands effective and interoperable systems for data exchange. The term Internet of Things (IoT) appeared in the literature in 2010's to highlight the not only the technology but also the networks required to connect the devices and people even the devices with themselves. Internet of Things has been defined as "things belonging to the Internet" involving sensor based data collection, data management, data mining and World Wide Web. The vision to interact anything and anytime is especially appealing in remote care [13, 14].

3. Case studies

The definitions provided in the previous section highlight the continual development of technologies and concepts as related to connected health. In this section, we describe examples from the literature to illustrate the diversity in modalities of connected health available today, from clinical settings, to the home, and within low-resourced settings.

3.1   From clinical settings

In clinical and acute settings, there have been efforts to improve communication among nursing and other health care professionals through the use of technology, beyond static computer stations and electronic health records. Among these efforts include exploring the potentials of mobile devices, environmental sensors, and in particular, the use of radio-frequency identification (RFID – a wireless Automatic Identification and Data Capture technology). As components of 'smart' hospital rooms, RFIDs enable ubiquitous computing and the collection of ambient data to inform and support the work of clinicians.

One example of such a study explored the use of RFID tags and readers worn by patients, healthcare workers, and placed in surrounding objects, as a means to track movement of persons and objects in real-time, as well as a means of collecting and using real-time data to support the work of health care providers and systems [15]. Multiple uses of RFID in a "smart hospital environment" were described. First, the ability to track and manage valuable assets such as expensive hospital equipment is made possible, reducing time spent searching for equipment and allowing for the ability to forecast requirements of future inventory. Another application is the ability – through wearable RFID tags and readers placed in the environment – to locate and track the positions, movement, and identities of health care workers and patients. This tracking function, combined with the ability to track certain physiological and biomedical patient data (e.g., heart rate, oxygen saturation, temperature, blood pressure, step count, etc.) serves as a powerful information source that can inform built systems of emergencies or adverse events. For example, an ambulatory patient whose movement is seen to abruptly stop combined with abnormal physiological conditions can trigger an emergency rescue process system, identifying the closest available health care worker who can attend to the patient. Similarly, Ariffin and colleagues proposed a system and provide recommendations for implementing a system that uses RFID tags and readers as an affordable way to monitor patients in a psychiatric ward, in an effort to reduce the numbers of patients who left without permission or formal discharge [16].

Other areas of interest in the acute care setting centers on the use of innovative communication technologies to facilitate communication and workflow among nurses and other members of the health care team, including telephones, various mobile technologies (e.g., pagers, mobile phones, personal digital assistants), and increasingly, wearable hands-free communication devices [17]. For example, Pemmasani and colleagues evaluated the use of a hands-free mobile voice communication system and assessed nurses' perceptions of advantages and disadvantages of this technology [18]. Results of the study were mixed. Although it was found that the technology successfully reduced the average distance that staff walked during a shift by nearly 20% -- in line with findings of other studies [19-22] – participants nevertheless expressed challenges and limitations related to signal reception and voice recognition [18]. Findings of this study suggests that hands-free communication technologies, with further development and refinement, have potential to free up nursing time and improve communication in inpatient acute care settings, although issues related to quality of the technology and connectivity need to be carefully considered [18].

Numerous studies suggest a positive potential in leveraging ICTs to support better communication in acute settings, however, limitations of past studies need to be considered in interpreting results. For instance, a systematic review of studies from 1996 to 2010 on ICT adoption among clinicians suggest that many studies were of lower quality; there remains limited evidence for improvement in communication effectiveness as a result of ICT adoption and the need for more robust evaluations [17].

3.2   At home: Gerontechnology

A recent review provided a narrative account of the of newly developed and implemented technologies in gerontechnology – "a term born in Europe just prior to the 1990s as a composite of a two words: 'gerontology,' the scientific study of aging, and 'technology'" [23]. Gerontechnology is concerned with research on the biological, psychological, social, and medical aspects of aging, exploiting the potentials offered by the progress of technology. [24]. The review sought to gain an understanding of technologies developed and implemented for older adults' home use, as well as to examine whether there is evidence to support the premise that these technologies can support independent living [25]. Of the 184 publications included in the review, the authors categorized devices as having three key target functions that addressed: (1) social isolation; (2) loss of autonomy and functional decline; and (3) cognitive disorders and behavioral and psychological symptoms of dementia. Many studies attempted to address specific health problems and limitations, with a dominance of issues related to chronic obstructive pulmonary disease, diabetes, heart failure, and other chronic conditions [25]. Currently, there is very limited evidence and few articles addressing the needs of the frail older person nor on upstream technologies that aimed to prevent physical disability or decline [25].

The review highlighted the diversity of technological approaches and devices being explored in gerontechnology. For instance, studies leveraging technology to address social connectedness of older adults employed the use of cell phones, computers, and innovative "sociometric" devices that can monitor interpersonal interactions and detect social isolation. One example was a wearable pendant that by detecting the presence of other pendants and analysis of the users' tone of voice, could quantify the quality and frequency of personal interactions of wearers [26]. Other approaches leverage tracking capabilities of mobile phones to determine patterns of movement and mobility as a way to quantify social networks.

Technological developments related to alarms and personal emergency response systems were a focus in gerontechnology studies [25] with the aim of monitoring risks, detecting acute and adverse events, and providing a sense of security for those living alone [27]. The use of various sensors were prominent ways of monitoring physical activity and abnormalities in movement. For example, the use of pressure sensors in "smart carpets", infrared sensors, and increasingly, wearable systems that make use of accelerometers, gyroscopes and inclinometers, were incorporated in devices to monitor falls and provide alerts to caregivers [28-30]. Other examples of developments to address functional and cognitive decline included: exploring the use of robotic systems to support the rehabilitation of disabled people [31], providing support for activities of daily living and provide companionship [32]; "intelligent" mobility aids with built-in safety features [33], that can facilitate the avoidance of obstacles and provide navigation [32, 34]; and computerized devices that use artificial intelligence to prompt and guide individuals through activities of daily living [35].

3.3   In low-resource settings: Liga Inan project in Timor Leste

In countries where penetration of more traditional communication technologies, such as telephone lines and broadband internet, are low, m-health in particular has been seen as a mechanism for connecting with patients who previously had limited access to the healthcare system [36]. One such example is the Mobile Moms, or Liga Inan project in Timor Leste. This project combines pregnancy stage-based text messages to expectant and new mothers with a means of requesting a call back from an on-call midwife as well as a clinical tool that midwives use for registering patients and tracking care [37]. Midwives reported overall job satisfaction with the tool including a perceived increase in communication with patients and a perceived increase in the use of skilled birth attendants. Midwives' perceptions of an innovative mHealth technology's impact on their work and job satisfaction Patients have given positive feedback about the program with 96% reporting satisfaction with the content of the messages [38]. The increase in demand in services, however, presented a challenge, as midwives reported being unable to arrange for transportation for patients to healthcare facilities [39].

Research on the impact of mHealth in low resource settings is showing improvements in delivery of care and access to the healthcare system to many challenges to successful implementation and sustainability remain [36]. While mHealth and other forms of connected health pose great promise towards strengthening and connecting patients with providers, new challenges can develop where staff lack the resources or the competencies to meet with new patient demands.

Table 1. Case study summary illustrating the variety of technologies described in these case studies in clinical, home, and low-resourced settings.

Setting	Technology
Clinical	Use of mobile devices, environmental sensors, and radio frequency identification (RFID) to collect real-time and ambient patient data, mobile technologies (pagers, mobile phones, personal digital assistants) and hands-free devices to support inter-team communication.
Home	Various sensors to monitor physical activity and abnormalities in movement, robotic systems to support the rehabilitation, communication devices to facilitate companionship, "intelligent" mobility aids with built-in safety features, navigation, and can avoid obstacles, computerized devices that use artificial intelligence to prompt and guide individuals through activities of daily living
Low-resource settings	Bi-directional text messaging to support communication, care coordination tools between community health workers and facility-based nurse managers

4. Competency recommendations and implications on the expected roles of nurses

The evolution of connected health technologies are moving towards multiple modalities and are taking innovative and diverse approaches to support health care workers, health systems, and patients, as illustrated in the above examples. Ultimately, the overarching intention of these diverse and innovative HIT developments is to support and deliver interventions and health care services that are better connected, integrated, and personalized. Unsurprisingly, these developments in connected health are accompanied by numerous implications for the provision of nursing care and require some new competencies of nurses to best make use of connected health technologies.

For one, the goal of having HIT facilitate patient-centered care, integrated care, and health care teams' communication can shift care team dynamics and patterns of care provision. For example, studies implementing HIT have described clinician concerns related to shifts in team dynamics and uncertainties as to whether the new technology should be adopted as a standard of practice or whether its use is up to the discretion of the health care provider [40]. In the same vein, new tasks and functionalities that are made possible with HIT also have the potential to restructure existing care models, support task shifting among various health care providers, and highlight the need for new and different ways of providing patient care [1]. For instance, a wider adoption of RFID tags and sensors in hospital settings will arguably change nursing workflows. For example, creating systems that are capable of continuous individual patient monitoring and aggregated data displayed in central nursing stations, the amount of time nurses need to spend physically checking on patients may be reduced. For such systems and new workflows to be successful however, the need to develop different nursing competencies and capabilities are made apparent. In the system described above, for example, nurses will need to have competencies related to data literacy in order to interpret and make use of ambient data that are collected. In the case of adoption of ambient sensing technology in smart homes, the ways that expectations and competency requirements of home care and community nurses need to similarly be thoughtfully considered. For instance, do nurses need to be more knowledgeable about mobility in the home, if the smart home is capturing data on obstructions that may cause increased risk for falls?

The rapid development and increasing diversity of connected health technologies will arguably influence patient expectations, which will have direct implications for nurses. For instance, rapid developments in HIT may create and promote patients' perceptions of extended provider capacity that may be unrealistic. The increasing push and marketing of innovative HIT, the public's increased and rapid access to HIT development news, and the "selling" of connected health technologies as being able to do more and more [1], may not be in line with actual levels of maturity and sophistication of connected health technologies. The mismatch between what HIT is purported to accomplish and what it is realistically able to achieve may be something that nurses may need to contend with, as related to patient expectations. Further, as HIT increasingly aims to facilitate ubiquitous connectivity, an important expectation that all health care providers will need to contend with is the potential expectation of 24/7 availability of health services.

Navigating the diversity and rapid development of technologies may be overwhelming for nurses in terms of learning and adopting technologies for their own work, as well as providing guidance for patients using HIT. These relate to two key aspects: 1) the actual use of new technologies; and 2) managing and make sense of the data produced. With regard to the first point, competencies that may need further development among nurses might be related to broad technological literacy and a foundational understanding of health and clinical informatics. The use of advanced technologies demands nurses to be familiarized with both synchronous and asynchronous messaging in terms of technology, psychology, and nursing aspect. It will be impossible for an individual nurse to know and master each piece of technology they come across. However, there may be fundamental aspects of all HIT hardware and software that can be identified as a foundational knowledge base. For instance, this may include the ability to recognize when the technology does not address end-user needs and understanding how this would ultimately influence decision-making around the appropriateness of HIT use and impacts on health outcomes. Another example may be the nurse's ability to identify when help is needed and knowing how and where to access additional resources to troubleshoot. Considering the increasing diversity of HIT, perhaps a goal in the future is to advocate for core features across all HIT devices (e.g. universally recognizable help button) to be incorporated in future HIT designs.

Finally, competencies related to managing and making sense of the masses of data produced by various HIT will be crucial for nurses. In addition to supporting the nurse's own work, it may be the case that nurses' responsibilities related to teaching and supporting patient self-care (e.g. diabetes management at home) will expand to include supporting patients' ability to navigate, use, and make sense of the data produced by HIT that they use. A crucial point of importance will be nurses' competencies around educating and guiding patients on privacy, confidentiality, safe data sharing, and ownership of data.

5. Conclusion

The challenges for nurses to provide connected health care services will focus on the environment where services are provided, which will vary based on patients' conditions and equipment and tools available. This means that nurses must have knowledge and skills to work with multiple technologies. As competencies, this involves basic understanding of data acquisition, information flow and exchange as well as archiving in nursing practice. In relation to connected technologies used in the context of nurses' own work, additional skills include the ability to use decision support systems in practice, data-based planning and decision making through the utilization & synthesis of HIT system data, quality assurance using technology, and the ability to articulate the application and significance of HIT to clinical practice. As HIT are increasingly taken up by patients, nurses require additional competencies to support patient teaching and self-care around connected health technologies and being able to make sense of the data produced. This includes the ability to synthesize data from more than one source and understand its relevance to practice, demonstrating awareness of and ability to access data and information from multiple sources, understanding of patient rights related to HIT and computerized patient data, and a conceptual understanding of data quality issues for HIT. Competencies related to understanding and interpreting research will also be important, as understanding the supporting literature and evidence upon which technologies are based on will serve as additional sources of knowledge to inform decision-making around HIT use and adoption.

References

[1]   Kvedar J, Coye MJ, Everett W. Connected health: a review of technologies and strategies to improve patient care with telemedicine and telehealth. Health Affairs. 2014;33(2):194-9.
[2]   De Vliegher K, Aertgeerts B, Declercq A, Milisen K, Sermeus W, Moons P. Shifting care from hospital to home: a qualitative study. Primary Health Care. 2015;25(9):24-31.

[3] Chouvarda IG, Goulis DG, Lambrinoudaki I, Maglaveras N. Connected health and integrated care: Toward new models for chronic disease management. Maturitas. 2015;82(1):22-7.

[4] Gagnon M-P, Ngangue P, Payne-Gagnon J, Desmartis M. m-Health adoption by healthcare professionals: a systematic review. Journal of the American Medical Informatics Association. 2016;23(1):212-20.

[5] IOM (Institute of Medicine). Capturing Social and Behavioural Domains and Measures in Electronic Health Records: Phase 2. Washington, DC: The National Academies Press; 2014.

[6] Blobel B, Sauermann S, Mense A. PHealth 2014: Proceedings of the 11th International Conference on Wearable Micro and Nano Technologies for Personalized Health, 11–13 June 2014, Vienna, Austria: IOS Press; 2014.

[7] ISO/TS 13131. Health Informatics—Telehealth Services—Quality Planning Guidelines. Geneva: Intenational Standards Organisation; 2014.

[8] Eysenbach G. What is e-health? Journal of Medical Internet Research. 2001;3(2):e20.

[9] Oh H, Rizo C, Enkin M, Jadad A. What is eHealth (3): a systematic review of published definitions. Journal of medical Internet research. 2005;7(1).

[10] World Health Organization. Assisting community health workers in India: Dimagi's CommCare. 2013.

[11] Murray PJ, Park H-A, Erdley WS. Nursing Informatics 2020: Towards Defining Our Own Future: Proceedings of NI2006 Post Congress Conference: IOS Press; 2007.

[12] Blobel B. Ontology driven health information systems architectures enable pHealth for empowered patients. International journal of medical informatics. 2011;80(2):e17-25.

[13] Hindia M, Rahman T, Ojukwu H, Hanafi E, Fattouh A. Enabling Remote Health-Caring Utilizing IoT Concept over LTE-Femtocell Networks. PloS one. 2016;11(5):e0155077.

[14] Singh D, Tripathi G, Jara AJ, editors. A survey of internet-of-things: future vision, architecture, challenges and services. Internet of Things (WF-IoT), 2014 IEEE World Forum on; 2014: IEEE.

[15] Sravani K, Kumar PS. Human Health Behavior Detection using Bio Sensors and Classification by Wearable Tags in Smart Spaces. International Journal of Innovative Technologes. 2015;3(6):851-6.

[16] Ariffin FNH, Wan AT, Suhaili WSH, editors. Psychiatric patients monitoring using RFID: An affordable approach. Computer and Communications (ICCC), 2015 IEEE International Conference on; 2015: IEEE.

[17] Wu RC, Tran K, Lo V, O'Leary KJ, Morra D, Quan SD, et al. Effects of clinical communication interventions in hospitals: a systematic review of information and communication technology adoptions for improved communication between clinicians. International journal of medical informatics. 2012;81(11):723-32.

[18] Pemmasani V, Paget T, van Woerden H, Minamareddy P, Pemmasani S. Hands-free communication to free up nursing time. Nursing times. 2013;110(13):12-4.

[19] Breslin S, Greskovich W, Turisco F. Wireless Technology Improves Nursing Workflow and Communications. CIN: Computers, Informatics, Nursing. 2004;22(5):275-81.

[20] Ernst AA, Weiss SJ, Reitsema JA. Does the Addition of Vocera Hands-Free Communication Device Improve Interruptions in an Academic Emergency Department? SOUTHERN MEDICAL JOURNAL. 2013;106(3):189-95.

[21] Kuruzovich J, Angst CM, Faraj S, Agarwal R. Wireless communication role in patient response time: a study of vocera integration with a nurse call system. Computers Informatics Nursing. 2008;26(3):159-66.

[22] Vandenkerkhof EG, Hall S, Wilson R, Gay A, Duhn L. Evaluation of an innovative communication technology in an acute care setting. Computers Informatics Nursing. 2009;27(4):254-62.

[23] Micera S, Bonato P, Tamura T. Gerontechnology. IEEE engineering in medicine and biology magazine : the quarterly magazine of the Engineering in Medicine & Biology Society. 2008;27(4):10-4.

[24] Micera S, Bonato P, Tamura T. Advanced Solutions for an Aging Society. IEEE Engineering in Medicine and Biology Magazine. 2008:11.

[25] Piau A, Campo E, Rumeau P, Vellas B, Nourhashemi F. Aging society and gerontechnology: A solution for an independent living? The journal of nutrition, health & aging. 2014;18(1):97-112.

[26] Sung M, Marci C, Pentland A. Wearable feedback systems for rehabilitation. Journal of neuroengineering and rehabilitation. 2005;2(1):1.

[27] Horton K. Falls in older people: the place of telemonitoring in rehabilitation. Journal of rehabilitation research and development. 2008;45(8):1183-94.

[28] Bourke A, Van de Ven P, Gamble M, O'Connor R, Murphy K, Bogan E, et al. Evaluation of waist-mounted tri-axial accelerometer based fall-detection algorithms during scripted and continuous unscripted activities. Journal of biomechanics. 2010;43(15):3051-7.

[29] Rimminen H, Lindström J, Linnavuo M, Sepponen R. Detection of falls among the elderly by a floor sensor using the electric near field. IEEE transactions on information technology in biomedicine: a publication of the IEEE Engineering in Medicine and Biology Society. 2010;14(6):1475-6.

[30] Lee Y, Ho KC, Popescu M. A microphone array system for automatic fall detection. Biomedical Engineering, IEEE Transactions on. 2012;59(5):1291-301.

[31] Carrera I, Moreno HA, Saltarén R, Pérez C, Puglisi L, Garcia C. ROAD: domestic assistant and rehabilitation robot. Medical & biological engineering & computing. 2011;49(10):1201-11.

[32] Robinson H, MacDonald B, Broadbent E. The role of healthcare robots for older people at home: A review. International Journal of Social Robotics. 2014;6(4):575-91.

[33] Paulo J, Peixoto P, Nunes U, editors. A novel vision-based human-machine interface for a robotic walker framework. Robot and Human Interactive Communication (RO-MAN), 2015 24th IEEE International Symposium on; 2015: IEEE.

[34] Rentschler AJ, Cooper RA, Blasch B, Boninger ML. Intelligent walkers for the elderly: Performance and safety testing of VA-PAMAID robotic walker. Journal of rehabilitation research and development. 2003;40(5):423.

[35] Czarnuch S. Advancing the COACH automated prompting system toward an unsupervised, real-world deployment [Ph.D.]. Ann Arbor: University of Toronto (Canada); 2014.

[36] Levine R, Corbacio A, Konopka S, Saya U, Gilmartin C, Paradis J, et al. mHealth Compendium, Volume Five. Arlington VA: African Strategies for Health, Management Sciences for Health; 2015.

[37] Mercer MA, editor Mobile moms: Design issues in the use of cell phones to improve maternal care in timor-leste. 141st APHA Annual Meeting (November 2-November 6, 2013); 2013: APHA.

[38] Health Alliance International. Liga Inan Program Preliminary Results: Follow-up Phone Calls with Enrolled Women from Sub-district Same. 2013 August 2013.

[39] Barnabee G, Harrison M, Mercer M, O'malley G. Midwives' perceptions of an innovative mHealth technology's impact on their work and job satisfaction. Annals of Global Health. 2014;80(3):214.

[40] Langhan ML, Riera A, Kurtz JC, Schaeffer P, Asnes AG. Implementation of newly adopted technology in acute care settings: a qualitative analysis of clinical staff. Journal of Medical Engineering & Technology. 2015;39(1):44-53.

Forecasting Informatics Competencies for Nurses in the Future of Connected Health
J. Murphy et al. (Eds.)

doi:10.3233/978-1-61499-738-2-183

Competences in Social Media Use in the Area of Health and Healthcare

Pirkko KOURI[a] and Marja-Liisa RISSANEN[a]
Patrick WEBER[b,], Hyeoun-Ae PARK[c]
[a] *Savonia University of Applied Sciences*
[b] *Nice Computing SA*
[c] *Seoul National University, Seoul, Republic of South Korea*

Abstract. In today's life, social media offer new working ways. People are increasingly expanding interactions from face-to-face meetings to online ways of communication, networking, searching, creating and sharing information, and furthermore taking care of patients/citizens via tweeting care, Facebook care, blogging care, vlogging care, infotainment care, gamification-care, infographic care, for instance. This chapter discusses the utilisation of social media in the healthcare domain including nursing education, practice and research. When in the current healthcare era, social media is used effectively and purposefully, it can give all of us a greater choice in how we live, how we take care of our health and how we learn and build both our professional competences and produce evidence-based, qualified data. Nurses need continuous education and proper tools to take the most of the benefits of social media, not forgetting privacy and ethical issues. This use of social media in professional nursing generates the need for new competences.

Keywords. Social media, health care, nurse education, practice, research

1. Introduction

We read news on the web, order tickets or shop and use different kind of services online. We can also make a doctor's appointment online, change dentist's appointment time and so on. Social media has become a part of our everyday life. Social media means participation, sharing same interests, interactive networking, working together, meeting people, and personalized connectivity between persons, groups and communities.

Social media offers opportunities to organize health care education all around the world for example in developing countries [1]. In addition, it provides a means for socialization [2]. The term Web 2.0 includes all the Internet media that are easily accessible, modifiable and in addition, can be easily published by an online community [1]. Existing Web 2.0 tools as for example Twitter, Facebook, YouTube, blogging, vlogging and WhatsApp are free and usable for example by mobile devices wherever you are - if you have an internet connection [2].

The use of open online solutions costs nothing for e.g. learning organizations meanwhile using a closed learning environment does. However, mixing different methods might be the most useful way to learn. Web 2.0 has been used in different ways in health education. Web 2.0 technologies incorporate as Cormode and

Krishnamurthy (2008) present "strong social component while encouraging user-generated content in the form of text, video, and photo postings along with comments, tags, and ratings" [3]. It fosters to take, share and to be in contact with other students but it also offers a platform for participation [2]. Using networks and social media diversifies student counselling and enhances the availability of support. Social media offers a chance both for the teacher and the tutor nurse to be present online. Furthermore, social media tools enable counselling and tutoring while student is in clinical practice, or abroad. The collaboration takes place smoothly when all users find suitable and user-friendly tools [4]. Counselling can be asynchronous e.g. emailing, electronic learning environment, Facebook, blogging, wikis, which are happening in different times or it can be synchronous counselling e.g. videoconferencing, instant messaging, chatting online at the same time [5, 6]. In web, counselling it is typical that the communication varies between asynchronous and synchronous [5]. In addition, we are discussing the concept Health Social Networks (HSNs) which are online health interest communities like PatientsLikeMe, ZocDoc or DrEd, where persons find and discuss information about conditions, symptoms, and treatments, give and get support, enter and monitor data, and join health studies [7]. The HSNs may be consumer/patient-focused or health care professional-focused.

The amount of scientific information focusing on health issues increases very fast and in addition, care provided has to be based on evidence-based knowledge. Therefore, it is important that healthcare staff and students have competences for example to find suitable information and in addition, to handle it by analyzing, sharing, discussing and creating new information with peers [2]. During two decades Health On the Net (HON) has a core mission, which is to promote transparent and reliable health information online. HON has developed both ethical standards, HON codes, in order to enhance qualified health information and tools to meet Internet users' needs [8].

2. Education with social media

Below are presented some common social media solutions in health care education. Twitter is a common and popular microblogging site that allows users to disseminate information in 140 characters of text or less. In nursing education, Twitter is used in classroom and embedded in nursing curricula and supports faculty-student engagement, enhances social support, reinforces course content, and advances critical thinking and reasoning skills, and increases a sense of connectedness among students and new graduates [9]. A study showed that during health care learning situations the students share their feelings and experiences openly and Twitter reveals "behind the scenes" conversations of the students which would have not been otherwise captured. This strengthens the learning process. For the nurse educators and tutors in clinical practice Twitter widens understanding the student role in learning classrooms or in clinical practice [10]. To obtain maximum benefit and most effective results, educators should have a theoretically driven pedagogical basis for incorporating Twitter [11].

Facebook (FB) was created in 2004 by a university student called Mark Zuckerberg with his group of other students for the college students [12]. Today FB [12] is a widely spread, global social networking environment in which people can create their personal virtual environment called profile. Via FB a user can exchange messages, post status updates and photos, share videos, use various applications and receive notifications when others update their postings. FB is well-known as a connector between people [13]. However, using FB in education for example as sharing information has not only advantages but also disadvantages, as problematic FB use is associated with a lower human well-being like subjective feeling of unhappiness, low vitality and low life satisfaction [14]. Therefore, both health professionals, educators and school counselors should develop interventions that focused on increasing well-being to decrease excessive use of FB. Additionally, social media literacy education may be a compulsory e.g. course for college students to increase their awareness of how overuse of FB or even FB-addiction may influence their wellbeing.

Learning should be fun. Infotainment is form of media how to combine educational or useful information and entertaining content. In healthcare simply content delivered via infotainment is designed to be informative yet entertaining enough to commit in learning, and in follow-up maintain the student's interest. This increases student satisfaction, too. Infotainment utilizes versatile techniques and a few of the features students can access on these all-in-one devices are e.g. Internet, video games, animations. There is a huge potential to combine health information with entertainment tools [15, 16].

There are social media platforms specifically designed to share e.g. ideas and research findings between researchers across the globe such as Google Scholar [17] and ResearchGate [18]. Google Scholar is a freely accessible Internet search engine, which helps to find e.g. scientific articles, theses, books and abstracts across many disciplines and versatile sources [17]. ResearchGate is more personalized and a person make his/her own research archive [18]. Furthermore via both services researchers can promote their profiles, view their citations, and network with others in the field by actively engaging in these type of social media.

LinkedIn is considered as business oriented social networking site, which connects registered members. They have personal profile page, which emphasizes skills, employment history and education. Furthermore the members build and document networks of people they know and trust professionally [19].

Visualized information sharing utilizing well-planned texts and clear graphics is called infographic [20].

Gamification is growing way of building services. It utilizes game mechanics and experience design to digitally engage and motivate people to achieve their personal goal. End users interact with computers, smartphones, wearable monitors or other digital devices [21]. Gamification serves students a possibility to approach knowledge and skills using the learn-by-failure technique without the embarrassment factor that often is a part of traditional classroom education. When implemented properly, gamification can be very powerful way to educate [22]. However, in assessing knowledge gamification is not as good as the traditional e-learning approach [23].

YouTube is a service that shares originally-created videos for multiple purposes, and provides a forum for people to connect, inform, and inspire people across the globe [24]. Also YouTube is used in numerous ways e.g. many-sided learning in all fields of education and understanding of complex issues, amusement and ways one can ever imagine [25].

A blog is a personal way of expressing your thoughts, observations, opinions and passions. It is also called a diary or journal on the Internet, for example. A blog user is called the blogger who adds text, photos, videos and links to interesting other websites. Originally, the blog term comes from the expression weblog [26]. A similar approach is currently taken with video on the web, called vlogging. Vlog is shortened from the video blog and it simply means using video distribution over the Internet. The vlog often combines embedded video (or a video link) with supporting text and images depending on what the vlog created wants to utilize. Well-known vlogging tool YouTube has created a platform for vbloggers to present their personal videos, which oftentimes are filmed using hand held point and shoot cameras.

2.1. Case Savonia and student blogging

In our organization, Savonia University of Applied Sciences (Savonia), social media has been taken into our learning, teaching and student-counselling, for instance. We have chosen several digital teacher's tools in which teachers can choose and are trained: Facebook, WordPress, Twitter, Padlet, ScreenCast. We have discussed about where and in which way both teachers, bachelor or master level students and other staff members can utilize different platforms and applications. The organization has its own social media policy and guidelines for using social media. Social media provides educators with an opportunity to engage students both in the online classroom, home or in clinical practice, and at the same time to support development of learning skills and competencies.

In Savonia every student creates her/his personal learning environment (PLE). The idea with PLEs is to put students in a more central position in the learning process by allowing them to design their own learning environments and by emphasizing the self-regulated nature of the learning. The nurse students (bachelor) learn the basis of blogging during the first learning period. The blog is created and maintained by each student who invites teacher, clinical nurse tutor, and if needed, other students to join her/his blog. Furthermore, the nurse students utilize the blog during international exchange period and during their clinical practice, also the WhatsApp is used in collaboration and communication with our students abroad. Via student blogs the teacher can see show how the student's competences have developed during their studies.

The case study in Savonia was realized due to the need to have first-hand information how our student blogs function in practice. On January 2016 the nurse teachers were invited to email experiences of student's blog usage and how the blog reveals nurses' competence development. Totally six nursing teachers wrote about their experiences. The data was formed of these experiences, and is analyzed by qualitative content analysis.

Preliminary results show that blogging mirrors the daily learning and increases the understanding of individual learning process, e.g. in nursing practice blogs reveal how the student develops from a task-focus beginner to an advanced holistic nurse student. Via blogging the student expresses development needs from the clinical practice setting. During the first week of creating their own blog students are confused of his/her role. He/she needs instructions and tutoring in order to learn reflecting how his/her learning objectives are developing. Gradually students learn to write, add links, photos and/or videos, and the students describe how they meet objectives during their clinical practice. The teacher and the tutor nurse evaluate using the student's blog environment. Along the time only a few tutor nurse have refused to use blog environment. In addition to, blogs show that the student writing improves the more they do it.

Furthermore, the communication and networking skills developed the more students used blogs and simultaneously the teacher and/or the nurse tutors commented on the blogs. The teachers expressed that blogging fits most of the students. However, some students are better in verbal reflection. Teachers suggest that there should be guidelines related to blog use, such how often the teacher or the other staff comment and/or evaluate the student blog. The teachers need to be notified when the students have added materials in their blogs. Also students need instructions how to create a blog in which learning objectives, realization and evaluation is scheduled. The advantage of the student blog is that both the learning process and the history are stored in one place. So along the nursing studies different teachers can see the development of each nurse student, not starting from 'empty table'. A blog is a personal product. And you can see student's competences in its breadth, depth, quality and it is in constant development. Utilizing the social media demands both ICT skills and awareness of one's own learning methods. The student needs to have reflection skills: how to reflect own learning by answering a question 'what have I learnt' instead of listing daily working tasks. The teacher's role is that of a facilitator.

Social media are often associated with breach of privacy of individuals and hence measures for data security are part of a schools or health care provider's social media policy. Paragraph 5 will discuss this in more detail.

3. Practice

Via social media tools vast amounts of data are being accumulated and processed to develop understanding of patients'/citizens activities, to encourage their health activities, to support their health decisions and to follow their motivation for healthy choices, and adding connectivity among social media users. There is a growing number of solutions available to be utilized in health care, such as analysis of virtual tools that are useful e.g. in distance communication, in consultation and counselling, in data gathering and in utilization of data for various purposes, such as sharing feelings, being open about health issues related to individual's daily living and asking questions [27]. Many hospitals use social media platforms such as Facebook, Twitter, or YouTube, and hospitals offer web-based broadcasting of health information, health related measurements e.g. body mass index or life style evaluations, and public information like guidelines or how to act in hospital surroundings [28].

3.1. Tweeting in health care

Tweeting care is using instant messaging. Twitter as an intervention delivery method is proved to be rapid and an effective means of information delivery to wide population [9], and to ask questions to be quickly responded [29]. Twitter is used for public health research [30]. There are findings that Twitter supports public health behavior and fits for sharing reliable information about unhealthy and healthy habits e.g. e-cigarettes and smoking cessation online [31]. Furthermore, there are e.g. Twitter communities in which healthcare staff and patients can share their interest in clinical research. Twitter enhances rapid connection between individuals globally, and people collaborate, share problems and find solutions. Both staff and patients share the same interest and enhance knowledge in order to improve patient care [32].

3.2 Facebooking in health care

FB is used in health purposes e.g. asking questions from health professionals, discussing with groups around different health problems e.g. mental health issues, encouraging groups for different purposes e.g. young mothers for the breast-feeding [33]. In addition, FB is used to stimulate a young cancer patient's physical activities [34], enhancing communication and collaboration between professionals and furthermore collaboration between professionals and patients/clients e.g. net clinic environment [33,35]. The flexible 'team' communication between professional and patients is effective because the patient and family experience also tends to improve with a high-functioning primary care [36].

3.3 Gamification in health care

Gamification is growing as a part of patient/client care. Gamification applies game mechanics and game design techniques to engage and motivate people to achieve their health or other wellbeing related goals. Creativity and fun support is enhancing people's health and wellbeing throughout life [37]. The health game can be used in numerous purposes e.g., child growth follow up, physical activity, dietary change, stress reduction and 'stroke rehabilitation' [38].

3.4 Infographic in health care

Infographic is utilized in health care related to literacy-sensitive information e.g. developing community health and address community needs, and aiming at better health and wellbeing for citizens [39].

3.5 Blogging in health care

The results of a three-year study related to health blogging [40] shows that the support from one's family and friends was related to improvements in the bloggers' health self-efficacy as well as reducing the bloggers' loneliness, particularly among those who also experienced increased support availability from blog readers. Furthermore, the bloggers' health-related uncertainty decreased. In health care blogger-patients participate more in their care path. Bloggers use many techniques like videos.

Using social media does not only have advantages, but also can spread negative news, or influence patients negatively. Witteman et al performed an experimental study in which they created a composite mock news article about home birth from six real news articles [41]. Witteman et al randomly assigned participants in an online study to view comments posted about the original six articles [41]. They found that exposure to one-sided social media comments with one-sided opinions influenced participants' opinions of the health topic regardless of their reported level of previous knowledge, especially when comments contained personal stories [41].

4. Research

Social media presents new opportunities for nurse researchers from exploration of research ideas to disseminations of research findings. In this section we describe how social media can be used at all stages of nursing research: from having ideas, finding information, collaborating, conducting the research, organizing and managing, disseminating, and evaluating. Here, social media includes not only social networking sites such as Facebook and Twitter, but also more narrow social forums such as Google Scholar and LinkedIn, and sites which store large amounts of socially generated data such as Google.

Nurse scientist are increasingly engaged in social media platforms, because it support discovery of new ideas, help to keep them up to date, allows easy following of the work of others and support publication [42].

Social media can be used as a method of study recruitment, especially snow ball recruitment. Snow ball recruitment, passing a research participant request from one person to another through a social media network can promote rapid dissemination of the request to the next level contacts. O'Connor et al were able to demonstrate Twitter as a low-cost method of recruitment for their online survey with 100 mothers of advanced maternal age [43].

User generated data on social media can be used for nursing researches. For example, social media can provide insights on consumers' information seeking behavior [44] or health behavior [45]. Social media can also provide indications of public opinion of specific topic, or reaction to specific event. Greaves et al used free-text comments posted on the Internet in blogs, social networks, and on physician rating websites to learn patient experience of their care using sentiment analysis [46].

Social media can be used as a dissemination strategy to get more citations and views of scholarly articles. For example, Nursing Research opened Facebook and Twitter accounts in 2010. Posts and tweets announce the current contents of the Journal. Nursing Research authors are showcased. Nursing Research sites serve as a hub for accessing research resources for nursing scientists. Information about critical and current health events from authoritative sources are shared and retweeted. Nursing Research combined social media with its traditional scholarly publication activities to support disseminating the best in nursing research to nursing scientist, scientist in related fields, nurses, health decision makers, policy makers, and people across the world [47].

It is important for nurse researchers to explore the potential and possibilities of social media for their researches in the future. With ready access to a vast range of people and data, social media offers much potential for conducting nursing research. However, social media research is in its early stages considering the research ethics, and many technical and methodological challenges in free data collection and analysis, and legal and ethical concerns inherent in using socially generated data remain.

Regarding technical challenges with researches using user generated unstructured social media, use of natural language processing (NLP) and ontology is important. NLP techniques have been used to structure narrative information from social media. NLP techniques have the capability to capture unstructured social media data, analyze its grammatical structure, determine the meaning of the information and translate the information so that it can be easily understood by the researchers [48]. In addition to NLP, unstructured content and data must be unified with structured data sources by a common ontological layer that allows users to understand and visualize important correlations between multiple data types and healthcare specific terms [49]. An ontology formally represents knowledge as a hierarchy of concepts within a domain, using a shared vocabulary to denote the types, properties and interrelationships of those concepts. Jung and Park used ontology to analyzed social media data on adolescents' depression [50]. For more knowledge on ontologies, please refer to section C chapter 1.

As more researchers use social media, protection of human subjects on social media needs to be developed. An important body is an institutional review board (IRB) which usually is a group of people that monitors research designed to obtain information from or about human subjects and how ethical issues are taken into consideration in research and development work, for instance [51]. However, IRB considerations relating to research using social media has not been very well-developed. Morenno, Goniu, Moreno, and Diekema reviewed the common risks inherent in social media research and made specific recommendations for researchers and IRBs for observational research, interactive research and survey/interview research. It is important for nurse researchers to check the latest requirements of the IRB when planning research using social media [52].

5. Safety, security, privacy, and ethics in the use of social media in healthcare

Healthcare professionals cannot be general users of social media. This means if you share information concerning health issue as a professional, you should use another account in your social media tool than the one you are using for your personal needs. In health related domain separate private and professional. The only way is to have separate accounts. Remember that what is published on social media tools is most of the time public domain and out of your control. Each of the tools like LinkedIn Facebook has private sectors where you can exchange information only to your target persons. Take into consideration that what you are exchanging in private sector may be reused by the receiver in public domain and all precautions taken are lost. To avoid trouble rules has to be defined between healthcare professionals and the receiver about what to do with information shared in the private sector through social media tools. The risk of misusing the ethical, privacy, safety or security rules is big. Part of this situation is bent with the country laws about these domains [53]. The main problem with the use of social media is the public aspect of the system as mentioned before. The adoption of the same code of conduct in place for patients and the institution is necessary. Recommendations are given in some countries for the use of social media. Never use personal tools for professional purposes. This must be separate. In the use of social media for healthcare only what is general, not related to patients, colleagues or institutions could be public domain [53, 54]. All the rest must be in the private domain and if it concerns a patient the rules must be clear and having the acceptance of the patient. The patient must be aware not to forward elements posted in the private section because as soon it is posted in public domain, it will be seen and may be misused.

Before publishing on social media tools a check is to be done about the subject and the confidentiality. Check if elements about a patient, or a colleague can be known? Can the message harm patients, colleagues or institutions? Is the reputation of the profession safeguarded? All material that could be published is concerned including photos, findings results, gene sequences i.e. The sender of social media information is responsible for safety, security and privacy [53,54,55,56,57]. Detailed information is available on Ventola's publication [57].

6. Conclusion

For the effective use of social media there are requirements. Firstly, the social media should be embedded carefully into care, education (including teaching and learning) process or other used processes. Secondly, there must clear instructions how and when one uses social media for versatile purposes. The user should have both information and communication (ICT) technical skills combined training with proper ICT-tools and health literacy skills. Thirdly, users of social media should recognize their responsibility to the other users and follow good ethical and privacy issues. Many online service providers use Netiquettes that covers both common courtesy online and rules of the Information highway. The risks related to social media are misuse, intimacy and privacy issues, data security issues especially in health care field. In personal level social media addiction should be taken into account. Depending on who creates the FB group, be that a public organization or a private person, there should be an understanding of the governance process, etiquette what this FB environment has and what the users should accept. The people should be instructed if the message or picture posted by a FB-user is considered offensive or inappropriate in any way, and any FB team member can delete it instantly they see it. Furthermore, the FB user's access can be denied. Due to rapid development of technical solutions, the use of social media requires constant education and training. In the future it is crucial to hear end-user voice and to ask what kind of social media tools and services are really wanted.

References

[1]   Amgad M., AlFaar AS., Integrating Web 2.0 in Clinical Research Education in a Developing Country, Journal of Cancer Education 29 (2014), 536–540.
[2]   McAndrew M., Johnson AE., The Role of Social Media in Dental Education, Journal of Dental Education 76 (2012), 1474-1481.
[3]   Cormode G., Krishnamurthy B., Key differences between Web 1.0 and Web 2.0, First Monday 13 (2008), 1–17.
[4]   Clark C., Student Growth in Asynchronous Online Environments: Learning Styles and Cognitive Development. Journal of the Indiana University Student Personnel Association (2012), 37-46. Retrieved 29.4.2016. Available at http://education.indiana.edu/graduate/programs/hesa/iuspa/4-%20Student%20Growth%20in%20Asynchronous%20Online%20Environments%20Learning%20Styles%20and%20Cognitive%20Development.pdf.
[5]   Obasa A., Eludire A., Ajao T., A comparative study of synchronous and asynchronous e-learning resources. International Journal of Innovative Research in Science, Engineering and Technology 2 (2013), 5938-5946.
[6]   Coleman A., Herselman M., Coleman M., Improving computer-mediated synchronous communication of doc tors in rural communities through cloud computing: a case study of rural hospitals in South Africa, International Journal of Computer Science & Information Technology (IJCSIT) 4 (2012), 13-22.
[7]   Swan M., Emerging Patient-Driven Health Care Models: An Examination of Health Social Networks, Consumer Personalized Medicine and Quantified Self-Tracking International Journal of Environmental Research and Public Health Health 6 (2009), 492-525.
[8]   Health on the Net Foundation (HON). Retrieved 29.9.2016. Available at https://www.hon.ch/.
[9]   Stephens TM., Gunther ME., Twitter, Millennials, and Nursing Education Research, Nursing Education Perspectives 37 (2016), 23-27.

[10] Sinclair W., McLoughlin M., Warne T., To Twitter to Woo: Harnessing the power of social media (SoMe) in nurse education to enhance the student's experience. Nurse Education in Practice 15 (2015), 507–511.

[11] Junco R., Elavsky C., Heiberger G., Putting twitter to the test: Assessing outcomes for student collaboration, engagement and success. British Journal of Educational Technology 44 (2013), 273–287.

[12] Zuckenberg M.. Bio. Retrieved 29.4.2016. Available at
      http://www.biography.com/people/mark-zuckerberg-507402

[13] Utz S., The function of self-disclosure on social network sites: Not only intimate, but also positive and entertaining self-disclosures increase the feeling of connection. Computers in Human Behavior 45 (2015), 1–10.

[14] Seydi A., Recep U., Well-being and problematic Facebook use. Computers in Human Behavior 49 (2015), 185–190.

[15] CDW Healthcare. Infotainment: Educate, Entertain, Empower, HealthcareCommunIT. 26.8.2013. Retrieved 29.4.2016. Available at http://www.cdwcommunit.com/technology/how-it-works/bedside-infotainment-technology/

[16] Gibbon C. Currie R, SONIC: Workbook evaluations from students using web-based resources. Nurse Education Today 28 (2008), 55– 61.

[17] Google Scholar. Retrieved 8.11.2016. Available at https://scholar.google.com/intl/en/scholar/help.html

[18] ResearchGate. Retrieved 8.11.2016. Available at https://www.researchgate.net/

[19] LinkedIn. Retrieved 8.11.2016. Available at http://whatis.techtarget.com/definition/LinkedIn

[20] English Oxford Dictionaries. 2016. Retrieved 8.11.2016. Available at
      https://en.oxforddictionaries.com/definition/infographic

[21] Gartner Blog Network. Retrieved 8.11.2016. Available at
      http://blogs.gartner.com/brian_burke/2014/04/04/gartner-redefines- gamification/

[22] Huang WHY, Soman D., A Practitioner's Guide to Gamification of Education. Research Report Series Behavioural Economics in Action. Rotman School of Management.University of Toronto. 2013.

[23] de-Marcos L., Domínguez A., Saenz-de-Navarrete J., Pagés C., An empirical study comparing gamification and social networking on e-learning. Computers & Education 75 (2014), 82–91.

[24] YouTube. Retrieved 8.11.2016. Available at https://www.youtube.com/yt/about/

[25] Pappas C. Why YouTube Should Be Part Of Your eLearning Course. eLearning Industry. Text written 14.9.2015. Retrieved 29.4. 2016. Available at http://elearningindustry.com/8-important-reasons-youtube-part-elearning-course

[26] Blood R., "Weblogs: A History And Perspective", Rebecca's Pocket. 7.9.2000. Retrieved 29.4.2016. Available at http://www.rebeccablood.net/essays/weblog_history.html

[27] Zandbelta L., Kanterb F., Ubbinkc D., E-consulting in a medical specialist setting: Medicine of the future? Patient Education and Counseling 99 (2016), 689–705.

[28] Gallant L., Irizarry L., Boone G., Kreps G. Promoting Participatory Medicine with Social Media: New Media Applications on Hospital Websites that Enhance Health Education and e-Patients' Voices. Journal of Participatory Medicine 3 (2011), e49.

[29] Sharoda A., Lichan H, Ed H. Is Twitter a Good Place for Asking Questions? A Characterization Study. 2011. Proceedings of the Fifth International AAAI Conference on Weblogs and Social Media.

[30] Paul M., Dredze M. You Are What You Tweet: Analyzing Twitter for Public Health. Human Language Technology Center of Excellence. Center for Language and Speech Processing. Copyright 2011. Johns Hopkins University Baltimore, MD 21218. Retrieved 29.4. 2016. Available at https://www.cs.jhu.edu/~mdredze/publications/twitter_health_icwsm_11.pdf.

[31] Tempel J., Noormohamed A., Schwartz R., Norman C., Malas M., Zawertailo L., van der Tempel J. Vape, quit, tweet? Electronic cigarettes and smoking cessation on Twitter. International Journal of Public Health 61 (2016), 249-256

[32] Gibbs A., Greaves B., Keeling M., Gaw A., O'Neill F. Clinical research benefits go viral via Twitter. Nursing Times 111 (2015), 16-17.

[33] Dion X., Using social networking sites (namely Facebook) in health visiting practice - an account of five years' experience, Community Practitioner 88 (2015), 28-31.

[34] Valle C., Tate D., Mayer D., Allicock M., Cai J. A randomized trial of a Facebook-based physical activity intervention for young adult cancer survivors. Journal of Cancer Survivorship 7 (2013), 355–368.

[35] Kouri P. Development of Maternity Clinic on the Net service – views of pregnant families and professionals. Dissertation. University of Kuopio. Social Sciences 131, 2006. Available at http://epublications.uef.fi/pub/urn_isbn_951-27-0501-X/urn_isbn_951-27-0501-X.pdf

[36] Gauthier J., Team-Based Care: Optimizing Primary Care for Patients and Providers. Institute for Health Improvement.   16.5.2014.   Retrieved   29.4.   2016.   Available   at

http://www.ihi.org/communities/blogs/_layouts/ihi/community/blog/itemview.aspx?List=0f316db6-7f8a-430f-a63a-ed7602d1366a&ID=29

[37] Luoto K., Suomen tietoyhteiskunta 2020 (Finnish Information Society 2020) Sitra article written 25.05.2011. Retrieved 29.4.2016. Available at http://www.sitra.fi/artikkelit/avoin-data/suomen-tietoyhteiskunta-2020.

[38] Baranowski T., Blumberg F., Buday R., DeSmet A., Fiellin LE. Green CS., Kato PM., Lu AS., Maloney AE., Mellecker R., Morrill BA., Peng W., Shegog R., Simons M., Staiano AE., Thompson D., Young K., Games for Health for Children—Current Status and Needed Research. White paper, Games for Health Journal 4 (2015), 1-12.

[39] CDC. Community Health Navigator. Retrieved 29.4.2016. Available at http://www.cdc.gov/CHInav/

[40] Keating D., Rains S., Health Blogging and Social Support: A 3-Year Panel Study. Journal of Health Communication 20 (2015), 1449-1457.

[41] Witteman H., Fagerlin A., Exe N., Trottier M., Zikmund-Fisher B., One-Sided Social Media Comments Influenced Opinions And Intentions About Home Birth: An Experimental Study. Health Affairs 35 (2016), 4726-4733.

[42] Cruzd A., Coertzen M.. Wired academia: Why social science scholars are using social media. Proceedings of the 36th Hawaii International Conference on System Sciences (HICSS), 2013

[43] O'Connor A., Jackson L., Goldsmith L., Skirton H, Can I get a retweet please? Health research recruitment and the Twittersphere. Journal of Advanced Nursing 70 (2014), 599-609.

[44] Smith B., Staci Smith S. Engaging Health: Health Research and policymaking in the social media sphere. Academy Health Retrieved 30.9.2016. Available at https://www.academyhealth.org/files/FileDownloads/AH_Translation%20Engaging%20Health%20report%20v5.pdf, 2015.

[45] Myslín M, Zhu S, Chapman W., Convay M., Using twitter to examine smoking behavior and perceptions of emerging tobacco products. Journal of Medical Internet Research 15 (2013),e174.

[46] Greaves F., Ramirez-Cano D., Millett C., Darzi A., Donaldson L. Use of Sentiment Analysis for Capturing Patient Experience From Free-Text Comments Posted Online. Journal of Medical Internet Research 15 (2013), e239.

[47] Henly S., Science Publishing, Social Media, and Nursing Research on Facebook and Twitter. Nursing Research 65 (2016), 169.

[48] Iroju O., Olaleke J. A Systematic Review of Natural Language Processing in Healthcare. International Journal. Information Technology and Computer Science 8 (2015), 44-50.

[49]. Kuiler E. From Big Data to Knowledge: An Ontological Approach to Big Data Analytics. Review of Policy Research 31 (2014), 311-318.

[50] Jung H., Park H., Song T., Development and Evaluation of an Adolescents' Depression Ontology for Analyzing Social Data. Studies in Health Technology and Informatics 225 (2016), 442-446.

[51] The Institutional Review Board (IRB): A College Planning Guide. Retrieved 8.11.2016. Available at http://www.apa.org/ed/precollege/undergrad/ptacc/irb-college-guide.pdf

[52] Moreno M., Goniu N., Moreno P., Diekema D., Ethics of social media research: common concerns and practical considerations. Cyberpsychology, Behavior, and Social Networking 16 (2013), 708-713

[53] BMA. Using social media: practical an ethical guidance for doctors and medical students. Retrieved 30.9.2016. Available at http://bma.org.uk/-/media/files/pdfs/practical%20advice%20at%20work/ethics/socialmediaguidance.pdf.

[54] NCSBN.White Paper: A Nurse's Guide to the Use of Social Media. Retrieved 8.8.2016. Available at https://www.ncsbn.org/Social_Media.pdf.

[55] Doctors' use of social media, General Medical Council 2013. Retrieved 8.8.2016. Available at http://www.gmc-uk.org/Doctors__use_of_social_media.pdf_51448306.pdf.

[56] Guidelines: Social Media and Electronic Communication Nursing Council of New Zealand Retrieved 8.8.2016 Available at http://www.waikatodhb.health.nz/assets/for-staff/social-media/A-nurses-guide-to-social-media-and-electronic-communication.pdf.

[57] Ventola C., Social Media and Health Care Professionals: Benefits, Risks, and Best Practices. Pharmacy and Therapeutics 39 (2014), 491-520.

Section D

Competencies for Nurses, Nurse Leaders and NI Specialists

Forecasting Informatics Competencies for Nurses in the Future of Connected Health
J. Murphy et al. (Eds.)
197

© 2017 IMIA and IOS Press.
doi:10.3233/978-1-61499-738-2-197

Nurse Leadership and Informatics Competencies: Shaping Transformation of Professional Practice

Margaret Ann KENNEDY[a], Anne MOEN[b]

[a] *Gevity Consulting Inc., CANADA*
[b] *Institute for Health and Society, Faculty of Medicine, University of Oslo, NORWAY*

Abstract. Nurse leaders must demonstrate capacities and develop specific informatics competencies in order to provide meaningful leadership and support ongoing transformation of the healthcare system. Concurrently, staff informatics competencies must be planned and fostered to support critical principles of transformation and patient safety in practice, advance evidence-informed practice, and enable nursing to flourish in complex digital environments across the healthcare continuum. In addition to nurse leader competencies, two key aspects of leadership and informatics competencies will be addressed in this chapter – namely, the transformation of health care and preparation of the nursing workforce.

Keywords. Leadership, digital competencies, professional practice, education, transformation

1. Introduction

Leadership and the technological revolution in today's dynamic healthcare sector are focal discussion topics both in the scientific and popular literature. Calls for development of informatics competencies among nurse leaders, while not new, are increasingly vocal and compelling [1-7]. Such demands are triggered by a variety of drivers including shifting population demographics, increasing burdens of chronic disease, spiraling health care costs, scarce resources, major shortages in qualified healthcare professionals, consumer demands for improved quality, transparency and self control, calls for person-centric integrated models of care, supported by the ubiquity of technology [7-11]. National reports call for significant reforms of existing healthcare infrastructure and leadership practices with tangible recommendations involving technology for the future [12-14]. In sum, this development exposes the need for leaders that don't simply react to suggested IT-solutions, but understand information management, digital trends, and future practice implications and are able to capitalize on opportunities in a digital era.

This chapter will highlight the skills required by nurse leaders such as Chief Nurse Executives (CNEs), Vice Presidents of Care services and other senior leadership personnel, to support authentic healthcare transformation, advance nursing roles in digital environments, and ensure workforce digital competence to provide professional, evidence-informed care in complex, connected health environments.

2. Leadership as a Characteristic of Nurse Executives

The 2010 Institute of Medicine & Robert Wood Johnson Foundation report [12] proposed a comprehensive map for the future of nursing in the United States with new roles to transform healthcare along three aspects - *leadership, education, and practice*. With broad and discipline-specific transformation as core principles, this report declared that nurses are essential to help shape and lead the future of a dynamic, integrated, patient-centric health care system. In response to the centrality of nursing in healthcare, new types of nursing roles are emerging to support leadership and transformation, including Chief Nursing Informatics Officers and Nursing Informatics Executives [12]. These innovative leadership roles are considered essential to effectively support transformational activities and enable new models of care in clinical practice with appropriate technology solutions [9-11]. Likewise, other international organizations, including the National Health Services (NHS), Organisation for Economic Co-operation and Development (OECD), Academy of Canadian Executive Nurses (ACEN), Norwegian Nurses Organization, and the Swedish Society of Nursing are highlighting that greater adoption of digital solutions requires nursing informatics competency among nursing leadership to leverage technological solutions that can support contemporary nursing practice, and advocacy for future optimization of nursing in technological environments [13-17]. Further, advocacy of nursing within key priorities includes but is not limited to data quality, evaluation metrics, data science/big data, eSafety, and strategic advocacy for clinical information system design, deployment and procurement aligned to meet patient and nursing needs [18-22].

Leadership, as both a professional descriptor and a commodity in practice, reflects skillful synthesis of a) capacities of the individual in the job, e.g., knowledge, skills, experiences, b) the frame of the role, e.g., purpose, perspective and position, and c) the agenda of the job, e.g., strategic and operating goals, care quality, resource utilization, and policy [5]. Clear expectations regarding nurse executive leadership and nursing informatics competencies are essential to move beyond simply 'being aware' of informatics while delegating responsibility to other specialists to create discrete learning opportunities targeting nurse executive preparation enabling effective practice of informatics knowledge and skills across executive environments [2-4, 9-11, 23].

While informatics specialists can be available for deep expertise, nurse executives require a "broad, working knowledge of IT to safeguard patient care outcomes" [3]. In his 2013 study of CNE competencies in nursing informatics, Simpson found that senior nurse executives experienced a competency gap in "awareness of societal and technological trends, issues, and developments as they relate to nursing" [3, p.6], resulting in self reports that most CNEs felt unable to effectively represent nursing needs in the technology discussion and evaluation processes dominated by physicians or other stakeholders. Further, nurse executives reported that their roles were relegated simply to review software functionality [3], and that nurse leaders may not even be invited to report nurse specific perspectives when assessing potential functionality [11].

Five common competency domains for nurse executives were identified by American Organization of Nurse Executives (AONE) [18]. Figure 1 illustrates the domains of communication and relationship management; knowledge of the health care environment; leadership; professionalism; business skills and principles. Within these domains, explicit competency statements are provided which support the broad skills required to effectively provide nursing leadership. These recently updated Nurse Executive Competencies [18] provide a robust example of explicit expectations around informatics competency. Development of these competency elements is critical to resolve some of the frustration historically encountered by nurse leaders.

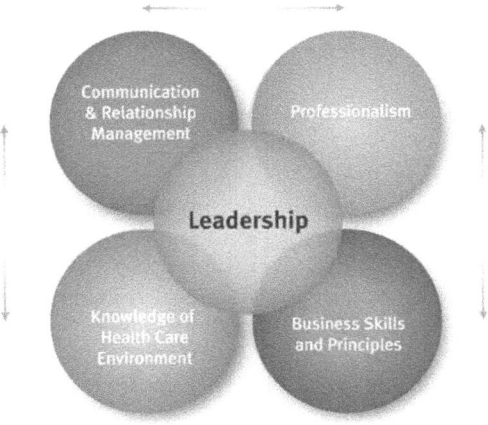

Figure 1 AONE Nurse Executive Competency Model (2015, p.2), copyright 2015, by the American Organization of Nurse Executives (AONE). All rights reserved.

Under Business Skills, AONE includes a subsection of Information Management and Technology, with seven key competency elements (Table 1).

Table 1 Business Skills excerpt, AONE Nurse Executive Competencies (2015, p. 10), copyright 2015, by the American Organization of Nurse Executives (AONE). All rights reserved.

INFORMATION MANAGEMENT AND TECHNOLOGY
Use technology to support improvement of clinical and financial performance
Collaborate to prioritize for the establishment of information technology resources
Participate in evaluation of enabling technology in practice settings
Use data management systems for decision making
Identify technological trends, issues and new developments as they apply to patient care
Demonstrate skills in assessing data integrity and quality
Provide leadership for the adoption and implementation of information systems

The following informatics competencies are recommended to extend the AONE list:
- Actively challenge boundaries within, across and outside the traditional care settings, to enable personalized, coordinated, and connected health care
- Foster nursing practice that maintains client advocacy in connected healthcare and empowers clients to effectively use the tools of connected health for supported self management to achieve desired health outcomes
- Identify data sources and data types that inform data driven clinical decisions that leverage clinical intelligence and practice-based evidence
- Demonstrate the ability to identify, filter, and use information to support strategic organizational and profession-specific decision making

- Balance the use of technology with the humanistic perspective of nursing practice
- Demonstrate effective change management skills to resolve resistance to change and further support digital enablement and clinical practice alike.

3. Transformation of professional practice environments

Healthcare transformation is reflected in shifting models of care, increasing use of interprofessional care teams, and the widespread adoption of clinical information systems (CIS) to support care provision. With many organizations investing in CIS, it is essential that nurses have an active role in contributing to the requirements gathering, evaluation, design, and ultimate selection of clinical systems [2-6, 11, 23-27].

Two core aspects of the ongoing transformation to *connected care*, include a) shifting from support of episodic to a more longitudinal perspective of care, and b) increasing opportunities for the individual and family's access and engagement with personal health information, which encompasses access to of all care settings, including the full scope of activities in primary care, home dwellings and specialized care [28].

As the largest group of users of and contributors to health information systems [26], nurses have enormous stakes in transformation of clinical environments. The availability of accurate, timely, and accessible data, collectively referred to as clinical intelligence, is essential in contemporary clinical practice environments. Nurses are ideally positioned to advance clinical intelligence and practice-based evidence through attention to data quality, guideline implementation, as well as design and selection of effective solutions [20].

When operating at their peak, innovative clinical systems provide users with accurate, readily accessible data supporting improved clinical decision making and nursing practice, outcomes and quality measurement, enhanced interprofessional communications, improved patient safety, and sophisticated analytics to inform all aspects of health care delivery and administration [2, 6, 9, 18, 21, 22]. However, when nurses are not engaged in design and procurement processes, they frequently find themselves working with systems that fail to meet clinical needs, and are subsequently compelled to find workarounds to maintain patient safety to compensate for system flaws or even failed implementations [4, 26, 36]. In these instances, nurse executives must "function as the voice of patient care" [3] in assertively advocating for functionality and workflows that effectively meet patient care needs and their safety.

As demands for data-driven decisions across healthcare systems continue to rise, the infrastructure supporting clinical information management will necessitate interoperable information systems seamlessly linked with financial, human resource, organizational systems. CIS that incorporate principles of data science and analytics to inform evidence-based decision making are critical elements of this demand [21, 22, 29]. However, in many instances, clinical information systems are the last to be deployed, after laboratory, radiology, financial, admission-discharge and transfer, and other modules have long been in use. Nurse executives can use tools like the AONE Guiding Principles [24,25] to develop capacities and prepare to advocate assertively to introduce solutions that are unambiguously patient-centric, and meet nursing needs with intuitive interfaces, clinical decision support solutions, and unrestricted access to databases in centers of excellence. Nurses and nurse executives are best positioned to represent nursing workflows and core nursing needs supporting patient care.

Where nurses are unable to provide leadership and clear requirements, other disciplines will emerge to drive change and procurement, such as physicians [3] or information system (IS) experts, who note that a "rare and remarkable opportunity has emerged for the IS community to leverage its in-depth knowledge to both advance theory and impact practice and policy" [29]. Further, in many practice settings, incongruence between existing clinical workflows and Commercial Off-The-Shelf (COTS) products necessitate additional customization and active nursing engagement to represent critical information flows and decision points in nursing workflows. With alignment to workflows being critical to securing an effective CIS, many IS resources recommend alignment to medical or generic workflows [29]. This is not an uncommon approach and illustrates necessity of nurse leaders being active participants in health information system requirements gathering, design, procurement, and implementation.

4. Transformation of the profession

Requirements identification and selection of a digital information system, whether a specific electronic health record (EHR), a clinical information system, a portal, or a selection of mobile apps, are often part of the organization's larger digital ecosystem (See section C chapter 1 for further explanations about the health ecosystem). Evaluations of systems and the vendors' offerings are often a procurement decision, influenced by a multitude of interests beyond those of the actual end users. Functional and non-functional requirements, and system choice are likely to reflect priorities and intentions of the organizational procurement division, but engagement and advocacy are important strategies to contribute clinician and end user perspectives.

Being a dependent adoption decision [30], procurement deliberations and decisions can generate challenging conditions for clinical practice. Gaps in clarity of or alignment with the scope of intended clinical transformation, and disrupted information flows within and among interprofessional teams often create challenges during and following implementation of CIS. For the existing workforce of registered nurses, physicians, and other health providers, starting to use a digital information system to document clinical encounters and professional decision making, becomes a process to adopt features and functionalities of already selected systems in the available digital ecosystem. Workforce preparation to maximize the abilities and advantages of the system will depend on the core features and identified problems a system sets out to solve. For example, a CIS can be perceived as invaluable in meeting specific professional requirements for one group of clinicians while it may be seen as very cumbersome to integrate for other professionals in another practice. Workforce preparations can therefore involve different activities.

The strategies required to achieve system transformation must include the strategic vision of what professional practice will be, identification of the necessary clinical and digital competencies, clear articulation of the program of activity with local clinical intelligence and required data needs supporting clinical practice and client outcomes, and overall alignment to organizational, regional/national, and disciplinary strategy and priorities [3, 9, 25]. Nurse leaders' capacities to shape future practice and ensure up to date competencies of the workforce to access information and apply knowledge are core contributions for the overall preparation of a workforce. This includes abilities to master available systems, support practice-based and data driven decision-making, maintain continuity of care, and ensure patient safety at all times [3, 9, 23]. Informatics overviews, anticipation and articulation of desired competencies, training requirements and education opportunities would ensure that the workforce has the necessary information technology (IT) skills and digital health literacy [23] to successfully practice and contribute to a transformed healthcare environment. Nurse executives are "in a prime position to bridge research, education, and practice" supporting workforce preparation [9]. Section A chapter 2 discusses the role of formal education in greater depth, and thus, the following section will highlight three core dimensions of workforce preparation: digital literacy, system, and practice.

4.1 Competency in health informatics - digital health literacy

A core challenge whenever health informatics and digital opportunities are introduced in health care is the development of workforce knowledge and articulation of specific competencies. A significant number of all health care professionals are digital immigrants [31], and as such, unfamiliar with many of basic features or functionalities of any digital system. Leadership is about facilitating and ensuring processes where nurses remain highly skilled professionals with added expertise in information technology and nursing. Therefore, digital health literacy or eHealth literacy is an important foundational topic for workforce preparation and in-service training. While often organized as part of deployment of any digital system, training should go beyond system specific introduction to ensure staff have demonstrable competencies to locate and act upon information in digital form [32].

Acquiring new skills and capacities to use and take advantage of the opportunities is a core issue in workforce preparation. Digital literacy or information literacy, informatics awareness or computer experience are connected to the professional use of information technology [33]. Few standards or guidelines are available to integrate broader nursing informatics competencies into either undergraduate or graduate level programs, making it difficult to design appropriate nursing curricula or provide competency guidelines [8, 23, 34, 35]. Defined and validated informatics competencies for nurses at four levels of practice have been available for more than a decade, and provide competencies for the beginner, experienced, Informatics Nurse Specialist and informatics innovator [7, 36]. These levels focus on different expectations regarding technology use, information system use and informatics-specific content issues to guide curriculum development. Educational resources that could apply for workforce preparation are discussed in section B chapter 1 - Informatics Competencies to Start Professional Life: A Global Perspective, and section B: What practicing nurses need to know about Health IT in order to practice today: Continuing education and certification. A collective challenge for nursing executives is to widely disseminate and adopt suggested competency–based training beyond formal academic programs to ensure timely, accessible workforce access.

For workforce preparations to advance digital health literacy a set of minimum level competencies will be necessary. There are suggested two levels of learning:

- *Understand:* demonstrated as a set of knowledge and skills related to actual use of any clinical information system, EHR, or eHealth/mHealth solution
- *Know:* familiarity with and ability to relate a topic in a clinical system to a specific aspect of work, for example laws, ethics and standards.

Therefore, workforce preparation could emphasize competence to access to information for continuous care and patient safety, confidentiality and privacy, conditions for exchange of health data, information use for different digital systems, and encourages health professionals to provide feedback and actively engage in processes to elaborate and expand the set of suggested competencies [11, 37].

Recommendations for leadership initiatives targeting workforce development include implementation of systematic processes to become digitally competent, and formalizing transitions to mandatory competencies with discrete education programs encompassing a full range of information [23]. This type of educational program would necessarily include foundational knowledge (e.g., data-information-knowledge-wisdom, data standardization, data quality) as well as core set of minimum data, to more advanced levels of information, such as that related to analytics [3, 9, 23]. As progress is made on core or 'classical' topics for nursing informatics for both the workforce and nurse executives, attention will need to shift to skills needed for connected care, where new actors join and the need will shift to even greater needs for data science and connecting people to health information [38].

4.2 Competency in information system procurements

An important area of workforce preparation relates to capacity for participation in procurement and customization of a system, where the selection of core features, emphasis on specific data elements or tailored information sequences or data subsets set the stage for local, practice-specific use [3, 9]. Ensuring appropriate workflow support, algorithms, patient safety and quality care when professional requirements and information systems assessment match up with little opportunity for harm is paramount for procurement and further customization of any CIS [24, 26, 39]. These are fundamental considerations leading to workable templates for documentation of professional deliberation and enactment, specifications of guidelines, selection of rules, and making decision support relevant.

As part of the nurse executive scope in procurement processes, it is critical that vendors understand and accept that they must consider more than one workflow to achieve transformation. Simply replicating a linear, generic "paper-based" workflow in a digital environment is insufficient to support authentic transformation and gain the true value of intelligent electronic systems. Nurse executives can challenge vendors to balance workflows, present data in multiple ways, and position the patient and clinical needs as their priorities – rather than forcing clinicians to accommodate to a system design. Further, requirements gathering must specifically include nursing as well as other clinical disciplines to ensure that both functional and non-functional requirements are explicitly captured, prioritized, and considered across the systems development lifecycle – and particularly in the design phase.

4.3 Competency in practice development, teamwork and workflow adaptation

A core challenge to workforce preparation is to learn how to work within CIS and broader digital health information ecosystems, and deal with changes introduced as a consequence of the CIS, either in the representation of professional practice or in the new opportunities to collaborate in hybrid teams. A key feature of current interprofessional teams is equity in contributions by health professionals combined with patient and family involvement. This is the prime example of transcending boundaries in connected health. Many opportunities exist to explore, and exploit information in CIS in concert with patient-generated data and reports of daily living.

Generating the clinical intelligence and practice-based evidence that drives improved patient outcomes through accurate and timely data provision to clinicians and interprofessional forums is only one dimension supporting best practice in transformation. Nurse executives are encouraged to adopt a systems perspective to ensure that such clinical intelligence is incorporated throughout care plans, assessments, and outcomes evaluations in ongoing, health-focused decision making that includes and supports patients. Nurse executives should also seek to include aspects of the following considerations to transformation:

- Prioritizing personalized care and new mechanisms of engaging individuals and families as partners in all aspects of connected health, where personal experience and preferences are incorporated into care delivery, appropriate analytics utilize multiple information sources ranging across clinical information systems; and self-care and clinical decisions are supported through access to Internet of Things-based personal devices;
- Accommodate changes in sites of care, developing models that are sensitive to multiplicity in spatial and temporal dimensions over longitudinal trajectories of care;
- Practice models of interprofessional teams where equity in contributions from the individual and family and health professionals are incorporated in the assessment, deliberations and enactment in ongoing, health related decision making;
- Challenging existing digitization of workflow and practice to support transcending traditional boundaries. Advocacy for transformation beyond simply placing "forms" into electronic environments and expecting clinical outcome improvements.

5. Implications for Leadership

Transformation sits in the convergence of drivers and enablers for a new digital health ecosystem, leadership, and workforce preparation. The layers of complexity within contemporary healthcare environments and the requisite skills needed to effectively lead professional nursing practice necessitate that nurse executives develop explicit informatics knowledge and skills for themselves and their workforce. While collateral competencies developed for effective organizational leadership and clinical information management can be scaled to support broader leadership across the profession of nursing and the healthcare sector, informatics knowledge cannot be delegated to informatics specialists, and nurse executives must prioritize this set of essential skills. Key competencies for nursing executives leading evolving connected care include:

- Fundamental understanding of core informatics concepts and their utility to nursing, professional collaboration and patient safety;
- Understanding how digital health information ecosystems either support or disrupt clinical workflows and the implications of any such changes;
- Ability to actively and accurately represent nursing needs in design and deployment as well and procurement and customization;
- Ability to facilitate/enable development of workforce preparation strategy and educational program, including mandatory competencies, additional competencies; and
- Change management skills to complement informatics skills.

Achieving these competencies will require nursing executives to examine a variety of educational forums, including formal academic programs, as well as entrepreneurial innovations that create opportunity within and beyond the organizations [40] using hybrid solutions for continuous education, such as digital learning environments (e.g., Massive Open Online Courses (MOOC), Small Private Online Course (SPOC), local eLearning courses). As enterprises across the globe continue to increase the pace of healthcare digitization in pursuit of greater quality and success, and the Internet of Things, mHealth, and data analytics continue to gain momentum, it is imperative that a coherent program of discrete opportunities are established to enable development of informatics competencies among nurse executives, and that nurse executives articulate their needs.

In this digital era of increasingly connected health, developing capacities and informatics competencies for nurses and nurses executives are an essential strategic enabler to the achievement of all other executive leadership competencies, including communication and relationship management, knowledge of the healthcare environment, business skills and principles, and supporting nursing practice.

References

[1]   Nagle L. The importance of being informatics savvy. Can J Nurs Leadersh. 2016;28(4):1-4.
[2]   Remus S. The big data revolution: opportunities for chief nurse executives, Can J Nurs Leadersh. 2016;28(4):18-28.
[3]   Simpson, R. Chief nurse executives need contemporary informatics competencies, Nurs Econ, 2013;3(6)1:277- 87.
[4]   Remus S., Kennedy MA. Innovation in transformative nursing leadership: nursing informatics competencies and roles, Can J Nurs Leadersh. 2012;25(4):14-26.
[5]   Moen A. (2002). Nursing leadership when an electronic patient record system is introduced in Norwegian hospitals. (Doctoral Dissertation), University of Oslo, Oslo.
[6]   Goeschel C. The future of nursing: leading change, advancing health stories to ignite the transformation, Nurs Crit Care. 2011;16(5): 217-19.
[7]   Staggers N., Gassert CA., Curran A. Delphi study to determine informatics competencies for nurses at four levels of practice. Nurs Res. 2002;51(6): 383-90.
[8]   Chang J., Poynton MR., Gassert CA., Staggers N. Nursing informatics competencies required of nurses in Taiwan. Int J Med Inform. 2011;80(5):332-40.
[9]   Harris C., Murphy J., Transforming nursing practice through technology and informatics: A position statement. J Health In Manag. 2011;25(3): 20-26.
[10] Hussey P., Kennedy MA., Instantiating informatics within nursing practice for integrated patient centered holistic models of care: A discussion paper, J Adv Nurs. 2016;75(5):1030-41.
[11] Moen A., Svarlien B., Berge M., Netteland G. Informatics competencies - necessary conditions for sustainable ehealth. Paper presented at the Scandinavian Health Informatics 2010, Copenhagen.
[12] IOM (Institute of Medicine). The future of nursing: leading change, advancing health. Washington, DC: The National Academies Press; 2010.
[13] National Health Service (NHS) Using data and technology to transform outcomes for patients and citizens. A framework for action; 2010. Available from: https://www.gov.uk/government/publications/personalised-health-and-care-2020.
[14] Organization of Economic Co-Operative Development (OECD) Improving health care efficiency: The role of ICT [eBook]; 2010. Available from: http://ec.europa.eu/health/eu_world/docs/oecd_ict_en.pdf.
[15] Meyer R.M., VanDeVelde-Coke S., Velji V. Leadership for health system transformation: what's needed in Canada? Brief for the Canadian Nurses Association's national expert commission on the health of our nation: The future of our health system. Can J Nurs Leadersh. 2011;24(4), 21–30.
[16] Swedish Society of Nursing (2013) EHealth: A strategy for nursing. Report ISBN: 978-91-85060-20-7. Available from www.swenurse.se.
[17] Norwegian Nurses Organisation (2013) Innovation and service development. Political platform 2013-2016. Available from: https://www.nsf.no/nursing-and-health-politics/artikkelliste/1218046

[18] American Organization of Nurse Executives (AONE), Nurse executive competencies. (2015) Available from: http://www.aone.org/resources/nec.pdf
[19] Westra BL., Clancy TR., Sensmeier J., Warren JJ., Weaver C., Delaney C. Nursing knowledge: big data science – implications for nurse leaders, J Nurs Adm. 2015;39:304-10.
[20] Brennan PF., Bakken S., Nursing needs big data and big data needs nursing, J Nurs Scholarsh. 2015;47(5):477-84.
[21] Harrington L. Clinical intelligence, J Nurs Adm. 2011;41(12):507-09.
[22] Harrington L. The Role of nurse informaticists in the emerging field of clinical intelligence, Proceedings NI2012: 11th International congress on nursing informatics, Montreal, QC, Canada (2012) 162-165.
[23] Oakes M., Frisch N., Potter P., Borycki E. Readiness of nurse executives and leaders to advocate for health information systems supporting nursing, Stud Health Technol Inform. 2015;208:296–301.
[24] American Organization of Nurse Executives (AONE) Guiding principles for defining the role of the nurse executive in technology acquisition and implementation, 2009. Available from: http://www.aone.org/resources/technology-acquisition-implementation.pdf
[25] American Organization of Nurse Executives (AONE) Guiding principles for the nurse executive to enhance clinical outcomes by leveraging technology, 2009. Available from: http://www.aone.org/resources/enhance-clinical-outcomes-leveraging-technology.pdf
[26] Harrington L., AONE creates new position paper: nursing informatics executive leader, Nurse Lead. 201;10(3);17-8.
[27] Lucius S., Nurse informatics executive: re-shaping the patient experience through technology, Nurse Lead. 2012;10(3):21.
[28] Karazivan, P., Dumez, V., Flora, L., Pomey, MP., Del Grande, C., Ghadiri, DP., et al. (2015). The Patient-as-Partner Approach in Health Care. Academic Medicine, 90(4), 437–441.
[29] Agarwal R., Gao G., DesRoches C., Jha A. The digital transformation of healthcare: current status and the road ahead, Information Systems Research, 2010;21(4):796-809.
[30] Rogers E., Diffusion of Innovation. New York: The Free Press; 1995.
[31] Prensky M. Digital natives, digital immigrants on the horizon. 2001.
[32] Monkman H., & Kushniruk AW., eHealth literacy issues, constructs, models, and methods for health information technology design and evaluation. Knowledge Management & E-Learning: An International Journal (KM&EL). 2015;74(4):541-49.
[33] Saranto K., Hovenga E., Information literacy - what is it about? Literature review of the concept and the context. International Journal of Medical Informatics. 2004;73:503-13.
[34] Canadan Association of Schools of Nursing, Entry-to-practice competencies for registered nurses, 2012. Available from: http://www.casn.ca/2014/12/casn-entry-practice-nursing-informatics-competencies/
[35] HIMSS, TIGER virtual learning environment, 2016. Available from: http://www.himss.org/professional-development/tiger-initiative/virtual-learning-environment.
[36] Peterson,vH.E., Gerdin-Jelger,U., (Eds.), (1988). Preparing Nurses for Using Information Systems: recommended Informatics Competencies.. New York, National League for Nursing
[37] Canadian Association of Schools of Nursing, Nursing informatics teaching toolkit: supporting the integration of the CASN nursing informatics competencies into nursing curricula, 2013. Available from: http://casn.ca/wp-content/uploads/2014/12/2013ENNursingInformaticsTeachingToolkit.pdf.
[38] Booth R., Informatics and nursing in a post-nursing informatics world: Future directions for nurses in an automated, artificially intelligent, social-networked healthcare environment, Can J Nurs Leadersh. 2016;28(4):61-9.
[39] Coiera E., Aarts J., Kulikowski C. The dangerous decade. JAMIA. 2012;19(1):2-5. doi:10.1136/amiajnl-2011-000674
[40] Wilson A., Whitaker N., Whitford D. Rising to the challenge of health care reform with entrepreneurial and intrapreneurial nursing initiatives, Online J Issues Nurs, 2012;17(2):Manuscript 5.

Forecasting Informatics Competencies for Nurses in the Future of Connected Health
J. Murphy et al. (Eds.)
207

© *2017 IMIA and IOS Press.*
doi:10.3233/978-1-61499-738-2-207

Opportunity and Approach for Implementation of a Self-Assessment Tool: Nursing Informatics Competencies for Nurse Leaders (NICA-NL)

Andrew PHILLIPS[a,d], Po-Yin YEN[b], Mary KENNEDY[c], and Sarah COLLINS[d,e]

[a] *Massachusetts General Hospital Institute of Health Professions, Boston, MA, United States*
[b] *The Ohio State University, Columbus, Ohio, United States*
[c] *AEGIS Informatics LLC, Barrington, RI, United States*
[d] *Partners Healthcare System, Wellesley, MA;* [e] *Brigham and Women's Hospital, Boston, MA, United States*

Abstract. The changing environment of healthcare and the increasing reliance on technology to drive and evaluate change requires efficient tools to assess and educate nursing leadership on the skills necessary to succeed in their leadership roles. Using the Nursing Informatics Competencies for Nurse Leaders (NICA-NL) Scale as an example, this chapter will explore how such a tool can be implemented and provide value to healthcare organizations, as well as advance nursing practice.

Keywords. Self-assessment tool, Nurse Leader, Informatics Competencies

1. Introduction

The role of the Nurse Leader is continuously demanding greater in-depth knowledge and skills related to nursing informatics, as discussed in section D chapter 1 of this book. Healthcare organization-based Nurse Leaders include Chief Nursing Officers, Directors of Nursing, and Nurse Managers. Individuals in these roles are engaged in a wide breadth of activities, ranging from planning EHR training curriculums to identifying strategic initiatives for innovation. Baseline knowledge of informatics is important to guide the Nurse Leader's work, particularly as advances in nursing practice become increasingly intertwined with innovation.

2. Background

The Nursing Informatics Competencies for Nurse Leaders (NICA-NL) Scale is a validated self-assessment competency tool for Nurse Leaders that has undergone extensive development and validation.[1]. The tool consists of 26 items that group into 6 factors (Strategic Implementation Management, Advanced Information Management and Education, Executive Planning, Ethical and Legal Concepts, Information Systems

Concepts, Requirements and System Selection).[1] The NICA-NL tool has been copyrighted and is available for use, and can be accessed here [1] or by contacting the authors. In previous work, our team identified that the majority of Nurse Leaders surveyed have learned informatics knowledge and skills 'on the job' or through 'self-learning'. Tools that can be applied to the Nurse Leader's practice, and are accessible as part of a suite of educational resources provided to the Nurse Leaders by his or her employer, have the potential for wide-spread adoption and impact.

3. Application of NICA-NL at health care organizations

3.1. Vision

Nurse Leaders comprise a large portion of middle to upper management leadership positions throughout healthcare organizations, with titles such as Nurse Manager, Nurse Director, and Nurse Executive. Given that the Nurse Leader's primary focus is not on nursing informatics, it is important to understand why we need a self-assessment tool focused on Nursing Informatics Competencies for Nurse Leaders. Nursing management and practice can no longer be separated from informatics and the pervasive use of technology and data to deliver, evaluate, and improve healthcare. Given the limited available time and resources of Nurse Leaders and their organizations, efforts to increase competency skills and knowledge need to be relatively low-intensity, scalable, and sustainable. Low-intensity interventions that can be delivered to large numbers of people may have a more pervasive impact than more efficacious interventions that require greater resources.[2]

In this chapter we provide an overview of one approach that can be used to implement a validated informatics self-assessment tool, the NICA-NL, and discuss opportunities NICA-NL could provide for healthcare organizations and more broadly nursing management and practice. The RE-AIM framework (Reach, Efficacy, Adoption, Implementation, and Maintenance) has been used to guide the implementation and evaluation of innovations in public health, informatics, and nursing. [2] The use of this framework provides an incremental path and guidance to achieve and measure increased informatics competency levels of Nurse Leaders at an organization.

3.2. Implementation Framework

The RE-AIM framework states that the impact and sustainability of an intervention should be evaluated based on its: 1) Reach, 2) Efficacy, 3) Adoption, 4) Implementation, 5) and Maintenance. Here we provide an overview of how the NICA-NL could be implemented at a healthcare organization using the RE-AIM framework. [2]

- Reach: Who is the intended, target audience for NICA-NL?
- Efficacy or effectiveness: What outcomes/impacts could you observe at your organization?
- Adoption level: How many Nurse Leaders have used the tool at your organization?

- **I**mplementation consistency, costs and adaptations made during delivery: What resources are needed to implement the NICA-NL?
- **M**aintenance of intervention effects in individuals and settings over time: How are NICA-NL re-assessments performed for new and existing Nurse Leaders?

3.2.1. Measuring potential for impact on organization

There are many nursing leaders at any given healthcare organization. Some Nurse Leader roles provide input into strategic plans for their organizations, others execute the management of staff nurses at the bedside. Understanding the varied Nurse Leader roles at your organization and clarifying the scope of efforts to increase nursing informatics competencies is critical. Small scale pilot implementations to only C-suite Nurse Leaders versus spreading the NICA-NL tool to all Nurse Leaders that make bedside nurse staffing and care process decisions will have different measures of success. Implementation of NICA-NL for C-suite Nurse Leaders may involve one-on-one sessions and individual guidance. NICAL-NL consists of six sections: 1) Strategic Implementation Management, 2) Advanced Information Management and Education, 3) Executive Planning, 4) Ethical and Legal Concepts, 5) Information Systems Concepts, 6) Requirements and System Selection. If identified as a low competency, the C-suite Nurse Leaders could be provided with one-on-one sessions and guided resources specific to these concepts. Evaluating effectiveness with C-suite Nurse Leaders could include individual follow-up via qualitative interviews to uncover perceptions of increased competencies related to Executive Planning, remaining gaps in knowledge, and demonstration of application of this new informatics knowledge into his or her responsibilities related to Executive Planning.

Implementation of NICA-NL across a broad swath of managers and directors of clinical units in a hospital could be achieved through recorded and live webcasts introducing the tool and how to access it and associated resources. Deployment using electronic survey software would allow for aggregated, de-identified data analysis to trend areas of low competency across the organization. Trending low self-assessed competencies areas could serve as high priority areas to identify and provide all Nurse Leaders within the organization links to existing educational resources or to design and provide nursing educational sessions and webinars. Process oriented metrics could be evaluated and aligned with the targeted areas for nursing informatics competencies. For example, one section in the NICA-NL tool is "Strategic Implementation Management". Identifying this as an area of need prior to a broad Electronic Health Record (EHR) system implementation or upgrade would provide data that additional training is needed in advance of the implementation. A re-assessment of the same Nurse Managers and Directors using NICA-NL post implementation of the EHR system combined with process metrics of system implementation success (e.g., decreased portion of help desk tickets related to lack of user knowledge) could provide important data on the effectiveness of training and resources on readiness of the end-user.

Measuring actual adoption level (how many people used the tool) is critical to understand what level of impacts could be expected and potential for further uptake and spread without additional resources. Technology typically follows an adoption curve consisting of: 1) use by a few Innovators, 2) use by a small minority of Early Adopters, 3) use by an Early Majority, 4) use by a Late Majority, and finally 5) use by Laggards, in that order.[3] Identifying characteristics of early adopters of NICA-NL may help identify motivated champions of Nursing Informatics at an organization.

3.2.2. Realizing value for an organization

A self-assessment tool is attractive to an organization precisely because it is of relative low-intensity, scalable, and sustainable. These qualities do not infer that there are no associated costs or overhead. Tracking costs, including individual's time and efforts, are important to be able to demonstrate that incurred costs, however small, are worth a sustained and budgeted investment for nursing. Resources may include use of electronic survey software and secure server access, time for nurse educators and informatics specialists to collate and/or develop resources or curricula to meet identified competency needs, and time for Nurse Leaders to complete the NICA-NL tool and use resources provided for professional development.

Incorporating the NICA-NL into orientation for new Nurse Leaders and/or yearly trainings for current Nurse Leaders at an organization could provide a sustainable path to improve competencies overtime. A culture change that recognizes the value of nursing informatics competencies as part of minimum competencies for the Nurse Leaders may be required at some organizations. Systematic implementation of the NICA-NL based on the RE-AIM framework provides steps and evaluation techniques that can be leveraged to encourage and evaluate adoption and demonstrate the value of increasing Nurse Leaders' informatics competencies for an organization.

3.2.3. Potential for impact internationally

Validated assessment tools are needed to identify gaps in knowledge and guide resource development to meet those gaps. Nursing management and practice are evolving worldwide, as described throughout this book. Our research team is currently expanding NICA for use by registered nurses (NICA-RN). Self-assessment tools can be used by the individual and with support by their organizations. The ability to evaluate trends in Nurse Leaders' informatics competency levels in the aggregate will enable the nursing profession to track improvements in knowledge and rapidly pivot resources to identified needs. With standardized validated tools these efforts can be realized at the local, regional, national and international level.

4. Conclusion

The NICA-NL is a validated self-assessment nursing informatics competency scale for Nurse Leaders. We described approaches to implementing NICA-NL at a healthcare organization using the RE-AIM framework as a path to evaluate and demonstrate value. Systematic measurement of competency levels is critical for the advancement of nursing informatics throughout the nursing profession.

References

[1]   Yen P-Y, Phillips A, Kennedy M, Collins SA. Nursing Informatics Competency Assessment for the Nurse Leader (NICA-NL): Instrument Refinement, Validation, and Psychometric Analysis. J Nurs Adm 2017; in press.

[2]   Glasgow R, Vogt T, Boles S. Evaluating the public health impact of health promotion interventions: the RE-AIM framework. Am J Public Health 1999;89:1322–7.
[3]   Rogers EM. Diffusion of innovations. 1995.

Forecasting Informatics Competencies for Nurses in the Future of Connected Health
J. Murphy et al. (Eds.)
© *2017 IMIA and IOS Press.*
doi:10.3233/978-1-61499-738-2-212

Evolving Role of the Nursing Informatics Specialist

Lynn M. NAGLE[a], Walter SERMEUS[b], Alain JUNGER[c]

[a]*Lawrence S. Bloomberg, Faculty of Nursing, University of Toronto, Toronto, Ontario, Canada*
[b]*Leuven Institute for Healthcare Policy, University of Leuven, Belgium*
[c]*University Hospital of Lausanne, Lausanne, Switzerland*

Abstract. The scope of nursing informatics practice has been evolving over the course of the last 5 decades, expanding to address the needs of health care organizations and in response to the evolution of technology. In parallel, the educational preparation of nursing informatics specialists has become more formalized and shaped by the requisite competencies of the role. In this chapter, the authors describe the evolution of nursing informatics roles, scope and focus of practice, and anticipated role responsibilities and opportunities for the future. Further, implications and considerations for the future are presented.

Keywords. Nursing informatics specialist, role function, connected health, data science, big data, personalized medicine, clinical intelligence, virtual care

1. Introduction

By 2018, 22 million households will use virtual care solutions, up from less than a million in 2013. Average (healthcare) visits among these adopter households will increase from 2 per year in 2013 to 6 per year in 2018, which include both acute care and preventive follow-up services in a variety of care settings—at home, at retail kiosk or at work. [1]

Nursing informatics roles have taken many forms in focus and function over the last decades; suffice it to say that they have not been consistently described or defined in terms of scope of practice. At the time of this writing it is clear that role of nursing informatics specialists will continue to evolve at an increasingly rapid rate in the coming years. The unfolding of new health care paradigms will bring greater connectivity between care providers and patients, include a wide array of emerging technologies and an increasing emphasis on data analytics will make the integration of informatics competencies into every area of nursing an imperative.

2. Brief history of roles of the past and present

The earliest and most common types of informatics work assumed by nurses has included: oversight of organizational workload measurement systems, project leadership, systems educator, and nursing unit or departmental information technology resource. In many instances, these roles were enacted on the basis of a specific identified organizational need and were often secondments to the Information Technology Department. It was not unusual for these roles to have the designation of

"IT nurse" [2]. As role responsibilities and job titles have been widely varied, so have the qualifications for each. The need for more specificity and consistency in nursing informatics roles has been recognized for several years [3, 4, 5].

The advent of formal education programs for nurses interested in specializing in informatics has occurred in conjunction with increasing sophistication in the use of information and communication technologies (ICT) in clinical practice settings. Today, nurses have the option to pursue specialization and credentials at a variety of levels including graduate specialization and specialty certification. Advanced credentials and certification (e.g., Certified Professional in Healthcare Information and Management Systems - CPHIMS) have afforded nurses the opportunity to achieve credibility and legitimacy regarding the specialty informatics knowledge and skills they bring to bear in nursing practice and academia and healthcare in general [6]. This credibility has been recognized with the development of executive level positions such as the "Chief Nursing Informatics Officer" (CNIO) in some countries. The position of the "Chief Medical Informatics Officer" (CMIO) is much more prevalent and deemed essential in medium and large health care organizations while the C-level nursing counterpart remains less common. Several authors [7-11] have described the role and competencies for these senior informatics positions, yet the valuing of these positions remains limited among health care provider organizations.

In addition to the evolution of formalized training programs for nurses interested in informatics, the specialty of nursing informatics has continued to evolve and has become recognized in local jurisdictions, nationally and internationally. Groups of like-minded nurses have organized into special interest groups affiliated with larger interdisciplinary organizations (e.g., International Medical Informatics Association - Special Interest Group on Nursing Informatics (IMIA-NI-SIG)). Organizations such as the Canadian Nursing Informatics Association (CNIA), the American Nursing Informatics Association (ANIA), the Nursing Informatics Working Group of the European Federation for Medical Informatics (EFMI-NURSIE) are examples of forums for nurses to network, collaborate and profile their work in informatics. The existence of these specialty organizations has served to further legitimize the work of nurse informaticians and provided a venue for advancing regional, national and international efforts in nursing informatics. Through conferences, meetings and the offering of educational sessions, virtually and face to face, these networks of nurse informaticists have collectively advanced the practice and science of nursing informatics. A case in point is the International Nursing Informatics Congress and post-conference, now held bi-annually and hosted by countries across the globe. Outputs of these meetings include publications such as this one; benefitting nursing informatics specialists and the nursing profession worldwide.

At the time of this writing, we find nursing informatics specialists in virtually every clinical practice setting. The roles and focus of their work endeavors are wide and varied. The titles of "informatics nurse", "nurse informatician", and "nursing informatics specialist" are but a few of the titles applied to nurses working in the field. Many of the roles of the past and present have been more extensively described elsewhere [2,12]. For the purpose of this chapter, the authors use the title of *nursing informatics specialist* to provide illustrations of the potential focus of these roles current and future.

Roles to date have largely focused on supporting acquisition, implementation and evaluation of clinical information systems in health care organizations. As noted by McLane and Turley [4], *"informaticians are prepared to influence, contribute to, and mold the realization of an organization's vision for knowledge management"* (p.30).

Nurses have been in pivotal roles at every step of the systems life cycle and instrumental in the success of deployments at every level of an organization. From the provision of executive oversight, project management, systems education and training, and analytics, nurses in clinical settings have become core to organizations' information management infrastructure and support.

In addition to health care provider organizations, nursing informatics specialists can be found in the employ of technology vendors, retail outlets, and consulting firms while many others have created their own entrepreneurial enterprise. Over the last few decades, technology vendors, hardware and software, have come to appreciate the invaluable contribution of nurses to the development, sales and deployment of their solutions. Throughout the world, nurses are also engaged in academic pursuits to advance the knowledge base of nursing informatics through the conduct of research.

Efforts are underway in many countries to advance the adoption and integration of entry-to-practice informatics competencies into undergraduate nursing programs. Notwithstanding some of the ongoing gaps in the provision of informatics content in undergraduate nursing education, many courses and programs have been taught in a variety of post-secondary education institutions over several years by nursing informatics specialists. In fact it is not unusual for many nurses to develop an interest in informatics through a single course and subsequently pursue further studies and employment opportunities.

Since the early 90's many graduate level courses and degrees, certificate and certification programs have been developed and offered world-wide. Nurses have pursued these opportunities recognizing the necessity of informatics knowledge and skills now and particularly into the future, as they face an increasingly connected world of digital healthcare. To a large extent, the core competencies of the nursing informatics specialist have become essential for all nurses and expectations of the specialist role will continue to evolve even further.

3. Emerging roles for nursing informatics specialists

The healthcare sector continues to evolve in the application and use of technologies to support the delivery of care. Factors including: a) rising health care expenditures, b) the increasing incidence of chronic disease, c) the ubiquity of technology, d) an aging demographic, e) personalized medicine, f) mobile and virtual healthcare delivery, g) the emergence of consumer informatics, h) genomics, i) big data science, and connected health are and will continue informing the evolution of nursing informatics roles.

One of the main challenges we have to cope with is the difference in growth rate that is exponential for the new technology and knowledge yet is still linear for changing human behavior, learning, organizations, legislation, ethics, etc, A linear growth rate is mostly represented by a function in a form like $y(x) = ax+b$. An exponential growth rate is mostly represented by a function in a form like $f(x) = ka^x$. For example: In an exponential world where the information is doubling every year, 5 exponential years would equal to 2^5 or 32 linear years which has a massive impact on the management of professional knowledge. In reality, we estimate that knowledge development in healthcare, which has doubled every century until 1900, is now estimated to double every 18 months. And the pace is getting faster. This means that when nurses finish their education, the knowledge they gained might be already outdated. The traditional way of developing procedures, protocols and care pathways, sometimes requiring a year to develop, are outdated when they are finalized and are insufficient to guide future practice. The only way forward is to integrate and embed the new knowledge in electronic patient records using algorithms and decision support systems so that practice remains aligned with new knowledge and insights. The impact might be that best practices can change very quickly and what is viewed as best practice before your holiday leave might be different upon your return to work. Making the connection between these different dimensions of time will be a key-role of the evolving role of the NI specialist.

A second challenge is that clinical practice in the future will be largely team based. The nature of teams will include interprofessional teams, patients and their relatives and a wide range of virtual devices (internet of things - IoT) that are all connected. Teams will work across boundaries of organizations and will be organized around a particular patient. We still have to come up with new labels for naming these temporary virtual interprofessional patient teams. Practically it will mean that nurses will be (temporary) members of different teams at the same time. This notion of teamwork is in contrast with what we normally see as teams organized in organizations, departments and units. It will challenge how teams will be managed, led, and evaluated. But it will also challenge the communication within teams and the exchange of information.

3.1 Virtual and connected care

The delivery of health services virtually is becoming commonplace in many places around the globe. Virtual care has been defined as: *"any interaction between patients and/or members of their circle of care, occurring remotely, using any forms of communication or information technologies, with the aim of facilitating or maximizing the quality and effectiveness of patient care"* [13, p 4].

The most common modalities of virtual care are currently in use in telemedicine. Telemedicine has been largely used to conduct remote medical consultations, assessments and diagnosis (e.g., teledermatology, telestroke, telepsychiatry) through the use of computer technology and associated peripheral devices including digital cameras, stethoscopes and opthalmoscopes, and diagnostic imaging. More recently, the tools of telemedicine have been extended to the provision of remote nursing monitoring and assessment particularly for individuals with chronic diseases such as congestive heart failure (CHF) and chronic obstructive pulmonary disease (COPD). The nurses providing these tele-homecare services are not necessarily informatics specialists but the design and management of the monitoring tools, infrastructure and support services may be provided by them in the future.

Another emerging area of nursing informatics practice will likely focus on the use of remote monitoring technologies such as sensors and alerts embedded in structures (e.g., flooring, lighting, furniture, fixtures) and appliances (e.g., stove, refrigerator) in the homes of citizens. These tools offer the promise of supporting seniors to maintain a level of independence in their own homes longer, particularly those with cognitive or sensory impairments. Such devices might trigger direct messaging to providers, lay and professional, flagging potentially harmful situations and affording early intervention as necessary. Different types of sensors (e.g., sleep, activity, falls, ambulation, continence, fluid and electrolyte) will also contribute new supplementary data to health information repositories, offering the possibility of linking to other data sets and provide new insights to the well-being of individuals in the community especially the aged and those living with chronic illness.

With the increasing use of consumer health solutions such as patient portals and smartphone apps for self-monitoring and management of health and disease, nurse informatics specialists will likely play a key role in their support and development. From the perspective of application design and usability, and training, nursing input and informatics expertise will be important to ensure appropriate and safe use of these tools. As individuals and their families become more active participants in their care through the use of applications and devices to connect with providers, they will likely also need expertise and support from the nursing informatics specialist.

3.2 Knowledge generation and innovation

The traditional ways of new knowledge generation is through research and the dissemination of findings in research journals. Knowledge is consumed by researchers and clinicians who transform it into relevant guidelines and care pathways. The time between the generation of research findings and application in the real clinical work can take several years. It is generally estimated that it takes an average of 17 years for research evidence to reach clinical practice [14]. Therefore clinicians are not always aware of existing evidence. In a landmark study, McGlynn et al. [15] evaluated the use of evidence-based guidelines in 30 conditions and 439 indicators for the use of the same. They showed that clinicians (doctors, nurses) only apply 50% of them in their daily practice. The use varied from 80% for structured conditions such as cataract to 10% for unstructured conditions such as alcohol addiction. There is also a lot of research demonstrating that nurses lack knowledge related to common procedures. Dilles study illustrated [16] that nurses lack sufficient pharmacological knowledge and calculation skills. Baccalaureate prepared nurses' pharmacological knowledge averaged between 60% and 65% of the level expected. Segal et al. [17] analyzed the use of hip arthroplasty care pathways in 19 Belgian hospitals finding a high variability in providing evidence-based interventions. While post-op pain monitoring is in 100% of the care pathways, pre-op physiotherapy was only present in 25% of the care pathways.

In the future of connected health, there will be direct links to knowledge generated by specialists from around the world. New knowledge will be automatically integrated and embedded into electronic patient records, and include new algorithms for decision support systems. It is interesting to note that Hearst Health Network, one of the largest media and communication groups in the world, is taking a leading role in healthcare. They started an intensive collaboration among strong health knowledge companies such as First Databank (FDB), Map of Medicine, Zynx Health and Milliman Care Guidelines (MCG). FDB is a United Kingdom company specialized in integrated drug knowledge to prescribe medication, follow-up drug interactions, improve clinical decision making and patient outcomes. Map of Medicine was created in the UK for clinicians by clinicians. It offers a web-based visual representation of evidence-based patient journeys covering 28 medical specialties and 390 pathways. Zynx Health offers a similar story from the US to provide evidence-based clinical decision support system solutions at the point of care through electronic patient records. MCG produces evidence-based clinical guidelines and software and is widely used in the US, UK and Middle East. Other examples of health information networks are CPIC (Clinical Pharmacogenetics Implementation Consortium) to help clinicians understand how available genetic test results could be used to optimize drug therapy, the International Cancer Genome Consortium (ICGC) which facilitates data sharing to describe genomic sequences in tumor types among research groups all over the world. In the information models, such as archetypes and Detailed Clinical Models (see section C chapter 1) offer summaries of evidence for specific clinical concepts.

Likely one of the most significant areas of focus for nursing informatics specialists in the near term is data science and the use of "big data". Big data has been defined as: *"large amounts of data emerging from sensors, novel research techniques, and ubiquitous information technologies"* [18, p. 478]. Access to big data unveils a whole new sphere of informatics opportunities related to health and nursing analytics. According to Masys [19], big data is *"that which exceeds the capacity of unaided human cognition and strains the computer processing units, bandwidth, and storage capabilities of modern computers"*. The future development of nursing capabilities in data science will essentially lead to an entirely new cadre of nursing informatics specialists whose work will focus on deriving new nursing knowledge from not only electronic health record data, but also the data from sensor and remote monitoring technologies, patient portals and mobile apps described above. The implications of -omics data such as genomics, metabolomics, and proteomics, being included as part of the electronic health record in the near future, should be taken into account. Nurse informatics specialists will be pivotal in assisting to identify potential ethical and practice implications in the use of these data.

Using big data, the knowledge generating process might be reversed into practice-based evidence where data from electronic health records, patient portals, sensors etc. are uploaded into large databases that identify patterns and clinical interesting correlations. An example of the power of analyzing large datasets is the Vioxx-case (rofecoxib). Although a clinical trial initially showed no increased risk of adverse cardiovascular events for the first 18 months of Vioxx use, a joint analysis of the US FDA and Kaiser Permanente's Healthconnect database of more than 2 million person-years of follow-up, the NSAID arthritis and pain drug was found shown to have an increased risk for heart attacks and sudden cardiac death. [20] After the findings were confirmed in a large meta-analysis, Merck decided to withdraw the drug from the market worldwide in 2004.

With the proliferation of these emerging data sources and databases, the nursing informatics specialist will play a key role in the use of these data to inform quality and safety improvements in every practice setting.

3.3 Sharing knowledge and communication

In the realm of the new normal of connected health, nurses will work in temporary teams around patients. Within these teams it will be essential that goals are clear and shared, that roles are defined and accepted and that the way of working is clear to everyone. It requires systems for coordination and communication to ensure the continuity of care. Reid et al. [21] defined continuity of care as: *"how one patient experiences care over time as coherent and linked; this is the result of good information flow, good interpersonal skills, and good coordination of care"*. They make a distinction between information continuity, relational continuity and management continuity. Information continuity consists on one hand in the exchange and transfer of information among health care providers and to patients and on the other hand how the knowledge of the patient is accumulated. It is about their specific knowledge, preferences, expectations, social network. With the existence of the new technology of the quantified self, it is important that these new data are effectively integrated and connected. Relational continuity consists of the trusted relationship between patient and healthcare provider. Increasingly advanced practice nurses are assuming this pivotal role within the health team. Management continuity is referring to a consistent and coherent approach to the health problem across organizations and boundaries. The Belgian healthcare system offers an interesting example of this: General Practitioners are stimulated (financially) to prescribe generic drugs. Hospitals are stimulated to negotiate discounts with pharmaceutical companies leading to brand named drug choices. Although they might chemically be identical, for the patient they often are not as they have different names. Like drugs may be different in size and color leading to more medication errors as patients may take two pills without being aware that they are the same drug.

Although nurses spend a lot of time documenting care, the accuracy of nursing documentation has been found to be poor. In a study within 10 Dutch hospitals, Paans et al. [22] found that within 341 patient records the accuracy of documentation of diagnoses was poor or moderate in 76% of the records. The accuracy of the intervention documentation was poor or moderate in 95% of the patient records. Only the accuracy for admission, progress notes and outcomes evaluation and the legibility were acceptable. The work of Connected Health should support the documentation systems of nurses and other health professionals. The use of structured documentation methodologies and standardized terminologies should improve the quality of the patient record and improve the capacity for comparability of care processes and outcomes across the care continuum and within patient care groups.

3.4 Impact of connected health on the Scope of Practice of Nurses and Advanced Practice Nurses (APN)

In Connected Health, the scope of practice of nurses will change. For example, based on time and motion studies, it has been shown that nurses spend 5-7% of their time [23, 24] collecting vital sign data. In the future this work will be assimilated by sensors and other devices. However, nurses' work will be more focused on analyzing the data and evaluating thresholds for action (e.g., alerting rapid response teams). Another example is the use of sensors for pressure ulcer monitoring [25]. The used sensors will provide information about patient temperature, skin humidity, pressure points and position. These data will generate a whole new set of information for review and action including pressure intensity map and humidity intensity maps. These data would lead to more precise management of pressure sores. Other examples of data gathering that will change the focus and processes of nurses' work include: barcode scanning for checking identity of patients, patient and device tracking systems, and robotic dispensing of medication.

Patient access to their own records and partnering in their own health will change the roles of physicians, nurses and hospitals drastically. The work of nurses will increasingly shift from a direct care provision to the role of knowledge broker in helping patients to understand care alternatives, manage their health, and navigate information access.

4. Impact of connected health on the evolving role of the Nursing Informatics Specialist

Connected health will alter the future role of the nursing informatics specialist and require a new set of competencies. To a large extent these competencies will build upon existing competencies but have an increasing emphasis on information use rather than technology use. Table 1 provides a summary of the anticipated new competencies and role responsibilities that are likely to be necessary for Nursing Informatics Specialists in the emerging world of connected health and the IoT.

Table 1. New competencies related to the future role of nursing informatics specialists

New Competencies	New Roles
Knowledge Innovation and Generation	• Provide guidance and support to others (nurses, patients) in the application and use of emerging knowledge (e.g., clinical decision support, Practice-Based Evidence (PBE), genomics, expert and patient/citizen knowledge) • Inform-teach others (clinicians, teams, patients) about new knowledge and knowledge innovations relevant to specific situations • Provide direction and support to others in the use of international guidelines and knowledge • Contribute internationally to new knowledge generation and innovations ensuring the inclusion of relevant team member and patient perspectives and expertise
Monitoring the use of new technology	• Monitor and maintain vigilance over data/technologies to identify those that add value to a given health situation. • Recognize that nurses, other clinicians and patients may engage and assume responsibility independently and or interdependently for specific data (e.g., remote monitoring, self-monitoring, wearables, appliances). • Recognize the emergence of patient self-service and relevance of patient expertise in specific situations.
Value judgement & quality assessment	• Provide guidance as to the value and relevance of specific data and information as derived from single or multiple sources for any given set of circumstances, or health situations.
Change Management	• Identify the broader scope and considerations for change management in the context of connected health (e.g., virtual and physical participants/partners) • Recognize the extended complexities of technology adoption in the context of connected health.
Communication & Documentation	With increasingly complex and personalized approaches to health care, participate in the identification and/or development of new: • models of clinical documentation • methods of communication • data standards • terminology standards • data sources • data models • data repositories
Data Analytics	In addition to traditional quantitative and qualitative analyses, support and participate in the development and use of new approaches and methods of data analytics for: • knowledge generation (e.g., natural language processing, experiential data) • reporting outcomes • demonstrations of value (e.g., patient-caregiver perspectives, health and financial outcomes) • predictive and retrospective analyses

5. Conclusion

The future Nursing Informatics Specialist will function in the context of virtual care delivery, be informed by data aggregated from a multiplicity of sources and real-time knowledge generation that will inform individualized care. In addition to the competencies required to date, they will be required to support other clinicians and patients and families as they assume new roles and use data analytics to interpret and appropriately apply new knowledge. With the IoT, connected care will pose as yet unknown challenges for the Nursing Informatics Specialist in the future; what is certain is that the role will continue to evolve from the role scope and responsibilities known today.

References:

[1]   Wang H. (2014). Virtual Health Care Will Revolutionize The Industry, If We Let It. April 3, 2014. Forbes.

[2]   Nagle LM. (2015). Role of informatics nurse. In K.J. Hannah, P. Hussey, M.A. Kennedy, & M.J. Ball (Eds.), Introduction to nursing informatics (pp. 251-270). London: Springer-Verlag.

[3]   Hersh W. (2006). Who are the informaticians? What we know and should know. J Am Med Inform Assoc 13(2):166-170

[4]   McLane S & Turley J. (2011). Informaticians: how they may benefit your healthcare organization. J Nurs Adm 41(1):29-35.

[5]   Smith SE, Drake LE, Harris JG, Watson K & Pohlner PG (2011). Clinical informatics: a workforce priority for 21st century healthcare. Aust Health Rev 35(2):130-5. doi: 10.1071/AH10935.

[6]   Health Information Management Systems Society(HIMSS) (2016). Health IT certifications. Retrieved September 28, 2016 from: http://www.himss.org/health-it-certification

[7]   Harrington L. (2012). AONE Creates New Position Paper: Nursing Informatics Executive. Nurse Leader 10(3): 17-21.

[8]   Remus S & Kennedy M (2012). Innovation in transformative nursing leadership : nursing informatics competencies and roles. Nurs Leadership 25(4):14-26.

[9]   Kirby SB. (2015). Informatics leadership: The role of the CNIO. Nursing 2015 (Apr):21-22.

[10]   Cooper A. & Harmer S (2012). Strategic leadership skills for nursing informatics. Nurs Times 108(20): 25-6.

[11]   Simpson R. (2013). Chief nurse executives need contemporary informatics competencies. Nurs Econ 3(6) 277-87.

[12]   Murphy J. (2011). The nursing informatics workforce: Who they are and what they do? Nurs Econ 29(3), 150-3.

[13]   Women's College Hospital Institute for Health Systems Solutions and Virtual Care (WIHV) (2015). Virtual Care: A Framework for a Patient-Centric System. Retrieved from: http://www.womenscollegehospital.ca/assets/pdf/wihv/WIHV_VirtualHealth Symposium.pdf on April 14, 2016.

[14]   Morris ZS, Wooding S, Grant J. (2011). The answer is 17 years, what is the question: understanding time lags in translational research. J R Soc Med 104(12):510-20.

[15]   McGlynn EA, Asch SM, Adams J, Keesey J, Hicks J, DeCristofaro A, Kerr EA. The quality of health care delivered to adults in the United States. N Engl J Med. 348(26):2635-45.

[16]   Dilles T, Vander Stichele RR, Van Bortel L, Elseviers MM. (2011) Nursing students' pharmacological knowledge and calculation skills: ready for practice? Nurse Educ Today 31(5):499-505.

[17]   Segal O, Bellemans J, Van Gerven E, Deneckere S, Panella M, Sermeus W, Vanhaecht K. (2011) Important variations in the content of care pathway documents for total knee arthroplasty may lead to quality and patient safety problems. *J Eval Clin Pract.*, Aug 23, p.11-5

[18] Brennan P. & Bakken S. (2015). Nursing Needs Big Data and Big Data Needs Nursing. *J Nurs Scholarship* 47(5):477–484.

[19]   National Institutes of Health Big Data to Knowledge. (2014). Workshop on enhancing training for biomedical big data. Retrieved from: http://bd2k.nih.gov/pdf/bd2k_training_workshop_report.pdf.

[20] Graham DJ, Campen D, Hui R, Spence M, Cheetham C, Levy G, Shoor S, Ray WA. (2005). Risk of acute myocardial infarction and sudden cardiac death in patients treated with cyclo-oxygenase 2 selective and non-selective non-steroidal anti-inflammatory drugs: nested case-control study. Lancet 365(9458):475-81.

[21] Reid R., Haggerty J., McKendry R. (2002). Defusing the Confusion: Concepts and Measures of Continuity of Healthcare. Canadian Health Services Research Foundation.

[22] Paans W, Sermeus W, Nieweg RM, van der Schans CP. (2010) Prevalence of accurate nursing documentation in patient records. J Adv Nurs. Aug 23, p. 1365-2648

[23] Mendonck K., Meulemans H., Defourny J. (2000), Tijd voor zorg: een analyse van de zorgverlening in de gezondheids- en welzijnssector, VUB Press, 126pp.

[24] Hendrich A, Chow MP, Skierczynski BA, Lu Z. (2008). A 36-hospital time and motion study: how do medical-surgical nurses spend their time? Perm J. 12(3):25-34.

[25] Marchione FG, et al., (2015). Approaches that use software to support the prevention of pressure ulcer: A systematic review. Int J Med Inform, 84(10):725-36.

Forecasting Informatics Competencies for Nurses in the Future of Connected Health
J. Murphy et al. (Eds.)
© 2017 IMIA and IOS Press.
This article is published online with Open Access by IOS Press and distributed under the terms
of the Creative Commons Attribution Non-Commercial License 4.0 (CC BY-NC 4.0).
doi:10.3233/978-1-61499-738-2-222

Integrating Health Information Technology Safety into Nursing Informatics Competencies

Elizabeth M. BORYCKI[a,1], Elizabeth CUMMINGS[b], Andre W. KUSHNIRUK[a]
and Kaija SARANTO[c]
[a]*University of Victoria, Victoria, Canada*
[b]*University of Tasmania, Tasmania, Australia*
[c] *University of Eastern Finland, Kuopio, Finland*

Abstract. Nursing informatics competencies are constantly changing in response to advances in the health information technology (HIT) industry and research emerging from the fields of nursing and health informatics. In this paper we build off the work of Staggers and colleagues in defining nursing informatics competencies at five levels: the beginning nurse, the experienced nurse, the nursing informatics specialist, the nursing informatics innovator and the nursing informatics researcher in the area of HIT safety. The work represents a significant contribution to the literature in the area of nursing informatics competency development as it extends nursing informatics competencies to include those focused on the area of technology-induced errors and HIT safety.

Keywords. Technology induced error, health information technology, safety, patient safety, nursing, competencies, nursing informatics

1. Introduction

Nursing informatics competencies are one of the most important types of competencies in a modernized health care system where the use of electronic health records, clinical documentation systems, telehealth systems and patient portals in the hospital, home and community are the norm. With the introduction of these technologies we have had a significant reduction in the number of medical errors. We have also seen the introduction of a new type of medical error (i.e. the technology-induced error) [1,2]. In this paper we outline a framework for introducing the topic of technology-induced errors and patient safety competencies involving health information technologies (HIT) into nursing curricula. Patient Safety was addressed earlier as a relevant topic for nursing during the 2003 Nursing Informatics post-conference, addressing the more general aspects of safe healthcare [3]. The competency work described here builds off Staggers and colleagues' framework in defining nursing informatics competencies for beginning nurses, experienced nurses, informatics specialists, informatics innovators, and nursing informatics researchers [4]. This work represents a significant contribution to the literature in the area of nursing informatics competency development as it

---

[1] Corresponding author: Elizabeth Borycki; email: emb@uvic.ca

extends these competencies to include those focused on technology-induced errors and HIT safety and includes those of a nursing informatics researcher.

2. Review of the Literature

2.1 Technology-induced Errors and Health Information Technology Safety

Technology-induced errors have emerged as a significant patient safety issue over the past decade. Technology-induced errors can be defined as errors that emerge from the complex interaction between individuals and technologies during real world work activities. They also include those errors that arise from the technology itself [1,2]. The root causes of these types of errors are many (see Figure 1) [6]. Some of them originate at the government level with changes in policy and legislation that are not mirrored in the technology used by clinicians. A lack of fit between policy, legislation and technology may lead to an error. For example, if there are differences between policies and procedures enacted by a technology and government policy or legislation, a technology-induced error may occur. If the model healthcare organization on which technology developers develop their technology has errors associated with its processes, those errors may be present in the technology, when it is implemented in another organization. This is especially the case when the model terminologies, workflows, policies and procedures found in the technology differ from those in the organization, where the technology will be implemented. Vendor organizations may also introduce new types of errors. Poor programming, requirements gathering, design and software testing may cause technology-induced errors at point of care (see Figure below). Local healthcare organizations may also be a source of technology-induced error. For example, mismatches between technology developed by the vendor and local organizational terminologies, workflow, policy and procedures and devices may lead to technology-induced errors. Also, local organizational customization of the technology to the local setting and poor organizational testing of these new customizations for error inducing properties may lead to a technology-induced error. Lastly, training and support, if insufficient, could lead to clinicians making such errors (see right side of Figure 1) [6].

Technology-induced errors have a number of origins in a health care system [6]. Today, researchers suggest that technology-induced errors range in frequency from 10-30 percent in organizations, regions and countries where there is a very high use of technology by health professionals [7]. In countries where there is use of hybrid paper-electronic patient care technologies these errors are much lower [8]. However, these errors are expected to increase as HIT becomes more widely used and deployed [9]. Over the past several years' researchers have documented the occurrence of these types of errors [1], reported on the types of errors that have arisen [7, 8], investigated the nature of their occurrence [1, 6-9], developed methods that can be used to evaluate the safety of technology [10], investigated/identified the root causes, and the role that technology has in leading to such errors [6]. In addition to this, researchers have identified and developed vendor and organizational strategies that can be used to mitigate technology-induced errors [10].

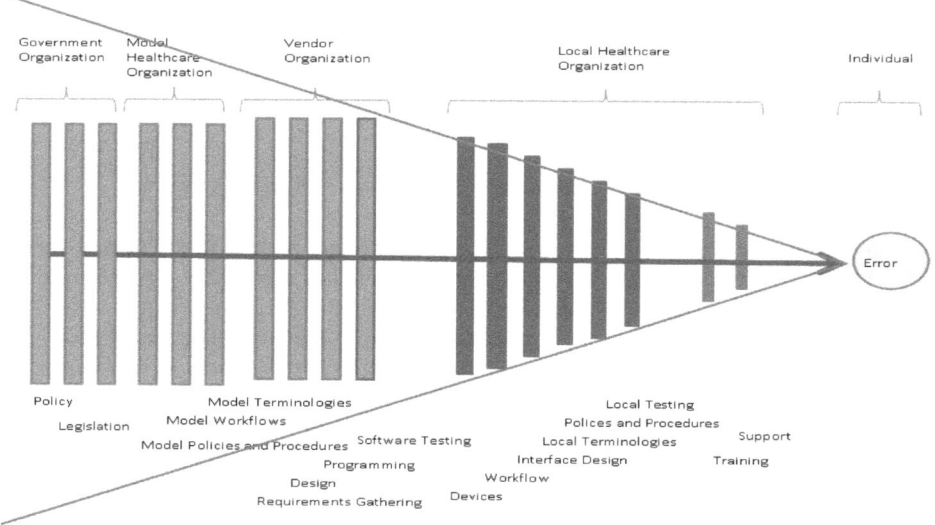

Figure 1. Root Causes of Error [see 6]

2.2 Nursing Informatics Competencies

Nursing informatics competencies remain an important aspect of nursing practice and investigation in nursing research. Over the past several years, researchers have developed nursing informatics competencies, evaluated their acquisition in response to educational interventions aimed at nurses, and described how these competencies can be extended among student and practicing nurses in health care organizations and across regional health authorities [12]. Even as nursing informatics competencies are being developed and incorporated into nursing curricula internationally, there is a need to extend these competencies to include new and emerging areas of health informatics practice, education and research and to reflect these changes in nursing informatics competency documents [13]. For example, technology-induced errors have emerged as a significant patient safety issue with the publication of the Institute of Medicine Report on *HIT and Patient Safety* [14] and the report on *Diagnostic Error in Health Care* [14], which not only outline how technology safety has become a significant public health issue, but how technology influences diagnostic error [15-17]. As well, there is recognition among the nursing informatics practice community that there is a need to extend nurses' knowledge about technology-induced errors to support the development and implementation of safer HIT [16]. Research by Saratan and colleagues [16] identifies that nursing informatics competencies need to be extended to include those that are specific to HIT safety. In a survey study of nursing informatics practitioners in British Columbia, Canada participants reported the need to add HIT safety competencies to already established nursing informatics competencies [16]. However, future nursing informatics competencies surrounding technology-induced errors and HIT safety need to be more fully defined at the undergraduate level and extended to the graduate level to include masters and doctorally prepared nurses in informatics.

In summary, with the advent of new findings arising from the health informatics literature and policy reports on technology safety, there is a need to acknowledge the relevance and importance of extending nursing informatics competencies to reflect these changes so that nurses who are practicing at point of care, expert nurse leaders, nursing informatics specialists and nursing informatics leaders develop these new competencies in the area of HIT safety.

3. Methods

There exist a number of nursing informatics competency frameworks. Staggers et al's [4] work in the area of nursing informatics competencies remains among the most cited of these works. Employing a modified version of Stagger's work as a fundamental framework, the researchers used this framework and extended it to include nursing informatics competencies with a focus on technology-induced errors and HIT safety. Using a modified version of Stagger's framework of nursing informatics practice, that of beginning nurses, experienced nurses, nursing informatics specialists, informatics innovators, and researchers, the authors of this work extended the reviewed literature on technology safety to the development of nursing informatics competencies at five levels to include competencies discussed in the HIT safety literature (See Table 1) [6].

4. Results

In this paper we were able to show that competencies can be developed for nurses that are specific to addressing and managing technology-induced errors and ensuring the safety of HIT. Current research regarding knowledge and skills aimed at reducing technology-induced errors and improving technology safety suggests that nursing informatics competencies at all of Stagger's [4] four levels are present with a focus on technology-induced errors and HIT safety (see Table 1). Nurses working at the point of care have an important role in ensuring that technology-induced errors are reduced by monitoring and reporting on these technology issues (see Table 1, Beginning and Experienced nurses) [7,17,18]. Nurses with graduate preparation can use their knowledge to develop safer software, test software for safety as well as implement these technologies in a safe manner. This work also includes educating point of care nurses about these types of errors and participating in the reporting processes around the technology as it is being implemented. Additionally, this may involve ensuring HIT training and supports are sufficient so that nurses can use the technology without introducing technology-induced errors (see Table 1, Nursing Informatics Specialists). Nurse innovators can contribute to this area of nursing informatics by developing and extending new software development approaches, methods and technologies that make health care safer (see Table 1, Informatics Innovators). Finally, nursing informatics researchers can study the factors or develop new research methods that can be used to enable the development of safe HIT, thereby further developing the nursing informatics research evidence base (see Table 1, Nursing Informatics Researchers).

Table 1. Mapping of Safety Competencies to Nursing Informatics Competencies

Level of Nursing	Nursing Informatics Competencies based on Level of Nursing	Health Information Technology Safety Competencies based on Level of Nursing
Beginning nurses	• Fundamental computer technology and information management skills • Use available information and information systems to manage their practice	• Defines a technology-induced error. • Identifies a near miss and observed technology-induced errors at point of care • Verbalizes how near misses and technology-induced errors may cause harm to patients and describes their impact upon patient safety • Reports near misses and technology-induced errors to regulatory bodies and to organizations where they work • Reviews safety alerts and incorporates suggested changes into their practice.
Experienced nurses	• Proficiency in their domain of practice • High computer technology and information management skills in their domain of practice • See data elements, trends in the relationships between data elements, see trends and patterns in the data • Collaborate with nursing informatics specialists	• Identifies near misses and observed technology-induced errors in their domain of practice. • Identifies technology-induced errors associated with data elements and their relationships at a unit, organizational or systems level. • Collaborates with nursing informatics specialists to remediate and rectify technology-induced errors with point of care staff • Educates point of care staff about how to prevent and incorporate changes to practice to prevent technology-induced errors
Nursing informatics specialists	• Graduate prepared nurses who have additional specialized knowledge about health informatics • Use "use critical thinking, process skills, data management skills, systems development life cycle knowledge and computer skills"	• Analyzes and evaluates technology-oriented incident reports for the presence of technology-induced errors (including how technology might have contributed) to near misses and observed errors. • Investigates technology-induced errors. • Applies error management investigation methods to understand how a technology-induced errors occur including the use of root cause analysis, case study analysis, safety heuristics, usability testing, clinical simulations, and computer based simulations • Develops technology, organizational and nursing practice strategies changes to prevent near misses and actual technology-induced errors. • Reports and works with vendors and health care organizations to address these types of errors • Educates health professionals and health information management professionals about risk mitigation and risk management techniques • Uses these techniques to prevent technology-induced errors
Nursing informatics innovators	• Conduct informatics research and generate informatics theory	• Develops new incident reporting methods for technology-induced errors • Analyzes data to identify new types of errors and develops classification systems for technology-induced errors

Level of Nursing	Nursing Informatics Competencies based on Level of Nursing	Health Information Technology Safety Competencies based on Level of Nursing
		• Develops methods for testing software and hardware to ensure the safety • Develops error investigation methods • Develops safety software and hardware • Develops methods that can be used to mitigate technology-induced errors • Develops policy, organizational strategies and vendor strategies that can be used to prevent technology-induced errors • Builds a nursing informatics evidence base for safe HIT.
Nursing informatics researchers		• Studies the factors that enable safe HIT development • Develops new research methods that can be used to study the safety of HIT • Extends the evidence-based research in nursing informatics.

5. Conclusions

It is clear that beginning and expert nurses are critical to ensuring technology is safe for use in the process of patient care as their role in identifying and reporting such errors is significant. The involvement of nursing informatics specialists in designing, developing and implementing software is fundamental. Nursing informatics specialists are responsible for employing the current knowledge base about creating, testing and implementing safe technologies. They also use the information provided by beginning and expert nurses to inform their work. Lastly, nursing informatics innovators, in the context, of a new field of study, focus on technology-induced errors and safety to develop new monitoring methods, design and development methodologies, and testing approaches (in addition to educating beginning, expert and informatics specialist nurses). Finally, nursing informatics research can build an evidence base to underpin such HIT safety research. However, simply developing competencies does not provide the skills to support identification and reporting of errors. Therefore, it is important that error reporting systems are developed and beginning level nurses are provided with training in the use of these systems. Again, as per the revised framework, identification and reporting of near misses is an important skill as is recognizing the need to follow up on reported errors or near misses.

References

[1] Kushniruk AW, Triola MM, Borycki EM, Stein B, Kannry JL. Technology-induced error and usability: The relationship between usability problems and prescription errors when using a handheld application. Int J Med Informatics. 2005;74(7):519-26.
[2] Borycki EM, Kushniruk AW. Where do technology-induced errors come from? Towards a model for conceptualizing and diagnosing errors caused by technology. In: Kushniruk AW, Borycki EM, editors. Human, social and organizational aspects of health information systems. Hershey, Pennsylvania: IGI Global; 2008. p. 148-65.

[3]   Van de Castle B, et al. Information technology and patient safety in nursing practice: an international perspective. Int J Med Inform. 2004 Aug;73(7-8):607-14.
[4]   Staggers N, Gassert CA, Curran C. Informatics competencies for nurses at four levels of practice. J Nurs Educ. 2001; 40(7):303-16.
[5]   Goossen, W., Hannah, K.J., (1991). A curriculum about nursing informatics for a nurse educator's educational programme. In: Hovenga, E.S.J., Hannah, K.J., McCormick, K.A., & Ronald, J.S., (Eds). Proceedings Nursing Informatics '91 conference. Melbourne Australia, 690-694.
[6]   Borycki EM, Kushniruk AW, Keay L, Kuo A. A framework for diagnosing and identifying where technology-induced errors come from. Stud Health Techol Inform. 2008; 148:181-7.
[7]   Palojoki S, Mäkelä M, Lehtonen L, Saranto K. An analysis of electronic health record-related patient safety incidents. Health Inf J. 2016; 1-12.
[8]   Magrabi F, Ong MS, Runciman W, Coiera E. Using FDA reports to inform a classification for health information technology safety problems. J American Med Inform Assoc. 2012; 19(1): 45-53.
[9]   Borycki EM, Househ MS, Kushniruk AW, Nohr C, Takeda H. Empowering patients: Making health information and systems safer for patients and the public. Yearbook Med Inform. 2011; 7(1):56-64.
[10] Borycki E, Keay E. Methods to assess the safety of health information systems. Healthcare Quart. 2010; 13:47-52.
[11] Kushniruk AW, Bates DW, Bainbridge M, Househ MS, Borycki EM. National efforts to improve health information system safety in Canada, the United States of America and England. Int J Med Inform. 2013; 82(5): e149-60.
[12] Cummings E, Borycki EM, Madsen I. Teaching nursing informatics in Australia, Canada and Denmark. Stud Health Technol Inform. 2015; 14; 218-223.
[13] Mather C, Cummings E. Mobile learning: A workforce development strategy for nurse supervisors. In HIC 2014; pp. 98-103.
[14] Institute of Medicine. Health IT and patient safety: Building safer systems for better care. Washington: National Academies Press; 2011.
[15] Institute of Medicine. Diagnostic error in health care. Washington: National Academies Press. 2016.
[16] Saratan C, Borycki EM, Andre W. Information management competencies for practicing nurses and new graduates. Knowledge Management & eLearning. 2015; 7(3); 378-94.
[17] Harrington L, Kennedy D, Johnson C. Safety issues related to the electronic medical record (EMR): Synthesis of the literature from the last decade, 2000-2009. J Healthcare Manage. 2011; 56(1): 31-43.
[18] Ensio A, Saranto K, Ikonen H, Iivari A. The national evaluation of standardized terminology. Stud Health Technol Inform. 2006;122: 749-752.

Forecasting Informatics Competencies for Nurses in the Future of Connected Health
J. Murphy et al. (Eds.)
© *2017 IMIA and IOS Press.*
This article is published online with Open Access by IOS Press and distributed under the terms
of the Creative Commons Attribution Non-Commercial License 4.0 (CC BY-NC 4.0).
doi:10.3233/978-1-61499-738-2-229

What Practicing Nurses Need to Know About Health Information Technology in Order to Practice Today: Continuing Education and Certification

Susan K. NEWBOLD[a]

[a] *Newbold Consulting/Nursing Informatics Boot Camp, Franklin, TN., USA*

Abstract. This chapter focuses on informatics and information management continuing education for all practicing nurses, as well as certification for informatics nurse specialists.

Keywords. Continuing education, certification, health IT competencies, informatics nurse, informatics nurse specialist, training, standards of nursing informatics practice

1. Introduction

Every nurse has a role working with informatics in healthcare as more aspects of care delivery are facilitated with technology. This chapter focuses on continuing education for the topics of informatics and information management for practicing nurses and informatics nurses, as well as certification for informatics nurses.

Continuing education related to informatics is vital for every level of nurse from the nurse practicing at the bedside, clinic or home - to administrators, educators and researchers. Opportunities for continuing education will be discussed.

Some informatics nurses choose to attain a professional milestone by seeking certification in nursing or healthcare informatics. The informatics nurse may look to certification as a way to validate knowledge and skills needed in order to deliver quality care and promote professional practice.

2. Continuing Education Opportunities in Nursing Informatics

Statistics are scarce regarding the extent of nurses who take advantage of nursing informatics continuing education. A 2010 publication [1] discussed the incidence of continuing education among registered nurses in the U.S. in 2000. Twenty one percent (21%) of the respondents reported continuing education in informatics the year prior to the survey. The authors surmised that the use of the internet would probably increase those numbers. They discussed some opportunities to increase the rates. Their data was derived from the National Sample Survey of Registered Nurses (NSSRN) which was discontinued in 2012.

The American Nurses Association (ANA) Scope and Standards of Practice: Nursing Informatics [2] supports lifelong learning in informatics. The standards of nursing informatics practice for education and leadership both promote lifelong learning. One way to attain education to promote lifelong learning is through continuing education (CE) courses. CE is usually needed to maintain certification or maintain nursing licensure.

There are numerous opportunities for continuing education in nursing informatics (NI). Although thirty-two (64%) states in the U.S. have mandatory continuing education for re-licensure [3], there are few requirements for informatics outside of health information privacy and security training. Most organizations require training to be proficient in the use of the facility electronic health record or electronic medical record.

A good way to find continuing education on informatics for nurses is to use an online search engine to explore the World Wide Web. A sample search could include, "nursing informatics continuing education." Nurses who do not have the money, finances or time to attend in person events can find online courses. Online courses may also support the learners learning style. Many continuing education opportunities are paid events, but some are free or low cost.

A variety of organizations offer continuing education for members often at no additional charge other than the membership fee. These organizations include the Healthcare Information and Management Systems Society (HIMSS) (www.himss.org) [4]; the American Medical Informatics Association (AMIA) (www.amia.org) [5], the American Nursing Informatics Association (ANIA) (www.ANIA.org) [6], the University of Maryland Summer Institute in Nursing Informatics (SINI) (http://www.nursing.umaryland.edu/sini/) [7], and the International Medical Informatics Association (www.IMIA.org) [8] with MedInfo and the International Congress in Nursing Informatics.

Specialty nursing organizations are beginning to interweave nursing informatics into their conferences and in webinars. The Association of periOperative Nurses (www.AORN.org) [9] is an example of an organization committed to continuing education and includes informatics content. Check with your specialty organization to see if continuing education in nursing informatics is offered.

There are stand-alone courses for nursing informatics like the Nursing Informatics Boot Camp (https://branded.me/susan-newbold) [10] and OnCourseLearning (http://www.nurse.com/focusedceseries) [11]. The Nursing Informatics Boot Camp is an intensive two day in person course which focuses on current informatics trends and issues in health. It includes content for nurses interested in becoming certified informatics nurses. It is held in various locations, primarily in the U.S.

The OnCourse Learning Nursing Informatics Certification Review Focused CE Series is a comprehensive learning experience that provides an extensive review of the nursing informatics board certification exam. In this six week web-based course, participants learn key concepts of NI including design, maintenance and support. Also, they discover how quality improvement is vital to patient and staff satisfaction from experts in the NI field.

PearlsReview overs a low cost, self paced, web based NI certification review course (http://www.pearlsreview.com/Informatics-Nursing-(RN-BC)) [12]. A Wolters Kluwer Journal – CIN: Computers Informatics Nursing (http://journals.lww.com/cinjournal/) [13] has occasional paid ANCC continuing education articles including a brief examination. See also http://nursing.ceconnection.com/default [14] to browse other continuing education by Wolters Kluwer.

3. Certification in Nursing and Healthcare Informatics

In the United States (U.S.), the American Nurses Credentialing Center (ANCC), a subsidiary of the American Nurses Association, offers Registered Nurse Board Certified credentials (RN-BC) for nursing informatics professionals who pass a computer-based examination. To qualify for board certification, individuals must be registered nurses with a U.S. license who have completed a baccalaureate degree as well as at least 30 hours of continuing education in nursing informatics within the last three years. There is a newly announced option for international nurses to become certified by the ANCC. The ANCC certification is valid for five years, and the nurse is required to complete professional development courses with a minimum of 75 contact hours and one or more of the eight renewal categories with 1000 practice hours or retake the examination in order to renew. For further information on the ANCC certification, see http://nursecredentialing.org/InformaticsNursing [15].

Certification in nursing informatics has been available since 1995 with 1837 nurses certified by the ANCC as of December 31, 2015 (http://www.nursecredentialing.org/Certification/FacultyEducators/FacultyCategory/Statistics/2015-CertificationStatistics.pdf) [16]. In addition to certification, an Informatics Nurse can seek a certificate, master's degree, post master's degree, doctorate of nursing practice (DNP), or doctor of philosophy (PhD) in Nursing Informatics. The ANCC certification is the most prevalent certification for informatics nurses, but others are available and viable. See Table 1 for a list of Potential Certifications for the Informatics Nurse. Nurses can be certified by The American Health Information Management Association (AHIMA), the ANCC, AMIA, Healthcare Information and Management Systems Society (HIMSS), Health IT Certification, LLC, the National Association for Healthcare Quality or the Project Management Institute (PMI).

4. Continuing Education and Certification in Development

The publishers of the free Online Journal of Nursing Informatics (http://www.himss.org/ojni) are currently exploring the possibility of offering CE credit. This could be another source of free or low cost continuing education in informatics.

The United States Government contracted with seven universities to update health information technology education previously offered by community colleges called the National Health IT Workforce Curriculum. In addition, new content has been added in the areas of population health, care coordination and interoperable health IT systems, value-based care, patient-centered care, and healthcare data analytics. Updated materials and newly developed materials will be available June 2017 at https://www.healthit.gov/providers-professionals/workforce-development-programs. This content is offered by five universities and two colleges at no charge and offers a certificate of completion.

Table 1. Potential Certifications for the Informatics Nurse

Certification & Reference	Requirements	Topics	Cost
American Nurses Credentialing Center (ANCC) Nursing Informatics http://nursecredentialing.org/InformaticsNursing	• RN License Hold a current, active RN license in a state or territory of the United States or hold the professional, legally recognized equivalent in another country. • Apply from Outside the U.S. Additional requirements for candidates outside the U.S. • Master's, Postgraduate, or Doctoral Degree Hold a bachelor's or higher degree in nursing or a bachelor's degree in a relevant field. Have practiced the equivalent of 2 years full-time as a registered nurse. Have completed 30 hours of continuing education in informatics nursing within the last 3 years. Meet one of the following practice hour requirements: • Have practiced a minimum of 2,000 hours in informatics nursing within the last 3 years. • Have practiced a minimum of 1,000 hours in informatics nursing in the last 3 years and completed a minimum of 12 semester hours of academic credit in informatics	For full outline see http://www.nursecredentialing.org/Informatics-TCO2014 I. Foundations of Practice (47.33% or 71 questions) A. Professional Practice B. Models and Theories C. Rules, Regulations, and Requirements II. System Design Life Cycle (26.00% or 39 questions) A. Planning and Analysis B. Designing and Building C. Implementing and Testing D. Evaluating, Maintaining, and Supporting III. Data Management and Health Care Technology (26.67% or 40 questions) A. Data Standards B. Data Management C. Data Transformation D. Hardware, Software, and Peripherals	• $270 Member American Nurses Association $395 non member • Valid 5 years then recertification

Certification & Reference	Requirements	Topics	Cost
	courses that are part of a graduate-level informatics nursing program. • Have completed a graduate program in informatics nursing containing a minimum of 200 hours of faculty-supervised practicum in informatics nursing.		
Healthcare Information and Management Systems Society (HIMSS) Certified Associate in Healthcare Information and Management Systems (CAHIMS) http://www.himss.org/health-it-certification/cahims	High School Diploma or equivalent	I. General 　Organizational Environment 　Technology Environment II. Healthcare Information and Systems Management 　Analysis 　Design 　Selection, Implementation, Support, and Maintenance 　Testing and Evaluation 　Privacy and Security III. Administration 　Leadership Support 　Management Support	HIMSS Individual Organizational Affiliate Member $140 U.S. HIMSS Regular, Corporate or Student Member $175 U.S. Non-Member $225 U.S.
Healthcare Information and Management Systems Society (HIMSS) Certified Professional in Healthcare Information and Management Systems (CPHIMS) http://www.himss.org/health-it-certification/cphims	Eligibility for the CPHIMS Examination requires fulfilling one (1) of the following requirements: • Baccalaureate degree from an accredited college or university plus five (5) years of information and management systems experience, three (3) of those years in a healthcare setting. • Graduate degree or higher from an accredited college or university plus three (3) years of information and management systems experience, two (2) of those years in a healthcare setting	I. General 　Organizational Environment 　Technology Environment II. Healthcare Information and Systems Management 　Analysis 　Design 　Selection, Implementation, Support, and Maintenance 　Testing and Evaluation 　Privacy and Security III. Administration 　Leadership Support	HIMSS Individual Organizational Affiliate Member $270 U.S. HIMSS Regular, Corporate or Student Member $300 U.S. Non-Member $375 U.S.

Certification & Reference	Requirements	Topics	Cost
Project Management Institute (PMI) Project Management Certifications Project Management Professional (PMP®) http://www.pmi.org/Certification/Project-Management-Professional-PMP.aspx	Prerequisite Skills: • Four-year degree, 4,500 hours in leading and directing projects, and 35 hours of project management education OR • Secondary degree (high school diploma, associate's degree, or equivalent), 7,500 hours leading and directing projects, and 35 hours of project management education	Management Support Exam Content Outline ©2015 Domain Percentage of Items on Test I. Initiating 13% II. Planning 24% III Executing 31% IV. Monitoring and Controlling 25% V. Closing 7% Total 100%	Computer-based exams: PMI member: $405 USD (retake $275) Non-PMI member: $555 USD (retake $375) Paper-based exams: PMI member: $250 USD (retake $150) Non-PMI member: $400 USD (retake $300)
Health IT Certification, LLC http://www.healthitcertification.com/overview.html Certified Professional in Health Information Technology (CPHIT) Certified Professional in Electronic Health Records (CPEHR) Certified Professional in Health Information Exchange (CPHIE)	No specific educational or experiential requirements for taking the CPHIT, CPEHR, CPHIE or CPORA certification examinations. It is recommended that individuals either have healthcare experience with plans to participate in health information technology (HIT), electronic health record (EHR), health information exchange (HIE) and/or operating rules administration (ORA) acquisition/implementation, use, and operations; or have information system experience with the intent of assisting healthcare organizations acquire and deploy an HIT, EHR, HIE or ORA.	Core Curricula for all exams: C-I. Overview of Health IT A. Flow and Nature of Data in the Health Care Delivery System B. Definition of Terms C. Conceptual Models of HIT, EHR, e-Rx, Administrative Simplification, and HIE D. Current Status of Adoption of EHR, personal health records (PHR), Transactions, and HIE in Various Health-related Settings C-II. Legal and Regulatory Aspects of Health IT A. Sources of Law and Standards B. Legal and Evidentiary Aspects C. Authentication D. Ethical Aspects of Health IT C-III. Goal Setting & Change Management for Health IT	Each examination $495 Two and a half day Curriculum Training Only for CPHIT, CPEHR, and CPHIE: $1,495 Two day Curriculum Training Only for CPORA: $1,095

Certification & Reference	Requirements	Topics	Cost

Certified Professional in Operating Rules Administration (CPORA)		A. Strategic Planning/Migration Path
		B. Visioning and Readiness Assessment
		C. Goal Setting
		D. Change Management Principles and Strategies
		C-IV. Workflow & Process Improvement for Health IT
		   A. Workflow and Process Improvement for Clinical Transformation
		   B. Workflow and Process Management
		   C. Workflow and Process Analysis
		   D. Workflow and Process Redesign
		   E. Complementary Techniques to Support Workflow and Process Improvement
		
		Additional curricula depending upon the examination.	

National Association for Healthcare Quality (NAHQ)
 	
Certified Professional in Healthcare Quality® (CPHQ)
 	
http://www.nahq.org/certify/content/index.html
	Self-assess readiness to take the examination. Two years of experience suggested.	1. Quality Leadership and Structure (20 Items)
		   A. Leadership
		   B. Structure
		2. Information Management (25 Items)
		   A. Design and Data Collection
		   B. Measurement and Analysis
		3. Performance Measurement and Process Improvement (52 Items)
		   A. Planning
		   B. Implementation and Evaluation
		   C. Education and Training
		   D. Communication
		4. Patient Safety (28 Items)
		   A. Assessment and Planning
		   B. Implementation and Evaluation
			NAHQ Member: $399
			Nonmember: $469

Certification & Reference	Requirements	Topics	Cost
The American Health Information Management Association (AHIMA) Registered Health Information Administrator (RHIA®) http://www.ahima.org/certification/RHIA	RHIA applicants must meet one of the following eligibility requirements: Successfully complete the academic requirements, at the baccalaureate level, of an HIM program accredited by the Commission on Accreditation for Health Informatics and Information Management Education (CAHIIM). OR •Graduate from an HIM program approved by a foreign association with which AHIMA has a reciprocity agreement.[2] The academic qualifications of each candidate will be verified before a candidate is deemed eligible to take the examination. All first-time applicants must submit an official transcript from their college or university.	1. Data Content, Structure & Standards (Information Governance) (18–22%) 2. Information Protection: Access, Disclosure, Archival, Privacy & Security (23–27%) 3. Informatics, Analytics & Data Use (22–26%) 4. Revenue Management (12–16%) 5. Leadership (12–16%)	$299 for members
The American Health Information Management Association (AHIMA) Certified Healthcare Technology Specialist (CHTS) Exams http://www.ahima.org/certification/chts Six focus areas: 1. Clinician/Practitioner Consultant (CHTS-CP) 2. Practice Workflow and Information Management Redesign Specialist (CHTS-PW) 3. Implementation Manager	None required.	See the candidate guide for the specific exam blueprint for the examination in question. http://www.ahima.org/~/media/AHIMA/Files/Certification/CHTS%20Candidate%20Guide.ashx	$299 each examination

Certification & Reference	Requirements	Topics	Cost
(CHTS-IM) 4. Implementation Support Specialist (CHTS-IS) 5. Technical/Software Support Staff (CHTS-TS) 6.Trainer (CHTS-TR) http://www.ahima.org/certification/chts			
American Medical Informatics Association, www.amia.org Advanced Health Informatics Certification (AHIC) [In development November 2016]	1) Practice focus on information and knowledge problems that directly impact the practice of healthcare, public health, and personal health, 2) Education in primary health fields and health informatics at the graduate level, and, 3) Significant experience in health informatics establishing an advanced level of real-world accomplishment.	In development November 2016.	In development November 2016.

AMIA is developing an Advanced Health Informatics Certification (AHIC) (https://www.amia.org/advanced-health-informatics-certification) which is thought to include nurses for an advanced level certification not offered by the ANCC. According to AMIA, the certification is intended for informatics professionals representing the spectrum of primary disciplines. Eligibility requirements include a practice focus, education, and significant experience in health informatics.

5. Conclusion

The ANA Scope and Standards of Practice: Nursing Informatics [2] encourages lifelong learning for self and others related to informatics. There are many opportunities for nurses for continuing education in healthcare information technology. There are also several opportunities for informatics nurses to seek voluntary certification.

References

[1]   Continuing Education in Informatics Among Registered Nurses in the United States in 2000 Manal Kleib, Anne E. Sales, Isac Lima, BA, Melba Andrea-Baylon, and Amy Beaith doi:10.3928/00220124-20100503-08 The Journal of Continuing Education in Nursing.· Vol 41, No 7, 2010
[2]   American Nurses Association. Scope and Standards of Practice: Nursing Informatics (2nd Ed.), 2015.
[3]   American Nurses Association© States Which Require Continuing Education For RN Licensure 2013. Available from: http://www.nursingworld.org/MainMenuCategories/Policy-Advocacy/State/Legislative-Agenda-Reports/NursingEducation/CE-Licensure-Chart.pdf
[4]   Healthcare Information and Management Systems Society (HIMSS). Available from www.himss.org
[5]   American Medical Informatics Association (AMIA). Available from www.amia.org
[6]   American Nursing Informatics Association (ANIA). Available from www.ANIA.org
[7]   University of Maryland Summer Institute in Nursing Informatics (SINI) Available from http://www.nursing.umaryland.edu/sini/
[8]   International Medical Informatics Association MedInfo and the International Congress in Nursing Informatics. Available from www.IMIA.org
[9]   Association of periOperative Nurses. Available from www.AORN.org
[10] Nursing Informatics Boot Camp. Available from https://branded.me/susan-newbold
[11] OnCourseLearning. Available from http://www.nurse.com/focusedceseries
[12] PearlsReview. Available from http://www.pearlsreview.com/Informatics-Nursing-(RN-BC)
[13] CIN: Computers Informatics Nursing published by Wolters Kluwer. Available from http://journals.lww.com/cinjournal/
[14] CE Connection. Continuing education by Wolters Kluwer. Available from http://nursing.ceconnection.com/default
[15] ANCC certification Nursing Informatics. Available from http://nursecredentialing.org/InformaticsNursing
[16] 2015 ANCC Certification Data. Available from http://www.nursecredentialing.org/Certification/FacultyEducators/FacultyCategory/Statistics/2015-CertificationStatistics.pdf

NOTE Other online reference links are available in Table 1.

Section E

Annotated Bibliography

Forecasting Informatics Competencies for Nurses in the Future of Connected Health
J. Murphy et al. (Eds.)
© *2017 IMIA and IOS Press.*
This article is published online with Open Access by IOS Press and distributed under the terms
of the Creative Commons Attribution Non-Commercial License 4.0 (CC BY-NC 4.0).
doi:10.3233/978-1-61499-738-2-241

Informatics Competencies in Connected Health: Annotated Bibliography

William GOOSSEN[a][1]

[a]*Results 4 Care BV, Amersfoort, the Netherlands*

Abstract. In this book it is of course impossible to be complete on all competencies publications, or all relevant subjects. For that reason the Post Conference Team decided to have some pages of the book reserved for annotations. An annotation is seen as a short reference to another topic or publication, not included in this book, and a brief motivation from one of us, why this might be of interest to the readers.

Keywords. Informatics, Competencies, Technology, Education, eHealth, Connected Health, Nursing, Annotated Bibliography

1. Introduction

During the discussions in the NI2016 post-conference the group came up with several suggestions for additional subjects to be included. However, once a specific theme is chosen, and all authors have contributed their work, it is has become too difficult to change it. And, in which direction would it have to be changed? There are so many options available. It is simply impossible to be 100% complete on the current health informatics topics, and given the targets for the post-conference to focus on connected health, some topics are simply out of scope.

In addition, due to the focus on the practicing nurse, and on nurse teachers and leadership who would facilitate the practicing nurses, this book could not include much for the nurse informaticians. In the past nursing informatics education was identified on four levels: level 1: the practicing nurse, level 2: advanced professional roles such as teaching, managing, advanced nursing practice, research, level 3: nurse informatics specialist and level 4: the PhD prepared nurse informatics researcher (1). In the context of this typology only levels 1 and 2 have been addressed, so not all competencies publications could be included.

For these reasons the Post Conference Team decided to have some pages of the book reserved for annotations. An annotation is seen as a short reference to another topic or publication, not included in this book, and a brief motivation from one of us, why this might be of interest to the readers. This way, it is possible to point to interesting new developments and to competencies that could not be included. Each of the participants was offered the opportunity to include a key reference.

---

[1] Corresponding author: William Goossen PhD, BSN, director Results 4 Care b.v., the Netherlands, email: wgoossen@results4care.nl

2. Annotated Bibliography, with references

2.1. Automation: Will it change nurse, nursing, or both?

Suggested by: Anne Moen, RN, PhD, FACMI:

Bibliographic data of the annotated reference: Peplau HE. Automation: Will it change nurse, nursing, or both ? Nursing Forum. 1962;34(3):31-6.

Summary of the content: This paper is among the first publications on automation, computers and medical technology for nursing. The paper points out the need for proactive leadership and future-oriented education to prepare, participate and embrace opportunities following "automation". Nurses should differentiate between types of technologies, acquire competencies to contribute developing and deploying solutions and take advantage of opportunities for transformation practices in line with the mission of nursing.

Reason to recommend this reference: A seminal paper, published 1962, calling for nursing leadership and nursing participation, raising a call to explore opportunities, prepare, ask questions and participate to prepare in shaping the informatics solutions that will support and not change the *mission* of nursing. We find inspiration and encouragement in this seminal paper and it gives a longer-term perspective to the nursing informatics community.

2.2. Nurse - patient relationship

Suggested by: Michelle Honey RN, PhD and Paula Procter RN, PhD:

Bibliographic data of the annotated reference: Nelson R, and Carter-Templeton HD . The Nursing Informatician's Role in Mediating Technology Related Health Literacies. Sermeus W et al (Eds) Nursing Informatics 2016: eHealth for All: entry Level Collaboration - From Project to Realization. IOS Press. 2016 pp 237-241. ISBN 978-1-61499-658-3 (online).

Summary of the content: The paper considers the link between informatics competencies that nurses develop within their programs and the digital engagement with patients.

Reason to recommend this reference: Some might argue that the link suggested in the paper between the nurse and patient through digital technologies is a little tenuous, it does however raise some key points around the role of nurses as we progress further into the 21st Century whilst at the same time remaining true to the core values of nurses and those in their care.

2.3. An Introduction to Nursing Informatics

Suggested by: Susan K Newbold, PhD RN-BC FAAN FHIMSS

Bibliographic data of the annotated reference: Houston, S., Dieckhaus, T., Kirchner, B., & Rookwood, R. (2015). An Introduction to Nursing Informatics: Evolution & Innovation. Chicago: HIMSS Media.

Summary of the content: This nursing informatics book was written as a primer for the nurse interested in informatics and considering entering the field. Informatics is defined and the evolution of nursing informatics is highlighted. The reader is invited to consider a career path in nursing informatics and is treated to a day in the life perspective of an educator, student, researcher, clinician, consultant, vendor, and government employee. The appendix includes four case studies and questions – for example – Career Options for Nurses working with Informatics.

Reason to recommend this *reference:*   A nurse who is considering nursing informatics as a profession can benefit from reading this primer on nursing informatics. The book could be a great investment in career planning.

2.4. Evidence-Based Health Informatics

Suggested by: William Goossen PhD:
Bibliographic data of the annotated reference: Ammenwerth E, Rigby M (Editors). Evidence-Based Health Informatics. Studies in Health Technology and Informatics, 2016, Volume 222. ISBN 978-1-61499-634-7 (print) | 978-1-61499-635-4 (online) Open Access.

Summary of the content: This book addresses the need for better understanding of the importance of robust evidence to support health IT and to optimize investment in it. The authors give insight into health IT evidence and evaluation as its primary source. They further promote health informatics as an underpinning science to demonstrate ethical rigor and proof of benefits in a similar manner that it is applied to other health technologies as medical devices and medicines. The three parts of the book cover: 1) the context and importance of evidence-based health informatics; 2) methodological considerations of evaluation of Healthcare IT; and 3) ensuring the relevance and the application of evidence in practice.

Reason to recommend this reference: There is an increasing understanding that health informatics technology (HIT) are not only beneficial to patients, providers or health care. Using scientifically sound methodologies to research the effects of HIT on patient care, professional work and healthcare is important so we learn and know what works and what does not. This book by Ammenwerth and Rigby is an important update to the existing knowledge in the field on the evaluation of health informatics. During the final weeks before the preparation for the NI 2016 Post Conference, the EFMI list for health informatics evaluation send out a message about its publication, but too late to be included as a subject, and also out of scope for our primary target audience.

2.5. Evidence based nursing informatics competencies

Suggested by: Michelle Honey RN, PhD et al:
Bibliographic data of the annotated reference: Desjardins KS, Cook SS, Jenkins M, Bakken S. Effect of an informatics for evidence-based practice curriculum on nursing informatics competencies. International Journal of Medical Informatics. 2005;74(11-12):1012-20.

Summary of the content: This article reports describes the effect of an evolving informatics for evidence-based practice curriculum on nursing informatics competencies in three student cohorts using a repeated-measures, non-equivalent comparison group design to determine differences in self-rated informatics competencies pre- and post- informatics evidence-based practice education. While no significant differences between cohorts were found, the importance of assessing informatics competency attainment so that curricula can be refined is emphasised.

Reason to recommend this reference: While this is a somewhat dated US based study from Columbia University School of Nursing, it is one of the few examples located that explores informatics within a curriculum. Despite none of the three nursing student cohorts studied achieving competence despite curricular revisions, this article demonstrates that nursing informatics competencies can be assessed against creating informatics competent graduates.

2.6. Practicing nurse competencies

Suggested by: Lynn Nagle PhD RN:

Bibliographic data of the annotated reference: Canadian Association of Schools of Nursing (CASN). Nursing Informatics Entry-to-Practice Competencies for Registered Nurses (2012). Author: Ottawa, ON Canada. Available at: http://www.casn.ca/education/digital-healthnursing-informatics-casn-infoway-nurses-training-project/

Summary of the content: This document provides a background and overview of the informatics entry-to-practice competencies developed for Canadian nurses. The competencies have been derived from previously developed competency frameworks. The 3 competency areas include performance indicators in the areas of: 1) information and communication technology use, 2) information and knowledge management, and 3) professional and regulatory accountability.

Reason to recommend this reference: This work may inform the nursing informatics competency development efforts of other countries. This document and other "how to" teaching materials are available at no cost from the above website (e.g., "Nursing Informatics Teaching Toolkit" and "Consumer Health Solutions Resource" for nurse educators).

2.7. TIGER Competency Synthesis Project

Suggested by: Joyce Sensmeier MS, RN-BC, CPHIMS, FHIMSS, FAAN:

Bibliographic data of the annotated reference: Hübner, U., Shaw, T., Thye, J., Egbert, N., Marin, H., Ball, M.J. Towards an International Framework for Recommendations of Core Competencies in Nursing and Inter-Professional Informatics: The TIGER Competency Synthesis Project. In Hoerbst, A. et al. (Eds.). Exploring Complexity in Health: An Interdisciplinary Systems Approach, 655-659. DOI 10.3233/978-1-61499-678-1-655. 2016 European Federation for Medical Informatics and IOS Press.

Summary of the content: Informatics competencies of the healthcare workforce must meet the requirements of the inter-professional process and outcome oriented provision of care. In order to help nursing education transform accordingly, the TIGER Initiative deployed an international survey, with participation from 21 countries, to evaluate and prioritize a broad list of core competencies for nurses in five domains: 1) nursing management, 2) information technology (IT) management in nursing, 3) interprofessional coordination of care, 4) quality management, and 5) clinical nursing. Informatics core competencies were found highly important for all domains. In addition, this project compiled eight national cases studies from Austria, Finland, Germany, Ireland, New Zealand, the Philippines, Portugal, and Switzerland that reflected the country-specific perspective. These findings will lead us to an international framework of informatics recommendations

Reason to recommend this reference: The TIGER Competency Synthesis Project continues to evolve with additional findings, publications and insights. This article was published subsequent to the NI 2016 Post Conference and is an important update to increase our understanding of the implications of the international competency synthesis.

2.8. Learning in nursing

Suggested by: Michelle Honey RN, PhD and Paula Procter RN, PhD:
  Bibliographic data of the annotated reference: Downes S. Connectivism and connective knowledge: Essays on meaning and learning networks [Internet]2012 [Available from: http://www.downes.ca/files/books/Connective_Knowledge-19May2012.pdf.
  Summary of the content: A self-published book that considers three major domains, knowledge, learning and community, each representing an aspect of network theory. He includes a critique of Siemens work, and also brings in use of the cloud and Massive Open Online Courses (MOOC) in education.
  Reason to recommend this reference: For those who are interested in reading more about Connectivism, this over 600 page self-published book provides views that will encourage consideration about what connectivism is and how it can impact education and learning.

2.9. Nursing informatics curriculum

Suggested by: Michelle HONEY RN, PhD and Paula PROCTER RN, PhD:
  Bibliographic data of the annotated reference: Cummings E, Shin EH, Mather C and Hovenga E. Embedding Nursing Informatics Education into an Australian Undergraduate Nursing Degree. Sermeus W et al (Eds) Nursing Informatics 2016: eHealth for All: entry Level Collaboration - From Project to Realization. IOS Press. 2016 pp 329-333. ISBN 978-1-61499-658-3 (online).
  Summary of the content: Following the mandate in Australia to include informatics in nursing curricula, this paper explains how one University has tried to meet this challenge even with a lack of nationally agreed competencies.
  Reason to recommend this reference: The paper raises a number of issues which remain unaddressed in a number of countries where there is a will to include informatics in nursing curricula particularly at first level education. It explores in a pragmatic way the decision steps that were followed in order to advance the knowledge for nursing students.

2.10. Online resources for nursing informatics

Suggested by: Lisiane Pruinelli, PhD, MS, RN:
  Bibliographic data of the annotated reference: Clancy, T.R. Integrating AACN Essentials, QSEN KSA's and TIGER Competencies for Nursing Informatics [Internet]. School of Nursing, University of Minnesota, US; 2016; [cited 2016 Sep 26] . Available from: https://www.nursing.umn.edu/outreach/nursing-informatics-educationand-resources/nursing-educators.
  Summary of the content: This repository contains resources from a collaborative effort of AACN, the University of Minnesota School of Nursing, and the University of

Maryland School of Nursing. Materials are freely available, featuring numerous sample assignments, links to informatics standards and professional Web sites, and instructional videos on a variety of subjects such as EHRs, standardized nursing languages, workflow, consumer informatics, telehealth, and other key emerging areas.

Reason to recommend this reference: This web page contains resources for students and educators in nursing informatics, aligned with national and international recommendations.

2.11. Assessment of nursing informatics competencies

Suggested by: Laura-Maria Peltonen, RN, MNSc:

Bibliographic data of the annotated reference: Choi J, De Martinis JE. Nursing informatics competencies: assessment of undergraduate and graduate nursing students. Journal of Clinical Nursing. 2013 Jul;22(13-14):1970-6. doi: 10.1111/jocn.12188.

Summary of the content: This article discusses informatics competencies of students in undergraduate and graduate nursing programs based on findings from a survey where data were collected regarding students' self-evaluation of informatics competencies from one state university in the USA. The authors discuss different aspects to be considered in informatics curriculum development of undergraduate and graduate nursing programs.

Reason to recommend this reference: The discussed aspects may be of use to nurse educators in determining specific areas to consider when developing nursing educational programs to ensure sufficient competence in nursing practice.

2.12. Structured Nursing Records

Suggested by: Ulla-Mari Kinnunen, PhD, RN:

Bibliographic data of the annotated reference: Saranto K, Kinnunen UM, Kivekäs E, Lappalainen AM, Liljamo P, Rajalahti E, et al. Impacts of structuring nursing records: a systematic review. Scandinavian Journal of Caring Sciences Nov (2013), 18: 1-19.

Summary of the content: The aim of this systematic review is to describe the impacts of different data structuring methods used in nursing records or care plans. It examines what kinds of structuring methods have been evaluated and the effects of data structures on healthcare input, processes and outcomes in previous studies. Various codes, classifications, terminologies or structured forms were most often used in the studies. Beside these or independently the nursing process model was used in 64 % of the analyzed articles. The unexpected impacts for healthcare inputs were a lack of resources, e.g. managerial support and education, and for processes negative attitudes because of lack of support. Vice versa the positive impacts to outcomes were secondary impacts, e.g. research, management, education.

Reason to recommend this reference: Review provides useful information about the knowledge of the needs of nursing practice and management as well as nursing informatics. Acquisition and dissemination of knowledge of the use, effects and benefits of standardized nursing languages is very much needed when its implementation is under planning or adoption already in process, and curricula for nursing schools are under development and update.

2.13. Personal Health Records

Suggested by: Kaija Saranto PhD, RN, FACMI, FAAN:

Bibliographic date of the annotated reference: Saranto K, Brennan Flatney P, Casey A (eds): *Personal Health Information Management Tools and Strategies for Citizens' Engagement* University of Kuopio, Department of Health Policy and Management, Kuopio, 214 pages, 2009.

Summary of the content: The publication is a summary of personal health information management tools and strategies for citizens engagement produced in the NI2009 post-conference congress. The publication gives several perspectives to personal health information management e.g. technology, usability, governance, clinical practice, confidentiality and safety. Reflecting our topic in 2016 a group of expert in 2009 also focused on competencies under the title: *The Personal Health Information Management Systems & Education: Preparing Nurses to practice in a Wired World*. It also provides descriptions of the situation in 16 countries.

Reason to recommend this reference: This publication reflects our post-conference theme *Forecasting Informatics Competencies for Nurses in the Future of Connected Health*. The publication from NI2009 describes the situation in personal health information management almost ten years ago. Thus it gives us perspectives how we have made progress during the years. The publication focuses on the development of tools, their use and implementations to practice. At that time we were probably more concerned about citizens' access to their data than the variety of tools providing the access nowadays. We also recognized the need for governance which still is sometimes our weakest link in implementations. However, most importantly without education there will be no progress. Thus we need to define and set the goals, contents and methods how to enhance nurses' informatics competencies needed in the future.

2.14. Competencies for Nursing Telehealth

Suggested by: Ybranda Koster MScN:

Bibliographic data of the annotated reference: C.T.M. van Houwelingen, A.H. Moerman, R.G.A. Ettema, H.S.M. Kort, O. ten Cate, Competencies required for nursing telehealth activities: A delphi-study, Nurse Education Today 39 (2016) 50-62.

Summary of the content: This study presents fourteen nursing telehealth activities to support patients and 32 'new' telehealth-specific competencies required for the provision of telehealth.

Reason to recommend this reference: The required telehealth competencies presented in this study can be used by nursing schools that are considering including or expanding telehealth education in their curriculum and may strengthen the development of telehealth education.

2.15. Patient Safety and Nursing Informatics

Suggested by: Elizabeth Borycki RN PhD:

Bibliographic data of the annotated reference: Borycki, E., Keay, E. Methods to assess the safety of health information systems. Healthcare Quarterly, 2010; 13: 47-52.

Summary of the content: There is growing evidence that health information systems, when not designed, developed, implemented and maintained properly, can cause health professionals to make errors (i.e. technology-induced errors). The article reports on the results of a review of the literature examining the methods that can be used to predict, prevent and evaluate the potential of health information systems to cause technology-induced errors. Such methods, if used appropriately, can reduce the likelihood of an occurrence of a technology-induced error and can improve the overall safety of health information systems.

Reason to recommend this reference: The reference outlines the main methods used to assess health information systems for safety and the presence of technology-induced errors. Identifying and addressing technology-induced errors will ensure the overall safety of systems over time. The article outlines the methods that should be used to identify technology–induced errors before, during and after the implementation of a health information system.

2.16. Competencies in social media use in the area of health and healthcare

Suggested by: Patrick Weber RN, MA

Bibliographic data of the annotated reference: Ventola CL. Social Media and Health Care Professionals: Benefits, Risks, and Best Practices. Pharmacy and Therapeutics. 2014;39(7):491-520.

Summary of the content: Many social media tools are available for health care professionals (HCPs), including social networking platforms, blogs, microblogs, wikis, media-sharing sites, and virtual reality and gaming environments. These tools can be used to improve or enhance professional networking and education, organizational promotion, patient care, patient education, and public health programs. However, they also present potential risks to patients and HCPs regarding the distribution of poor quality information, damage to professional image, breaches of patient privacy, violation of personal–professional boundaries, and licensing or legal issues. Many health care institutions and professional organizations have issued guidelines to prevent these risks.

Reason to recommend this reference: This paper is a very good overview of the use of social media for healthcare professionals. It takes into account the healthcare professional person, the patient, the institution. It gives information about a number of social media tools. It goes through some legal aspects.

2.17. Genomics relevance for nursing

Suggested by: Kathleen McCormick RN, PhD:

Bibliographic data of the annotated references: McCormick, K.A. and K.A. Calzone, The impact of genomics on health outcomes, quality, and safety. Nurs Manage, 2016. 47(4): p. 23-6.

Summary of the content: This recent publication highlights the importance of integrating genetics and genomics into nursing care to improve outcomes, quality, and safety.

Bibliographic data of the annotated references: McCormick, K.A., Calzone, K.A. , Big Data Initiatives: Genomics and Information Technology for Personalized Health, in Essentials of Nursing informatics, 6th Edition. Saba,VK &. McCormick,KA Editor. 2015, McGraw-Hill: New York. p. 707-725.

Summary of the content: This book chapter summarizes the initiatives ready for use throughout the continuum of care, the resources available, implications for nursing informatics, and the Blueprint for Nursing Research needed in genetics/genomics.

Bibliographic data of the annotated references: Relling, M.V. and W.E. Evans, Pharmacogenomics in the clinic. Nature, 2015. 526(7573): p. 343-50.

Summary of the content: Describes the new evidence in CPIC guidelines ready for implementation into clinical practice.

Reason to recommend these references: This set describes the state of the art of genomics with respect to nursing care. First serves as an introduction, second as in-depth chapter. The third moves it to the multidisciplinary care guideline for practice.

2.18. Nursing leaders

Suggested by: Charlene Ronquillo, RN, MSN:

Bibliographic data of the annotated reference: Collins S. ANI emerging leaders project: Clinical informatics governance & nursing leadership. Computers Informatics Nursing. 2014 Sep 1;32(9):420-3.

Summary of the content: This paper provides a discussion of the integral link between nursing leadership and clinical informatics governance, informed by a survey administered to leading nursing informatics leaders in the United States. The importance of nursing informatics leaders' roles in representing and communicating the relevance and added value of innovations in health informatics is highlighted, along with the need for organization's informatics governance to support the full extent, education, and training of nursing informatics leaders.

Reason to recommend this reference: This paper describes a key organizational factor to consider in supporting the visibility of nursing practice in healthcare organizations' clinical informatics systems.

2.19. Nurse executive competencies

Suggested by: Margaret Ann Kennedy RN PhD:

Bibliographic data of the annotated reference: American Organization of Nurse Executives (AONE), *Nurse executive competencies*. (2015) Retrieved from: http://www.aone.org/resources/nec.pdf

Summary of the content: This recently updated publication from the AONE specifically sets forth a comprehensive model for nursing leadership competencies. The recommended competencies encompass all aspects within broad topics of nursing leadership including communications and relationship management, knowledge of the health care environment, leadership, professionalism, and business. Within the business section, information management and technology competencies are explicitly defined.

Reason to recommend this reference: Nurse executives require clearly defined competency expectations regarding informatics within leadership and executive roles. Additionally, nurse executives require support and resources in order to effectively incorporate these competencies into their day to day activities.

2.20. Collaborative practice

Suggested by: Raji Nibber BSN, RN:

Bibliographic data of the annotated reference: Christopherson TA, Troseth MR, Clingerman EM. Informatics-enabled interprofessional education and collaborative practice: A framework-driven approach. Journal of Interprofessional Education & Practice. 2015 Mar 31;1(1):10-5.

Summary of the content: This article summarizes the work of more than 346 rural, community and university settings in the United States towards developing and implementing a framework-driven approach (as opposed to project-driven) to address the gap between education and practice in delivering safe, efficient and quality care. Six models were created as a part of the framework along with processes, tools, and infrastructures to support the use of health information technology and promote interprofessional education and collaborative practice.

Reason to recommend this reference: This framework can be used by organizations to improve and achieve sustainable outcomes. Nurse leaders and educators specifically can address and bridge the gap between education and practice to improve interprofessional integration and collaboration of informatics across health professions.

2.21. Health Informatics: An Interprofessional Approach

Suggested by: Bickford, Carol J. PhD, RN-BC, CPHIMS, FHIMSS, FAAN:

Bibliographic data of the annotated reference: Nelson R, Staggers N. Health Informatics: An Interprofessional Approach. St. Louis, MO: Elsevier Mosby; 2014.

Summary of the content: This textbook provides an interprofessional perspective and comprehensive presentation of health informatics content. Thirty-one chapters are categorized into nine units: Background and Foundational Information; Information Systems in Healthcare Delivery; Participatory Healthcare Informatics and Healthcare; Project Management: Tools and Procedures; Quality, Usability, and Standards in Informatics; Governance and Organizational Structures for Informatics; Education and Informatics; International Informatics Efforts; The Present and Future. The detailed robust content provides extensive evidence of the diversity and complexity of contemporary health informatics practice. Additional learning materials and supplemental faculty resources augment and enhance this textbook's value.

Reason to recommend this reference: Industry experts beyond the nursing informatics community provided key insights about issues and trends within their specialty areas. Frameworks and theories are referenced to guide the reader's understanding of health informatics.

2.22. Improving Health Care through Informatics

Suggested by: Daragh Rodger RGN, RNP, RANP, MSc & PhD student:

Bibliographic data of the annotated reference: Botin L, Bertelsen P, Nohr C. Challenges in Improving Health Care by Use of Health Informatics Technology. In: Botin L, Bertelsen P, Nohr C. 215 Techno-Anthropology in Health Informatics Methodologies for Improving Human Technology Relations. IOS Press: Netherlands, 2015:3 – 11.

Summary of the content: This chapter introduces Techno-Anthropology as the study of the relationship between humans and technology and how they interact. Within an eHealth and health informatics agenda, this topic is emerging as a facilitator to the provision of quality holistic healthcare through interdisciplinary engagement. It outlines the need for and identifies support strategies to meet the challenges faced by health care providers, patients and their relatives to be competent users and developers of health technology. The book further presents how adopting a Techno-Anthropology approach can enhance health informatics and eHealth agendas.

Reason to recommend this reference: The overarching aim of connected health involves the patient being central to healthcare service delivery. This chapter provides an introduction to the relevance of Techno-Anthropology on eHealth and in particular on patient-centric health informatics. It also demonstrates how Techno-Anthropology can support new ways of conceptualizing and developing systems that embrace patient-centered needs, values and perspectives for a quality orientated health care system.

2.23. Nursing Informatics Research Priorities

Suggested by: Maxim Topaz PhD, RN, MA:

Bibliographic data of the annotated reference: Peltonen LM, Topaz M, Ronquillo C, Pruinelli L, Sarmiento RF, Badger MK, Ali S, Lewis A, Georgsson M, Jeon E, Tayaben JL, Kuo CH, Islam T, Sommer J, Jung H, Eler GJ, Alhuwail D. Nursing Informatics Research Priorities for the Future: Recommendations from an International Survey. Stud Health Technol Inform. 2016;225:222-6.

Summary of the content: This paper provides a discussion of the future nursing informatics research priorities, based on analysis of a study conducted by the International Medical Informatics Association- Nursing Informatics Special Interest Group (IMIA-NISIG) Student Working Group. 373 responses from 44 countries were analyzed. The identified top ten nursing informatics research trends were big data science, standardized terminologies (clinical evaluation/implementation), education and competencies, clinical decision support, mobile health, usability, patient safety, data exchange and interoperability, patient engagement, and clinical quality measures. Acknowledging these research priorities can enhance the successful future development of nursing informatics to better support clinicians and promote health.

Reason to recommend this reference: This paper describes ten key research areas recommended as a focus for nurse informatics researchers in the coming years.

References

[1]   Goossen, W., Hannah, K.J., (1991). A curriculum about nursing informatics for a nurse educator's educational programme. In: Hovenga, E.S.J., Hannah, K.J., McCormick, K.A., & Ronald, J.S., (Eds). Proceedings Nursing Informatics '91 conference. Melbourne Australia, 690-694.

Forecasting Informatics Competencies for Nurses in the Future of Connected Health
J. Murphy et al. (Eds.)
© 2017 IMIA and IOS Press.

Subject Index

Forecasting Informatics Competencies for Nurses in the Future of Connected Health
J. Murphy et al. (Eds.)
© *2017 IMIA and IOS Press.*

255

Author Index

www.ingramcontent.com/pod-product-compliance
Ingram Content Group UK Ltd.
Pitfield, Milton Keynes, MK11 3LW, UK
UKHW022221170526
471099UK00001B/113